The Link: Pediatric History-Taking and Physical Examination

Disclaimer

Both the authors have taken all possible measures to reference the work quoted in the chapters in the texts within this book. Additionally, we have also felt that we should recommend books and journals as relevant reading material meant for greater understanding of the text, for deeper scientific knowledge on the topics covered and for wider clinical integration of the facts and data presented. Should there be any reference that has been inadvertently missed, the authors would be more than happy to include it in this book.

The Link: Pediatric History-Taking and Physical Examination

Prameela Kannan Kutty
MBBS (Hon) MRCP (UK) FRCP (Edin) MSc (Lon) DTM&H (UK)
Professor, Department of Pediatrics
Deputy Dean of Postgraduate Studies
MAHSA University
Kuala Lumpur, Malaysia

Co-author
Gauri Krishnaswamy
MBBS (Ind) MRCGP (INT) (UK) MMed (S'pore) MFOM (Ire) FFOM (Ire) MMed (Aust)
Associate Professor and Head
Department of Primary Care Medicine
MAHSA University
Kuala Lumpur, Malaysia

Foreword
Tan Sri Dato' Seri Dr. Hj. Mohd Ismail Merican

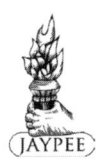

The Health Sciences Publisher

New Delhi | London | Philadelphia | Panama

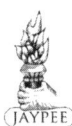

Jaypee Brothers Medical Publishers (P) Ltd

Headquarters

Jaypee Brothers Medical Publishers (P) Ltd
4838/24, Ansari Road, Daryaganj
New Delhi 110 002, India
Phone: +91-11-43574357
Fax: +91-11-43574314
Email: jaypee@jaypeebrothers.com

Overseas Offices

J.P. Medical Ltd
83 Victoria Street, London
SW1H 0HW (UK)
Phone: +44-20 3170 8910
Fax: +44 (0) 20 3008 6180
Email: info@jpmedpub.com

Jaypee Medical Inc
325 Chestnut Street
Suite 412, Philadelphia, PA 19106, USA
Phone: +1 267-519-9789
Email: support@jpmedus.com

Jaypee Brothers Medical Publishers (P) Ltd
Bhotahity, Kathmandu, Nepal
Phone: +977-9741283608
Email: kathmandu@jaypeebrothers.com

Jaypee-Highlights Medical Publishers Inc
City of Knowledge, Bld. 235, 2nd Floor, Clayton
Panama City, Panama
Phone: +1 507-301-0496
Fax: +1 507-301-0499
Email: cservice@jphmedical.com

Jaypee Brothers Medical Publishers (P) Ltd
17/1-B Babar Road, Block-B, Shaymali
Mohammadpur, Dhaka-1207
Bangladesh
Mobile: +08801912003485
Email: jaypeedhaka@gmail.com

Website: www.jaypeebrothers.com
Website: www.jaypeedigital.com

© 2016, Jaypee Brothers Medical Publishers

The views and opinions expressed in this book are solely those of the original contributor(s)/author(s) and do not necessarily represent those of editor(s) of the book.

All rights reserved. No part of this publication may be reproduced, stored or transmitted in any form or by any means, electronic, mechanical, photocopying, recording or otherwise, without the prior permission in writing of the publishers.

All brand names and product names used in this book are trade names, service marks, trademarks or registered trademarks of their respective owners. The publisher is not associated with any product or vendor mentioned in this book.

Medical knowledge and practice change constantly. This book is designed to provide accurate, authoritative information about the subject matter in question. However, readers are advised to check the most current information available on procedures included and check information from the manufacturer of each product to be administered, to verify the recommended dose, formula, method and duration of administration, adverse effects and contraindications. It is the responsibility of the practitioner to take all appropriate safety precautions. Neither the publisher nor the author(s)/editor(s) assume any liability for any injury and/or damage to persons or property arising from or related to use of material in this book.

This book is sold on the understanding that the publisher is not engaged in providing professional medical services. If such advice or services are required, the services of a competent medical professional should be sought.

Every effort has been made where necessary to contact holders of copyright to obtain permission to reproduce copyright material. If any have been inadvertently overlooked, the publisher will be pleased to make the necessary arrangements at the first opportunity.

Inquiries for bulk sales may be solicited at: jaypee@jaypeebrothers.com

The Link: Pediatric History-Taking and Physical Examination

First Edition: **2016**

ISBN: 978-93-5152-512-7

Printed at Sanat Printers

Dedicated to

Our beloved students
It is hoped that this book will help you
understand the little ones better

Foreword

It is with great pleasure that I share some of my thoughts in this unique book written by Dr Prameela Kannan Kutty and Dr Gauri Krishnaswamy.

The book, aptly titled *The Link: Pediatric History-Taking and Physical Examination*, is obviously the result of many years of experience in teaching students at MAHSA University, Kuala Lumpur, Malaysia, by the authors and reflect the passion and zeal they both have in perfecting the art of managing pediatric patients. Medical students should consider themselves fortunate to have this book as their companion. It will steer them well during their clinical interaction with pediatric patients who may pose a challenge to students who are unprepared and uninitiated. Special skills are required to ensure that students or doctors do not miss important details during history-taking and physical examination of their patients.

One can sense that the contents of the book are carefully structured and formatted to motivate readers to grasp the essentials of history-taking and physical examination, infuse their own thinking and analytical skills and link all of these with vital relevant information with the ultimate goal of providing the best diagnostic and management strategy for their patients.

Both undergraduate and postgraduate students will benefit from this excellent book, which has been imbued with information on the humanistic aspects of medicine. Dr Prameela has put her vast clinical experience as a pediatrician to good use in the preparation of this book and in today's world, where technology may dictate the way we think and practise medicine, soft skills must be nurtured from the beginning of a doctor's career so that such important attributes will not get lost or perish in his or her pursuit to acquire knowledge and clinical skills and embrace technology. This is well amplified in this book, which also stresses on compassion and ethics in our interaction with patients and their parents.

I would like to congratulate the authors for their sterling efforts in producing this book. I know it involves lots of sacrifice, hard work, energy and determination to produce such a book.

We in MAHSA University are proud that both Dr Prameela and Dr Gauri are part of our teaching team and hope others will follow their footsteps and produce books that will help students achieve more during their training.

It is with great pleasure that I recommend this book to all those pursuing a course in medicine, those who aspire to become good pediatricians and those who are involved in teaching. This book will also be of tremendous benefit to doctors in general.

Professor Tan Sri Dato' Seri Dr. Hj. Mohd Ismail Merican
PSM DGPN PJN SIMP DPMS DMPN DSPN JSM KMN PKT AMP
MBBS (Mal) FRCP (Lond) FRCP (Edin) FRCP (Glasg) FRCS (Ire)
FACP (Hon) FRACP (Hon) FAMM (Mal) FAFP (Mal) FASc FMSA
Pro-Chancellor & Chairman, MAHSA University
Kuala Lumpur, Malaysia

Preface

The students of clinical medicine, whether undergraduate or postgraduate, must be impressed that a good history and a complete physical examination are essential tools in arriving at the diagnosis. The art of eliciting the clinical history and conducting the physical examination in the different age groups spanning the pediatric discipline should not be dismally relegated to the background as may happen these days when investigations are easily available and occasionally callously done. Nothing is compromised and much in fact is valuably gained in taking your time towards a gentle and caring approach to the young patients, carefully listening to the problems of the patients, the parents or the caregiver, and conducting a gentle but meticulous physical examination.

The approach to both the history-taking and the physical examination in children must be oriented towards care and compassion for the pediatric patients and respect towards the parents. Such an approach at any stage of one's career cannot be overemphasized. These are distinctly time-tested tools that even the most experienced medical practitioners cannot do without.

Genuine human empathy may come naturally for many; however, it is our feeling that as teachers of a clinical discipline that imposes an extreme obligation of the display of compassion, the clinical students must be taught such methods, inculcated and instilled the possession and modest exhibition of such emotion. Adequate bedside teaching and time must be spent in highlighting a compassionate approach and giving it the importance that it rightfully merits.

While many books are available on methods of approach to pediatric patients, we have, in this book, chosen to emphasize a path to help the students think and link. Sound preclinical knowledge has to be harnessed in all of our analysis toward the patient's problems. Comprehension of the foundation and core knowledge must be brought to the forefront of the thinking process. The route to thinking is to link and indeed the course to linking is because we think. Students must be encouraged to utilize self-searching questions and teachers must stimulate thinking and clinically meaningful linking. Linking factual knowledge to the clinical setting is that which cannot be simply procured at face value from any book, nor can it be learnt and committed to memory.

A method to analyze, form hypothesis, test and question the hypothesis and retest with analytic and critical thinking must commence early in history-taking as essential developmental milestones that every student of medicine must conscientiously achieve.

I am deeply indebted to numerous illustrious experts, such as Stuart Mason, Michael Swash, Marcdante K, Kliegman RM, Jenson HB and Berman RE and many others whose publications were freely reviewed, referenced and frequently quoted. This has infused in us enormous confidence in preparation of this book, which is appropriately entitled *The Link: Pediatric History-Taking and Physical Examination*. Much of what has been embodied herein may need rethinking in the future as pediatrics, like any other discipline in medicine is evolving continuously. I am fully aware that with time, the necessity for revision of the approach both in style and content may be felt but, as of now, I am gratified to respond to the clarion call of interested students who had time and again expressed their desire to see a book of this nature.

Prameela Kannan Kutty

Acknowledgments

I owe the positive attributes that my students may gain from this book to my father Professor Dr Methil Kannan Kutty, who has been a source of inspiration ever since I can remember. His magnanimity in all things that he has done or partaken in is engraved in me as a lifetime's lesson.

I thank my husband and my mother for their patience and kind endurance of my long hours of work, my two children who allowed me time and space despite their missing me very much during the hours I spent writing the book.

I thank all my students in MAHSA University, Kuala Lumpur, Malaysia, particularly Kong Liang who drew all the pictures, Arravindh and Chandni, for their tireless efforts in organizing the pictures, Eric, Edris, Selvarani, Solomon and others who helped with the photography; Azhar as well as all my wonderful students who, due to space constraints, I am not able to singly name, but who surely and selflessly helped in so many different ways. It is an honor for me to have taught such students.

I also extend my appreciation to my student Deborah Shobana Das for her willingness to help in proofreading much of the text and for her ungrudging help whenever asked of her.

I thank Associate Professor Dr Loh Keng Yin for kindly allowing us to use some of his clinical photographs.

I thank Associate Professor Haresh Kumar Kantilal who gave his valuable suggestions in the writing of the book.

I thank Vishnu Raj Kumar for his views on IT and on some important and enlightening perspectives that he gave towards the writing of the book.

I thank Vidhya Raj Kumar for her kind support in my every effort.

I thank Associate Professor Dr Gauri Krishnaswamy who willingly co-authored the book, and who also spent many hours with computer work and the adjustments to the text.

Prameela Kannan Kutty

First and foremost, I would like to thank Professor Dr Prameela Kannan Kutty for inviting me to co-write this book with her. I would also like to express my gratitude to the many people who saw me through this book; to all those who provided support and guidance and talked things over.

Above all, I would like to thank my daughter, Anusia, my parents, Dato and Datin M Krishnasamy and sister, Anu, who supported and encouraged me in spite of all the time it took me away from them. It has been a long and difficult journey for them, especially my daughter.

Last but not least, I would like to thank my cousin, Stanley Jeyapalan Ramakrishnan for supporting and encouraging me to give this book my very best.

Gauri Krishnaswamy

CONTENTS

SECTION 1: PEDIATRIC HISTORY-TAKING, BREASTFEEDING AND IMMUNIZATION

1. **Rationale of the Pediatric History**   3–12
   Pediatric History—Salient Feature   4
   Points to Think Through for Effective History-Taking   5
   Things to Do for Effective History-Taking   6
   Symptoms   7
   The Cardinal Ten (Historical)   8
   Historical Link   8
   Activities of Daily Living in Children   9
   Pertinent Negatives in the History   10

2. **History of the Presenting Problem and the Past Medical and Surgical History**   13–18
   Clarification of the Pediatric History Under Specific Headings   13
   Chief Complaint and History of the Presenting Complaint (HPC)   13
   History of the Presenting Problem   13
   History of Past Medical or Surgical Problems   17

3. **Review of Systems**   19–57
   Core Objectives   19
   Symptomatic Enquiry of Systems   19
   Review of Systems Spreadsheet   20
   Symptomatic Enquiry using the Cardinal Ten (Historical) and the Historical Link   24
   Respiratory System   24
   History of Cough and Its Characteristics   24
   Distinguishing Features in the History of Wheezing   27
   Ear, Nose and Throat (ENT)   28
   Gastrointestinal Tract   30
   Abdominal Pain   30
   Gastrointestinal Manifestations of Allergies to Cow's Milk Protein   34
   Gastrointestinal Links   34
   Cardiovascular System   35
   Congenital Cardiac Lesions with Increase in Pulmonary Blood Flow   36
   Congenital Cardiac Lesions with Decrease in Pulmonary Blood Flow   37
   Links to Cardiac Failure   37
   Genitourinary System   38
   Nonspecific and Specific Symptoms   39
   History in Hematuria and Suggested Diagnosis   39
   Central Nervous System   41
   Links of Onset to Neurological Event   41
   Syncope   41
   Seizures   42
   Musculoskeletal System   45
   Musculoskeletal Pain   45
   Limb Abnormalities or Deformities   47
   Child With a Limp   48
   Endocrine System   48

XIV *The Link*: Pediatric History-Taking and Physical Examination

    Enquiry and Links 49
    Neonatal History in Thyroid Disorders 50
    Child with Ambiguous Genitalia 51
    Skin 52
    Dermatological Links to the Diagnosis of Allergy to Cow's Milk Protein 53
    Hematological System 54
    Link History to Hematological Abnormality 54

4. **History of Pregnancy, Delivery, and the Neonatal Period**   58–68
    History of Events Relevant to Birth and Delivery 58
    Relevant Prepregnancy History 58
    History of Pregnancy and Delivery 59
    History of Events Related to Labor and Delivery 62
    Apgar Score 62
    Neonatal History 64
    History of Neonatal Jaundice 65

5. **Other Components of the Pediatric History**   69–95
    Developmental History 69
    An Approach to the Developmental History 70
    Links in the Feeding History 80
    Historical Importance of Inheritance 83
    Link to Diseases 83
    Other Historical Points 85
    Link Between the Social History and Health 86
    Specific Behavioral Problems and Temper Tantrums 88
    Links to Behavioral Disorders 90
    Factors in Drug Allergy 91
    Importance of Drug Interactions in the Drug History 92

6. **Clinical Links Relevant to Breastfeeding**   96–105
    Reasons as to Why Breast Milk Protects from Diseases 96
    Breastfeeding History 102

7. **Immunization**   106–119
    Immunizing Agents 106
    Active and Passive Immunization 107
    Vaccines and Vaccination 107
    Counseling on Optional Vaccines 116
    Vaccination and Breastfeeding 118

8. **Analysis and Deduction in the Layout of a Complete Pediatric History**   120–125
    Process of Analysis 120
    History-Taking Requires Practice and Practice Makes Perfect 122
    Layout of a Complete Pediatric History 124
    Some Points to Reiterate 124

SECTION 2: COMPREHENSIVE PEDIATRIC PHYSICAL EXAMINATION

9. **An Approach to the Pediatric Physical Examination**   129–136
    Building A Rapport 129
    The Cardinal Ten (Physical) 131

Physical Link 132
Pertinent Negatives 134

10. Pediatric Physical Examination 137–210
Measurements 138
General Observation 149
Specific Observation and Examination 156
Systemic Examination 168
Thorax 168
Compare, Contrast, Capture and Consolidate (CCCC) Your Findings 171
Abdomen 172
Cardiovascular System 178
Nervous System 181
Correlate, Compare, Capture and Confirm 185
Musculoskeletal System 200
Ear, Nose and Throat (ENT) Examination 202
Skin 204

11. Layout of a Complete Pediatric Physical Examination 211–220
Physical Examination 212
Systemic Examination 216

SECTION 3: NEWBORN: HISTORICAL AND PHYSICAL LINKS

12. Newborn 223–237
Terms and Definitions 223
Normal Full-Term Neonate 224
Premature Neonate 224
Postmature Neonate 225
Important Physical Features of the Newborn 228

SECTION 4: DIFFERENTIAL DIAGNOSIS AND PROVISIONAL DIAGNOSIS WITH SELECTED CASE STUDIES

13. Formulation of Differential Diagnosis and Provisional Diagnosis 241–267
Process of Formulation of the Provisional Diagnosis 241
Analytic Thinking During the Process of Formulation of the Diagnosis 243
Case Studies 244
Case Studies on Fever 244
System: Cardiovascular 254
System: Gastrointestinal Tract 257
System: Hepatobiliary 258
System: Nervous System 262
System: Development 264
System: Musculoskeletal 266

SECTION 5: 'THE KNOW' FACTS

14. Factual Knowledge 271–300
Factual Knowledge Categorized As 'Must Know', 'Good to Know' or 'Nice to Know' 271
System: Fever in Children 271
System: Skin 272

XVI *The Link*: Pediatric History-Taking and Physical Examination

    System: ENT   275
    System: Respiratory   277
    Pattern of Wheezing: Clarify with the Cardinal Ten Historical and Physical Links   278
    System: Cardiovascular   281
    System: Gastrointestinal   283
    System: Hepatobiliary   284
    System: Renal   286
    System: Blood   289
    System: Childhood Malignancies   290
    System: Endocrine   290
    System: Central Nervous System   292
    System: Musculoskeletal   297

Index

    301

SECTION 1

PEDIATRIC HISTORY-TAKING, BREASTFEEDING AND IMMUNIZATION

- Rationale of the Pediatric History
- History of the Presenting Problem and the Past Medical and Surgical History
- Review of Systems
- History of Pregnancy, Delivery and the Neonatal Period
- Other Components of the Pediatric History
- Clinical Links Relevant to Breastfeeding
- Immunization
- Analysis and Deduction in the Layout of a Complete Pediatric History

Chapter 1

Rationale of the Pediatric History

The pediatric specialty is unique as it spans across a range of age groups.[1-10] Age variation is perhaps its most distinguishing feature. Most patients who are seen in pediatric wards and out-patient departments are babies or young children; hence the history is usually obtained from the parents or guardians of the patient and not directly from the patient. Today, in many countries around the world, an increasing number of families have dual incomes where the mother is expected to work to help support the family. Consequently, children are left in the care of relatives or at nurseries or daycare centers.[1-5]

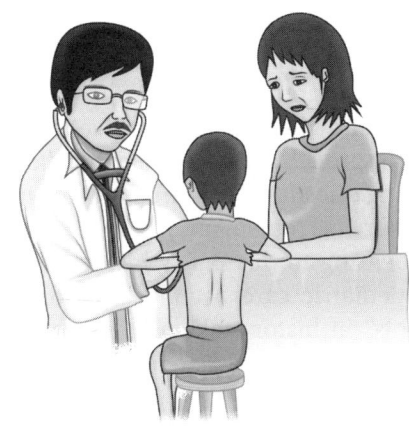

In many countries, children form a large proportion of the population that attend the out-patient clinics

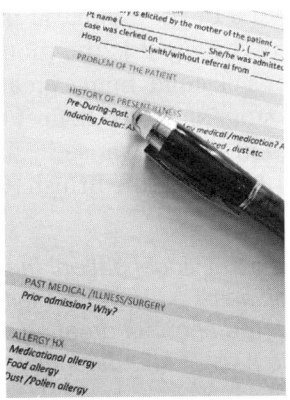

Hence, children across the world require meticulous care and universal concern regarding their health and well being and because of this, doctors dealing with children must show interest, be equipped with basic knowledge of childhood illnesses and be empathetic towards their problems. The statistics in some countries indicate that approximately a third of the population importantly consist of young citizens below the age of fifteen years.[6]

Parents, grandparents, older siblings, extended family members, the babysitter or the social worker will give the history. Consequently, the history is usually one of perception, one that 'is felt to be' by reliable observers. The taking of the pediatric history that is often attained 'second hand' requires a skill that must be learnt and indeed fostered.

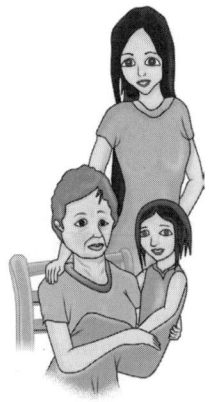

Parents and grandparents are often the best historians

Mothers are often astute observers of their young ones and the maternal history often reveals many clues to the underlying disorder or disease. A good history taker is one who listens attentively and then interjects with appropriate questions.

4   The Link: Pediatric History-Taking and Physical Examination

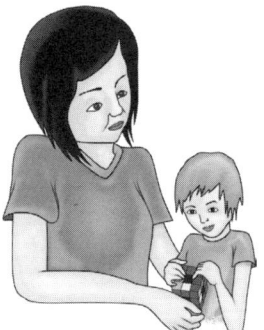

Mothers are astute observers

Unfortunately, a small number of parents cannot recall many events pertaining to vital facets in the lives of their children. Dealing with these parents is both difficult and challenging. In these circumstances, a different approach may unavoidably be used; like asking leading questions that directly bring forth events that may otherwise remain untold. These incidents may have vital bearing to the child's history of disorder or illness. In pediatric care, a good clinician uses some special "tools" in history-taking to help parents recall distant events.

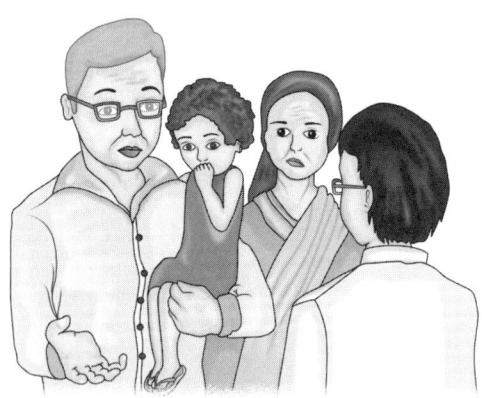

When eliciting the history from grandparents and siblings, one needs to ask if they are involved in caring for the child. Obtain all possible information during that visit. Sometimes, one making an appointment with the parents to retake the history or fill in on details is necessary.

If the child is at an age capable of relating his or her own story of himself or herself, it is mandatory to talk to the child, asking the history in a lingo that is simple, practical and understandable. Remember, the first-hand information from the patient is free from the prejudice of perception. Questioning must be uncomplicated and direct. Leading questions are useful in this situation. Tact must be exercised in a non-alarming fashion, neither hurting nor embarrassing the child. Needless to say here too, historical details should also be taken from the parents or guardians present.

In the adolescent, discretion and wisdom is always necessary. Some questions are best left to the last. More detailed information may be ideally explored with the adolescent alone. Beforehand, ask if that is what he or she prefers before raising specifically personal details. Yet other queries may be asked in the presence of the parent or guardian which are alright by the adolescent.

It is thus clear that pediatric history-taking is a skill where versatility in thought, care of the patient and consideration of all matters that relate to the patient are important. Indeed it is a skill to be mastered with diligent practice and patience. Thus, even in an age where many investigative methods are readily available in many parts of the world, the art of history-taking in pediatrics as an essential tool to the accurate diagnosis, clearly cannot be dismissed.

PEDIATRIC HISTORY—SALIENT FEATURES[1-5,7-10]

In pediatrics, great reliance is placed on the mother's history. About 70% of the pediatric diagnosis comes from the history. Usually it is the mother who nurses and cares for her sick child, hence great attention must be given to the story she tells. Reflect on the depth of meaning and good clinical sense in this quote by Sir William Osler (1849–1919) the British (Canadian-born) physician.

"Care more for the individual patient than for the special features of the disease. . . . Put yourself in his place . . . The kindly word, the cheerful greeting, the sympathetic look — these the patient understands."

Approach to the Mother and Child[1-5,7-10]

This is perhaps the most important part of the interview. First impressions count. Often they last.

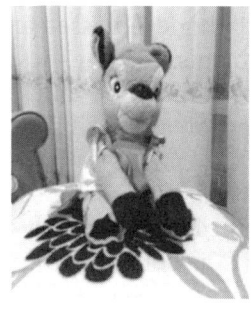

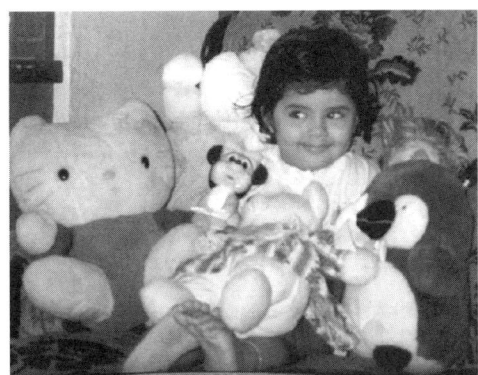

The happy child plays with the cuddly toys (Reprint with kind permission from VRK)

A warm smile and a cuddly toy in one's hand will help in one's approach towards a child. These little objects immediately help to put the child at ease and in good cheer.

A Physician's Approach[1-5,7-10]

- Politely introduce yourself
- Politely request permission from the mother or caretaker
- Gently request permission from the older patient
- Ask keenly what the child is called at home and greet the child by that name (i.e. his pet name or home name)
- Be genuinely interested and concerned when speaking to the parents and patient
- Appear keen to interview both the parent and an older child and show empathy towards the patient and the parents and keenness to make an accurate diagnosis. This is best done by establishing eye contact with the historian
- Allow the mother who has the infant or toddler on her lap to continue to do so as you take the history in her position of comfort. Do not force a change in her comfortable routine unless she herself chooses to do so
- Know that young children may need a little time getting to know you; give a safe toy to the child to allay anxiety lest he or she may be uncomfortable in your presence
- Make the child and parents feel that you have the time, interest and competence to help them. As a consequence of all the above, develop and nurture a good doctor–patient relationship starting from the history-taking. The mother often reveals to you many a hidden secret if she trusts you and has some confidence in you
- Exercise tact and discretion when taking history in front of the child; always weigh the pros and cons of what you say and ask
- Do not forget to give due respect to the child by asking some questions, if the child can understand you. Children aged four years old and above must be included in history-taking
- Allow the child to speak. This is especially important if the child is able to understand and give his or her version of the problem. This will nurture a sense of self-esteem in the young child
- At times where sensitive questions must be asked, and understood by the child, realize that it may be necessary to interview the parents alone
- Likewise, in an adolescent patient and according to the wishes of the patient, it may be necessary to interview the patient alone.

POINTS TO THINK THROUGH FOR EFFECTIVE HISTORY-TAKING[1-5,7-10]

- Use all your senses for observation including your eyes and ears while you take the history
- Observe parent-child interactions which may give you clues to diagnosis
- Recognize specific sounds produced by the pathology in some illnesses (e.g. stridor in upper respiratory diseases) or even be aware of peculiar or distinctive odors that may lead you to ask related questions (e.g. the sweet smell of urine in maple syrup disease)
- Be aware that parental distractions which could practically occur during history-taking can interfere with the quality of the given history; however never show impatience
- Likewise parental feelings of guilt or extreme anxiety may interfere with their perception of some or many historical events
- Be aware that the reliability of parental observation varies
- Be aware that in the younger child you are depending on the parental interpretation of signs and symptoms which you may be compelled to rationalize

> **Reflect upon the History**
> THINK
> WATCH
> LISTEN
> TALK
> THINK AGAIN

- Start mentally processing the story and truthfully organize the history for clear and succinct comprehension both to yourself as well as to the listener—giving a truthful, clear, chronologically correct meaningful history which conveys the story briefly yet accurately
- You must yourself think maturely and this must be reflected in the history
- You are responsible for the history you take and the message you convey by it.
- Utilize history-taking as an effective and accurate patient management tool.

Issues of Child Protection[1,3]

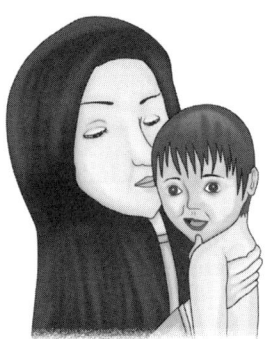

As mentioned, in taking the pediatric history, the mother or carer is heavily relied upon and trusted as they have the advantage of having spent many hours with the sick child. A large part of the diagnosis depends on their history.

However, in pediatrics, one must also realize that occasionally some parents or carers do not have the child's best interest at heart. This may or may not be a deliberate act of parental unkindness towards their offspring.

For example, when parents are disabled by the "burden" of nurturing as a result of physical, emotional or financial stresses, the welfare of children can be neglected.

When problems within a family are as immense as to endanger the normal physical, developmental, emotional and psychological well-being of their child, various difficulties towards the child can potentially arise. In these instances, the child needs to be protected and doctors, the social worker and child protection agencies must intervene.

In much situations, when the child is unwell and if brought for medical advice, parents or caregivers may not reveal the aspects of the history that may be vital to make a diagnosis of the illness. Important facts are deliberately concealed. In these cases, one must be clear that the duty of the doctor is towards the safety and health of the child. If this is suspected during the process of history-taking, various concerns regarding child protection must be considered.

These include:

Some concerns in issues pertaining to child protection[1,3]

• Involve a team with multiple disciplines including the local social health worker in your team
• Consult a senior child specialist
• Seek medicolegal advice from your medical indemnifier
• Consult child protection teams for up to date advice
• Consider the latest policies and guidelines in child protection

THINGS TO DO FOR EFFECTIVE HISTORY-TAKING[1-5,7-10]

• Remember that in most cases involving smaller children, the information is from someone other than the patient, usually the mother
• Remember that the mother perceives the symptoms; she does not herself experience them
• Observe the infant while taking the history from the mother
• The older child must be given the opportunity to talk to or to present symptoms. Ask the child if the illness interferes with school and how the child feels about the illness in simple terms
• Establish a rapport with mother and child by being kind and sincere
• Speak the language she is most comfortable with, if you too know the language
• Speak in non-medical language that she easily understands, not in medical jargon
• All information that is later related in the history must be absolutely and completely truthful
• Detailed and accurate documentation of the history is important

Consider these matters too............

While at the patient's bedside, in the hospital setting, the following issues must be given due thought before you approach the mother for historical questioning and physical examination: [1-5,7-10]

• Should the question(s) be asked to the mother or the patient?
• Terminology you use
• Respect privacy of both mother and child
• Care when discussing certain issues with the mother

• Care when discussing certain issues with the patient
• In the older child or the adolescent, would you want to question the child alone on certain matters?
• Tact when discussing issues with colleagues
• Tact as to where to present concerns regarding some of your patient's more personal problems to the team of doctors in charge of the patient
• The most appropriate place to present the history if you are given the choice as certain historical details may require utmost confidentiality

SYMPTOMS[1-5,7-10]

It is vital to understand symptomatology as your history is entirely based on the patient's symptoms.

What are Symptoms?

Symptoms form the basis and the core of the pediatric history. This commences from the presenting (chief) complaint. Symptoms are clinical expressions of underlying pathophysiology that are vital to the understanding of the patient's illness.

Characteristics of a Symptom

A symptom[1-5,7-10]

• Is what the patient feels
• Is what the mother or caretaker is perceived to feel about the child to the best of their knowledge
• Is what the patient complains of as a feeling or sensation
• Is what the mother or caretaker complains of as a perceived problem to the best of their knowledge

Symptoms the mother perceives may be as follows:[1-5,7-10]

• My baby seems to be crying in pain
• She is having ear pain because she keeps rubbing her ear

Symptoms the mother has observed may be as follows:[1-5,7-10]

• He is not as active as before
• She does not want her solids but takes the milk feeds as usual
• She is one-year-old now and has not walked or talked yet; her brother did at 10 months

The doctor then enquires in detail about the symptom(s) and asks about other relevant related symptoms. Hence, it is important that your questions are in a language that the mother or caretaker understands and that both you and the historian are speaking about the same thing.

Symptoms are supported by the following:[1-5,7-10]

• The general description of clinically important event(s)
• The accurate description of clinically relevant event(s) in order of chronology that have led to the complaint(s)
• Relevant and detailed symptomatic enquiry that will shed light on the clinical problem and differential diagnosis
• Relevant and complete details of all supporting evidence based on the various important facets and features of the patient's day-to-day living

What you should do when told of symptoms:[1-5,7-10]

• Clearly and legibly document the symptoms with an ink pen
• State from whom the symptoms were obtained (i.e. the relationship of the historian to the patient)
• Document the date and time that you took the history
• Document in chronological order when and how the symptoms occurred
• Document all details of the symptoms
• Try your utmost to link and associate symptoms together so that they may relate to each other rather than thinking of them as separate entities
• Think through the symptoms and the sequence of events and form a logical impression on how the disease has brought the child to medical attention and how it has affected the child and the family
• Ask anything else relevant about the symptoms that you may have left out before leaving the patient by polite direct questioning
• Needless to say documentation is of paramount importance in today's practice of medicine as patients are more aware of their rights

Enquiry of Symptoms

Give the patient a chance to talk, be a good and attentive listener : open ended questions and closed ended questions

• In the early part of the history the questions are mainly open ended, starting with how, when, why, etc. Open ended type of questions require more than a simple "yes" or "no" answer. Hence listen carefully to the patient's history
• When you have got a fair idea of the problem, you may also ask closed ended type questions which are more focused, where you limit choices to the answers and patients or parents may answer "yes" or "no"
• At times, you may want to bring the patient or the mother back on "track" (or redirect) to the illness. Historians can get carried away because of their fear of their illness or extreme concern for their child. Gentle "redirection" comes with practice in history-taking, and one must remember to be patient, tactful and very polite at all times

The establishment of normal patterns and the need for historical comparison

- Establish normal patterns

- The enquiry of symptoms must establish the normal pattern of events first.
- This is important as:
  - There are wide variations to some normal patterns of symptoms in children of different ages.
  - The symptoms that are perceived by the guardian to be abnormal must be re-examined (with humility and respect) by further questioning in the light of this wide normal variation in children to better understand the symptoms related to you so that you can ask closed ended questions during history-taking.

So for example,

a. You must determine the child's normal bowel pattern before proceeding with a history of diarrhea.
b. You must ask what the normal number of changes of nappies is before deciding on reduced urine output.
c. Ask whether the infant normally regurgitates his food and differentiate it from the perceived symptom of vomiting.

Compare with Siblings

Comparison with siblings is a form of enquiry that is important in pediatrics. This is particularly important when asking about development, appetite and growth. Comparison gives the mother the opportunity for recall and often enables the discovery of other relevant information in the history.

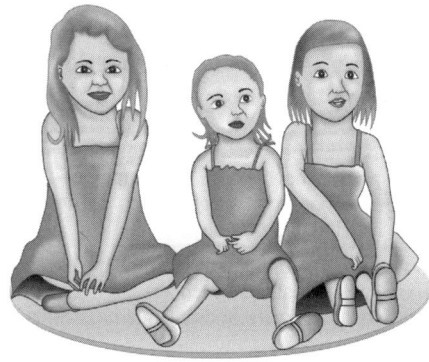

Comparison with siblings—a form of important pediatric enquiry

An example of the importance of comparison at arriving at a cause for the diagnosis would be:

a. If on comparison with siblings of a child who is deemed to be small-for-age other siblings were also small, a familial or genetic cause may be considered. Further enquiry of this would then be necessary.

b. The age at which the child walked or said the first meaningful word may not be remembered by the mother but comparison to the siblings may reveal "that they were no different from the others" enabling you to form some impression of the developmental milestones of the patient.

THE CARDINAL TEN (HISTORICAL)

The Cardinal Ten (Historical) describes and enquires into essential features of the history by analysis of important symptoms. **The Cardinal Ten (Historical)** asks ten important and relevant questions. The enquiry of each of these actually describes the symptom with entirety and clinical significance. Study these points and bear them in mind.[1-5,7-10] Use them as a quick reference pertaining to questioning symptomatology.

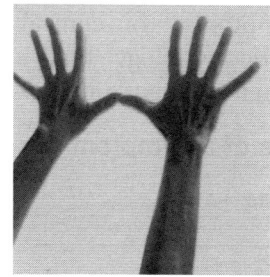

The Cardinal Ten (Historical)

1.	**T**ime of onset	When
2.	**N**ature of onset	What
3.	**T**rigger of onset	How
4.	**I**ntensity at onset	How much
5.	**D**uration of symptoms	How long
6.	**C**hange in intensity	How much less or how much more
7.	***A**ssociated factor(s)	**What else
8.	**E**xacerbating factor(s)	Worsened by
9.	**R**elieving factor(s)	Lessened by
10.	**A**ction factor(s) or intervention(s)	What was done?

*Associated factors or **what else explores in the clinical history the possible related or relevant links

HISTORICAL LINK

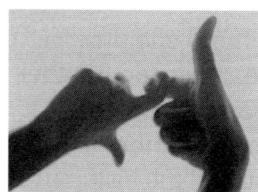

The historical link is good to ask!

This mainly attempts to link the pathophysiological connection that occurs in the human body as a result of interactions of known physiological processes.

The historical link is a bridge between the presenting complaint and many relevant factors that are vital to making an accurate clinical diagnosis:

The historical link links the history to:
• The clinical facets of the disease and its differential diagnoses
• The pathophysiological processes of the disease
• The possible etiological diagnosis
• The activities of daily living of the index patient and the activities of daily living of the family
• The social impact of the disease to the patient, family and community.

To elicit questions to form the link of clinical events, remember that these events are often told to the history taker by the mother in one way or the other so listen attentively.

Think, watch, listen, talk and think again.

When asking **The Cardinal Ten (Historical)** bear in mind that the "what else" can link you to significant events in the history. New events that emerge in the history which may have relevance to the disease or its differential diagnosis may also be elicited.

The associated factor(s) or the "what else" for each symptom is different, base it on your existing knowledge of the pathophysiology of the symptom. Here, you will form a link of related symptoms; the more histories you take the easier this will become.

In any underlying health condition enquire about how the illness has affected the **activities of daily living.**[10]

In the history of the **more acute presenting complaint,** enquire for example if the cough disturbed sleep; if the breathlessness interfered with feeding or if the fever kept the child away from school.

In a chronic problem, activities of daily living are important.

Ask if the repeated cough in a case of chronic cough caused frequent vomiting and if this interfered with weight gain; also ask if the cough was associated with dyspnea or if the dyspnea interfered with the child's attendance at school or playing of games. In an asthmatic child on inhaler therapy, ask if the child could play games like other children and if inhalers were necessarily taken before a game at school. In case of a diabetic child, for example, ask if the child knew to take a sweet in response to dizziness (due to hypoglycemia) and hence was always made to keep a sweet in the pocket.

In **chronic diseases**, the **social impact of the disease and the activity of daily living involving the family** are also very important.

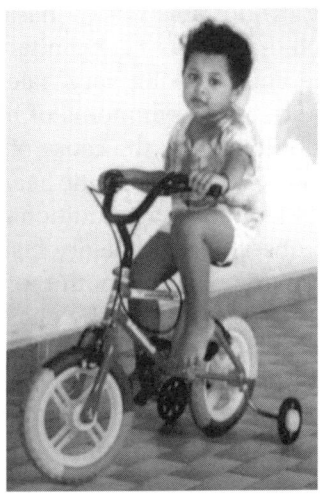

A young boy enjoys cycling which is an activity of daily living. Remember that the activities of daily living are as important to the child as they are to the adult. Emphasize its relevance and reflect it in your good clinical history. (Reprint with kind permission from VRK)

ACTIVITIES OF DAILY LIVING IN CHILDREN[1,2,4,5,7-10]

In the clinical history, enquiry into the activities of daily living that reflect the quality of the patient's **life** is an important component of the practical history because it:
• Makes the history more meaningfully related to the patient's daily life
• It gives relevance to the differential diagnosis
• Makes it a practical history relating the disease to the influence of his or her daily activities
• Makes it a clinically useful history that relates to the pathophysiology of the disease
• Is an important component for a more focused diagnosis of the underlying condition
• Is reflection for treatment issues of the underlying condition and its influence on other aspects of the patient as a whole
• Is a means of prioritizing management issues and where needed appropriate referral of patient and family to a multidisciplinary team.
• A support network for coping with pertinent emotional issues, patient and family support as a support tool for up-to-date patient information and education

The Link: Pediatric History-Taking and Physical Examination

The links in history-taking through observation and pathophysiology (observe the things around the patient as you take the history)

As the first example....... The link to activities of daily living reflects the severity of disease

During history-taking from the mother, you must also observe the surroundings and the patient. While taking the history you notice that the young child is sitting up in bed looking comfortable but on nasal oxygen. The mother tells you that he has a congenital heart disease. You notice the child looking very pale. In this case you must enquire on all symptoms of heart failure at that age, attempt to deduce the cause of the condition knowing that cyanotic and acyanotic heart diseases can cause heart failure at that age. Additionally, due to the striking pallor observed, the dietary history including all questions on type and amount of feeding and difficulties during feeding must be elicited. Details of growth and developmental milestones must be asked. Be aware about pathophysiological processes like the expression of cyanosis: if the hemoglobin is less than 5 g/dL, the cyanosis will be difficult to clinically detect.

The links are:
- To ascertain all historical details of heart failure, the underlying cause of heart failure. The past history of illnesses and chest infections will be important in forming a diagnosis.
- Peripheral vasoconstriction in heart failure can make a child look pale. Bearing this in mind, you will later examine the cardiovascular system thoroughly to exclude this. But in this comfortable child, do not assume that the pallor is only due to heart failure. Determine the cause of the pallor by asking about difficulties in feeding and in going into the nutritional history. Remember also that poor nutrition includes not only intake but all conditions that interfere with absorption and assimilation of nutrients.
- Enquire about the activities of daily living like playing, getting up and down stairs, attendance to nurseries and many others. Ask about how this illness has affected the family. Appreciate how activities of daily living give you a clue to severity of the underlying condition. The social history of the family also gives you an idea of how the disease has impacted living activities of the family.

A second example ....The link to the onset of the disease helps narrow the diagnosis

During history-taking of a child with stridor, you must enquire from the mother about its onset, whether sudden or insidious and the child's activity prior to the episode. Enquire also if accompanied by other symptoms like choking, vomiting or cyanosis. This may reveal the cause which may be acute bacterial in origin with the history of drooling of saliva, being very ill or of refusing to feed or on the other hand, of a slightly more insidious viral etiology. A sudden onset in a previously healthy child must immediately alert one to possible foreign body inhalation. In foreign body aspiration, quickly ask, if the child was playing on the carpet with small toys. The age and developmental history would tell you if the child has already developed a pincer grip.

Notice how the mode of onset links you to other questions to determine the etiology of the stridor. Appreciate in the above examples how knowledge of the pathophysiology of the disease helps in forming a chain of relevant questions which are clues for an informed clinical guess and with the physical examination, basis for a sound clinical diagnosis.

PERTINENT NEGATIVES IN THE HISTORY

Pertinent negative history has often not been emphasized enough. During history-taking you ask many questions that you feel can directly take you to a possible diagnoses or a list of differential diagnoses. You ask questions and may find that the patient is experiencing illness in one particular system. You proceed to ask important questions of that system. You also ask about related symptoms. You ask more questions on the diagnosis considered while asking to exclude symptomatology that could overlap with other diseases. The negative responses or the absence of such symptoms helps you reaffirm the positive answers and make a case in strengthening your provisional diagnosis.

When you have got a fair idea of the problem, you may also ask many closed ended type questions which are more focused, where you limit choices to the answers

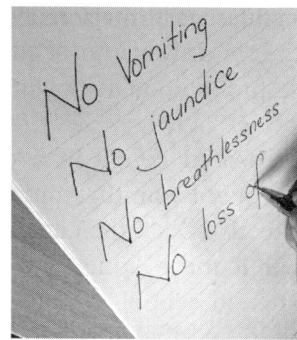

Negative symptoms have as much diagnostic value as the positive ones

and patients or parents may answer "yes" or "no". Usually, during closed ended type questioning, positive symptoms and negative symptoms are elicited. These negative symptoms have as much diagnostic value as the positive ones.

Pertinent negatives
• Negative symptoms of either the system affected by the illness or of another system that overlap with the symptoms of the system that is affected by the disease
• These symptoms reduce the possibility of other systems involved and the need to consider these systems in the differential diagnosis
• These symptoms give greater credence to the positive symptoms experienced and help for greater accuracy in the diagnosis
• Help eliminate unlikely etiological diagnosis

Remember that in linking an important clinical symptom to another based on pathophysiology and pattern of diseases, you will have to ask many direct questions. The mother too may volunteer much vital information which you understand by attentive listening. This is the importance of the historical link and it elicits many questions that are answered in the affirmative. This line of questioning strengthens your most probable diagnosis.

While the astute mother herself may have told you many things that did happen in the history, she cannot tell you things that did not happen but may be deemed highly relevant. Hence you ask these questions, by direct questioning, whether such important events occurred. When armed with sufficient knowledge about diseases that occur in children these questions will help in excluding the more unlikely differential diagnosis. They give weight to the diagnosis that you feel is most likely. Hence given the importance of these events (or the lack or absence of such events), these pertinent negatives must be written down and narrated to the listener who can then make his or her own clinical judgment.

Remember that when a good history is taken, the need for superfluous and sometimes unnecessary investigations is reduced. A good clinician asks sharp important questions that quickly eliminate unlikely diagnoses.

As an example........The link of a symptom to other systems with similar symptomatology
A child of three years and who is not thriving well, has a cough of two weeks' duration. The child has a history of rhinorrhea and fever and other family members have any history of an upper respiratory tract illness. You mentally formulate that the problem involves infection of the respiratory system. You ask about how the cough started, the precipitating factors and relieving factors. If the mother says that the cough worsens when the child lies down, you may think of a postnasal drip. But in view of the poor growth of the child, you may also want to exclude "orthopnea". You ask if there is exercise intolerance, a history suggestive of paroxysmal nocturnal dyspnea. These questions are asked to exclude cardiac failure as a cause of the cough. You later review the relevant systems well. If these questions have negative answers, you decide that a cardiac cause of the cough is unlikely and consolidate your opinion of a respiratory problem. You continue to ask other relevant questions to focus the pathological and etiological diagnosis.

You proceed to ask if the fever was high grade or low grade to determine an etiological diagnosis. You ask if there were chills. The absence of chills in an active child with fever supports a viral etiology whereas high grade fever with chills in an inactive child suggests a bacterial etiology.

You may ask about travel or immunization. Based on the history of travel to endemic regions for some diseases, or the absence of specific immunization, a more specific etiological cause may be suspected and you further narrow down the differential diagnosis.

Another example is the links in the history to search for an etiological cause
In a child diagnosed with bronchial asthma, the mother may tell you that the child usually has an attack of cough and wheezing when he or she has flu or a running nose. You must also ask about other precipitating factors like animals, furry toys, cigarette smoke, aerosol sprays, exercise, cold weather, excitement and fizzy drinks. Even if the answer is "no" to all these triggers, it tells you importantly that the asthma attack is triggered by infection and not due to allergens, irritants exercise, excitement, colored or fizzy drinks. These trigger factors are important to elicit and to eliminate by the history. Your knowledge of etiology and a spectrum of variable disease triggers may prompt you to bring these possible triggers to the attention of the mother when counseling about management, treatment and prevention of such diseases.

REFERENCES

1. History-taking. Available at http://medicaltextbooksrevealed.s3.amazonaws.com. Accessed April 2013.
2. Goel KM, Gupta DK. Hutchinson's Pediatrics (1st edn). India: Jaypee Brothers Medical Publishers (P) Ltd; 2009.
3. Marcdante K, Kliegman RM, Jenson HB, Behrman RE (Eds). Nelson's Essentials of Pediatrics (6th edn). Saunders Elsevier, 2010.
4. Pediatric history and physical examination (Children are not just little adults). Available at http://www.ped.med.utah.edu. Accessed April 2013.
5. The pediatric history. Available at http://www.patient.co.uk/doctor. Accessed April 2013.
6. Website of Ministry of Health, Malaysia. Available at www.moh.gov.my. Accessed April 2013.
7. Mason S, Swash M (Eds). Hutchinson's Clinical Methods (17th edn). A Baillere Tindall Book Published by Cassell Ltd; 1980.
8. Milner AD, Hull D. Hospital Pediatrics. 3rd edn. ELBS with Churchill Livingstone. 1998.
9. Richard E. Behrman (comps). Robert M Kliegman, Waldo E Nelson, Victor C Vaughan III (eds). Nelson's Textbook of Pediatrics (14th ed). Philadelphia: WB Saunders; 1992.
10. Stephenson T, Wallace H (Eds). Clinical Pediatrics for Postgraduate Examinations. UK: Churchill Livingstone; 1991.

The essence of the relevant chapters in the following books have also been numbered as references in this chapter. We recommend for further reading, the rich text in these books for greater integration and deeper understanding.

1. Goel KM, Gupta DK. Hutchinson's Pediatrics, 1st edn. Jaypee Brothers Medical Publishers (P) Ltd, India. 2009.
2. Marcdante K, Kliegman RM, Jenson HB, Behrman RE (Eds). Nelson's Essentials of Pediatric, 6th edn. Saunders Elsevier. 2010.
3. Mason S, Swash M (Eds). Hutchinson's Clinical Methods, 17th edn. A Baillere Tindall Book Published by Cassell Ltd. 1980.
4. Milner AD, Hull D. Hospital Pediatrics, 3rd edn. ELBS with Churchill Livingstone. 1998.
5. Behrman RE (comps), Kliegman RM, Nelson WE, Vaughan III VC (Eds). Nelson's Textbook of Pediatrics, 14th edn. Philadelphia: WB Saunders. 1992.
6. Stephenson T, Wallace H (Eds). Clinical Pediatrics for Postgraduate Examinations. UK: Churchill Livingstone.1991.

Chapter 2

History of the Presenting Problem and the Past Medical and Surgical History

CLARIFICATION OF THE PEDIATRIC HISTORY UNDER SPECIFIC HEADINGS

The pediatric history is an important tool for diagnosis.[1-8] The history commences with the chief complaint and continues with the history of the presenting complaint.

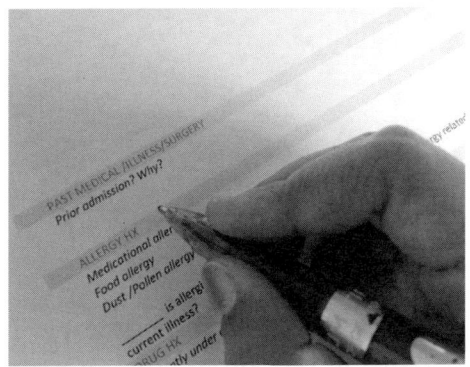

CHIEF COMPLAINT AND HISTORY OF THE PRESENTING COMPLAINT (HPC)[1-4]

Features of the Chief Complaint

The first part of the history must be recorded in the historian's exact words. This will include the reason for seeking medical attention and the last clinical event that triggered the seeking of medical attention. This is what worried the mother most and is the reason that prompted her to bring the child to the doctor. The chief complaint is recorded in the mother's own words. The duration of the complaint must be clearly mentioned.

Where there is more than one symptom, set them out separately with space in between to document the details of how it developed and the relationships between the symptoms.

The chief complaint is:

• The reason for the visit to the doctor
• The clinical event that worried the mother most
• Recorded in the mother's, caretaker's or patient's own words
• Stated with a time duration (if it is a symptom)
• Stated separately with the duration of each symptom in case of more than one symptom

The following are examples of chief complaints:

a. In a child who has been unwell with symptoms of flu for a week and a fever of a day's duration, one must ask what made the mother bring the child to the doctor; the chief complaint here is likely to be as follows:
"High fever of one day duration associated with flu of a week's duration".

b. In a child who may be a slow walker, the chief complaint may be "she is not walking yet even though her sisters walked at her age and I am quite worried".

HISTORY OF THE PRESENTING PROBLEM[5,6]

It is best to use non-medical terms, describing every symptom that is mentioned to you in simple and accurate terms without changing the essence of the information given to you. Document when the symptoms started and their duration. In case of more than one symptom, observe their sequence and chronological order.

After attentively listening to the symptom(s) in the presenting problem, it is necessary to further enquire in depth or in detail about the symptom (s). Use **The Cardinal Ten (Historical)**. When did the symptoms

14   The Link: Pediatric History-Taking and Physical Examination

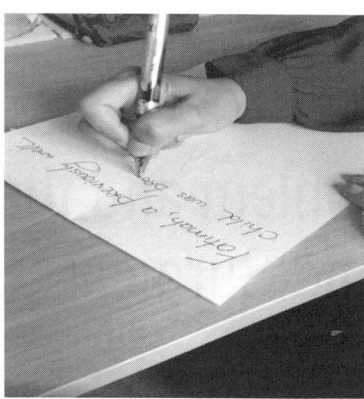

It is important to establish when the child was last well

The history of the presenting problem[1-8]

• Reviews the chief complaint in detail
• Includes the reason for the visit, **what** the concerns were and **why** the concerns were present
• Asks a **focused history** based on:
– Generally, starting off the history by asking when the child was last well
– Listening to the patient's story
– Asking open ended questions
– The ten important questions (referred to as **The Cardinal Ten (Historical)** with all relevant historical links
– Asking more precise questions when there are some clinical clues
• Conducts a **focused review** of the system involved in the chief complaint
• Relates the presenting problem to important activities of daily living

begin, what were the nature of events of clinical relevance, how those events happened, how severe they were at onset, how long the symptoms lasted, did the symptoms improve or worsen (i.e. how much less or how much more intense did they get) what other symptom(s) was associated, factors that worsened the symptoms, factors that improved the symptoms, and what was done, i.e. seek medical attention, resorted to home remedies, etc.

Remember that in the initial part of the history, the questions are mainly open ended, starting with how, when, why, etc. Open ended type of questions are not to be answered with a simple "yes" or "no". Hence listen carefully to the patient's history. Take care to listen to the symptoms told to you. Observe facial expressions and body language like despair, anguish or hopelessness and try to understand the untold part of the story as well. Sometimes, you may have to put yourself in the mother's shoes to begin to understand some of her genuine worries.

When you have got a fair idea of the issues, you may also ask closed ended type questions which are more focused, where you limit choices to the answers and patients or parents may answer "yes" or "no". The "what else" question in **The Cardinal Ten (Historical)** often leads you to links to ask closed ended questions.

Remember to be courteous and polite at all times.

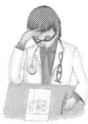

"I must get the history of the presenting problem right as much of the rest of the history is based on this!"

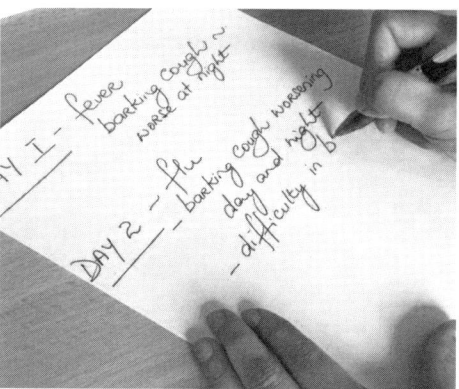

In an acute problem, start narrating from the onset of the most recent symptom on a day-to-day basis. Mention all relevant positives and pertinent negatives

When asking about the symptoms not already volunteered to you by the historian, think of the pathophysiology of the presenting issues and ask all possible questions in relation to it. Be aware that some of these associated symptoms may not readily be told to you as the mother may not have perceived them to be important or simply, may have forgotten the details. Rarely these symptoms are not related deliberately. Try to obtain as much information as possible about these symptoms by using comparison to siblings, establishing normal patterns and so on.

You may bring in other relevant components of the history here (refer to appropriate section for details).

The following example illustrates this point:
In taking the history of a child with fever and rash, the behavioral and feeding history can be narrated in

this section. Family history, if relevant to a particular problem, could be narrated here briefly. Alertness, irritability, lethargy, feeding, vomiting, diarrhea and sleep pattern can be relevant. Additionally, history of other family members having fever or rash and history of contact with the patient are all pertinent here. Remember! Where a positive lead is given, detail that with **The Cardinal Ten (Historical)**.

In a chronic problem where the presenting symptoms are a part of the continuum of the disease, after explaining the reason for the presenting problem and going into the sufficient details of the presenting symptoms, you should also narrate the history with relevant details of the long standing illness from when it started. This gives meaning and depth to the history. It helps put things into perspective and provides a systematic approach to the patient's problems.

Example 1

A good example can be illustrated in the history taking of a child with nephrotic syndrome in relapse. After going into details of the presenting causes for the relapse, you must mention briefly about the initial diagnosis of nephrotic syndrome and that this is not the first time of such an illness. The disease progression since the initial diagnosis and greater details must all be told in the past medical illness that will soon follow after the history of present illness (HOPI) in this case.

Example 2

A second example could be a history from the mother of a known asthmatic who presents with symptoms of acute exacerbation of bronchial asthma. After elucidating the presenting symptoms in detail with the help of **The Cardinal Ten (Historical),** which will include the possible reasons for the present exacerbation or trigger of onset, mention that this is not the first time of such an episode. State with clarity about the overall trend or pattern of the illness thus far. Describe all other asthma attacks clearly in chronological order, mentioning its severity and presentation, reviewing them using **The Cardinal Ten (Historical)** as a guide. Narrate this in detail in the past medical history which will follow soon after the HOPI in this case.

For example, after describing the reasons for this admission in the HOPI, you may also add, "the child was well until a year ago when he developed breathing difficulties and cough following a game of badminton. He had a sudden onset of dyspnea, lasting about ten minutes. Despite treatment, the child continued to have nocturnal cough, exercise-induced cough and dyspnea on exertion. From then on, he had about two attacks a month. Most of these attacks were precipitated by exercise and relieved by nebuliser therapy as an out-patient. There was never any need for hospitalization until this presenting episode".

A questionnaire guide to the history of the presenting problem[1-8]—(remember to use the questions in **The Cardinal Ten (Historical)** and to enquire about how the illness influences the daily activities of the child.

- When did the illness start?
- Was your child well before that?
- Were there similar symptoms as in the current illness before?
- What triggered the onset of the current symptoms or how did the current illness develop?
- Have there been any noted factors that aggravate the current symptoms?
- Have there been any noted factors that relieve the current symptoms?
- What was done by way of intervention like seeking out-patient treatment or treatment from a general practitioner for the current symptoms?
- Has there been any similar symptom among any family member? The importance of this is that most infective illnesses in children are spread from siblings or family members
- Have there been any similar illnesses or outbreaks in the nursery?
- Has the illness affected the child's activity?
- Has the illness affected the child's feeding?
- Has the illness affected the child's attendance at playschool/nursery/school?
- How has the illness affected other family members?

The Trend of the Illness[5]

When observing the details of symptoms, it is important not to forget the trend of the illness. The trend of the illness refers to the onset, the progression and then the present state. The trend of the illness is often as important if not more important than the details. Ask yourself if it is something that began insidiously or acutely? Has it gradually worsen till present time? Ask yourself if it is intermittent in nature or whether it is an acute illness that has improved but has not completely disappeared. Ask yourself if the overall health of the child is related to the clinical outcome. Consider the influence of interventions on the overall trend of the illness.

At the end of the history of the presenting problem, you must try to mentally form an impression of the problem which will then help you formulate a few reasonable differential diagnoses.

16 *The Link*: Pediatric History-Taking and Physical Examination

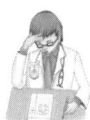

This is good advice. I must stand back and consider the trend of the illness. An overall idea of the pattern of the events is as important as the details of the individual symptoms

---

Remember! The Formulation of the Hypothesis

Cause
- What are the possible causes of the patient's problem(s)
  Think laterally or broadly on the various possible causes to the patient's problem(s)

Determine system involved
- Determining the main system involved remembering that in pediatrics some symptoms can be nonspecific hence you may have to sometimes include more than one system

Consider the history volunteered to you; then the open ended questions and the guided or close ended questions
- Consider all the symptoms that have been told by the patient to you on his or her own accord. Then consider your open ended questioning, and similarly your more focused questioning. Review this information in a balanced and logical manner

Hypothetical diagnosis
- Form hypotheses of the problem

Question the hypothesis
- Proceed to further focused questioning on the hypothesis formed
- Formulate an early clinical impression of the problem and make about 3–5 reasonable differential diagnoses
- Then proceed with history taking; asking further questions in the review of systems and under other components of the history (refer to Chapter 3 and Chapter 5)

Remember many more focused or closed ended questions in the other components of the history will constitute important positive or negative historical facts which would reduce the number of differential diagnosis formulated after the history of the presenting complaint. Other parts of the history must be used to give you a clearer idea on your initial impression and sharpen your clinical impression logically.

These questions may strengthen one diagnosis and weaken another so that at the end of the history you are able to make a more focused differential diagnosis of the patient's problem. This will guide you in the physical examination after which you will come to a possible diagnosis—directing appropriate examination and investigations.

Schematic formulation of the hypothesis and the differential diagnosis

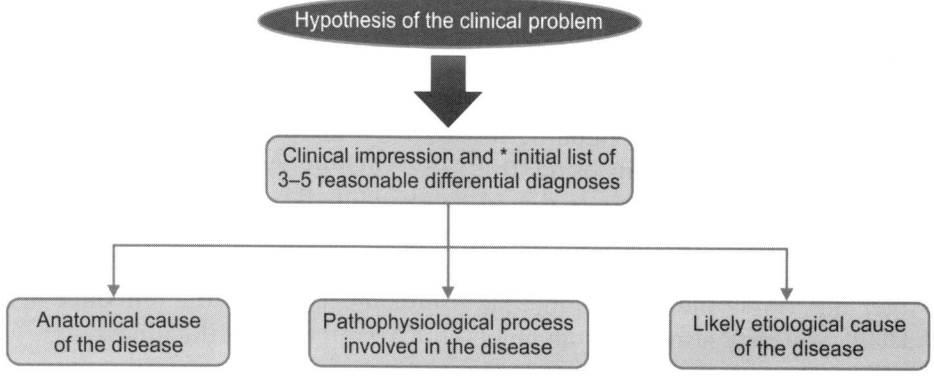

*These become more-likely or less-likely as you use each component of the history to strengthen the most-likely differential diagnosis

HISTORY OF PAST MEDICAL OR SURGICAL PROBLEMS

(All past medical and surgical problems must be documented here)

Past Illnesses

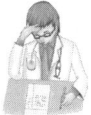

Always try to ascertain diagnosis of past illnesses yourself rather than naively believing "diagnostic labels" rendered to you by the historian. Think critically and explore the symptoms and signs of the past illness and convince yourself of the possible past disease.

Comment on the child's previous general health. Explore specific areas listed below.[1-5,7,8]

Past health problems[1-5,7,8]	Details[1-5,7]
Infections • Viral, bacterial	Age Types Numbers Severity
Contagious diseases • Viral exanthems	Age
	Complications following infectious diseases such as rubella, mumps, pertussis, diphtheria, scarlet fever
Chronic diseases	Age of diagnosis
Rarer in pediatric age groups • Nephrotic syndrome • Bronchial asthma • Hypertension • Cardiac diseases • Diabetes mellitus • Malignancy • Skin diseases	**Symptoms:** Symptoms of exacerbations or relapse, specific pathognomonic symptoms, inter-episodic (attack) symptoms, influence of disease to daily life **Medications:** Types, methods of use, time periods, rapidity and completeness of response, in-patient or out-patient treatment **Follow-up**
Past hospitalizations	Medical/surgical (indication and type of surgery) Age Drugs given Duration of treatment and follow-up

As examples

In a case of nephrotic syndrome in relapse, the disease progression since the first diagnosis, the details of the symptoms that led to the first diagnosis (so that you are convinced of the initial diagnosis and attempt to elicit details of the type of nephrotic syndrome) and details of treatment, complications if any and urine examination results, must all be told in the past medical illness that will soon follow after the HOPI. It is vital to know if a relapse has occurred and why it occurred.

In a case of diagnosed bronchial asthma, the description of all asthma attacks clearly in chronological order, mentioning its severity and presentation, night time symptoms, daily activities, condition between attacks, treatment and response, using **The Cardinal Ten (Historical)** must be done. It is then important to classify asthma according to frequency, severity and response.

If the patient had previously been admitted to the hospital, write a brief summary for each hospitalization.

Remember also, following hospitalization, in the past history, that you must enquire about the condition of the child from the time of discharge up to the time of readmission. Ask about medications given on discharge. These are especially vital if these medications are prescribed for long-term use. Any subsequent illnesses, surgeries, accidents or trauma must be asked in this part of the history.

Some examples of trauma to children[1-5,7,8]

• Accidental injuries
• Accidental falls
• Road traffic accidents
• Drowning or suffocations
• Flames and fires
• Car accidents
• Poisoning
• Non-accidental injuries

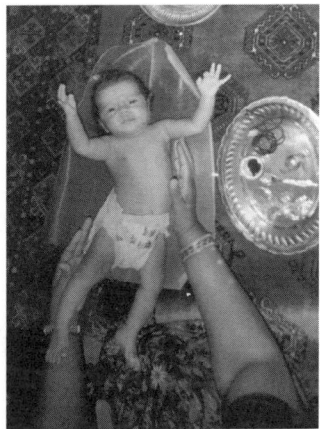

The 28th day marks the end of the neonatal period and is an auspicious occasion for celebration and thanks giving in some Asian cultures (Reprint with permission from VRK)

Screening tests results or concerns must be reviewed here[1,4,7]

Newborn screening includes:
• Metabolic screening
• Hemoglobin electrophoresis where indicated
• Hearing evaluation
• Developmental screening

Some screening tests that are done in the newborn period and in infancy[1-5,7]

• Developmental screening including developmental dysplasia of the hip
• Congenital hypothyroidism
• Critical congenital heart disease (CCHD)
• Hemoglobinopathies (sickle cell anemia)
• Fatty acid oxidation disorder
• Biotinidase deficiency
• Cystic fibrosis
• Amino acid disorders
• Galactosemia
• Congenital adrenal hyperplasia
• Homocystinuria
• Maple syrup urine disease (MSUD)
• Phenylketonuria (PKU)
• Organic acid disorders
• Medium chain acyl CoA dehydrogenase (MCAD) deficiency

REFERENCES

1. Richard E. Behrman (comps), Robert M Kliegman, Waldo E Nelson, Victor C Vaughan III. (Eds). Nelson's textbook of pediatrics (14th ed). Philadelphia: WB Saunders; 1992.
2. Elizabeth KE. Clinical Pediatrics for Undergraduates. India: Jaypee Brothers Medical Publishers (P) Ltd. 2009.
3. Goel KM, Gupta DK. Hutchinson's Pediatrics (1st edn). Jaypee Brothers Medical Publishers (P) Ltd. 2009.
4. Marcdante K, Kliegman RM, Jenson HB, Behrman RE (Eds). Nelson's Essentials of Pediatrics (6th ed). Saunders Elsevier, 2010.
5. Mason S, Swash M. Hutchinson's Clinical Methods, 17th edn. A BAILLLERE TINDALL book published by Cassell Ltd, 1980.
6. The pediatric history. Available at http://www.patient.co.uk/doctor. Accessed April 2013.
7. Milner AD, Hull D. Hospital Pediatrics. 3rd edn. ELBS with Churchill Livingstone; 1998.
8. Stephenson T, Wallace H (Eds). Clinical Pediatrics for Postgraduate Examinations. UK: Churchill Livingstone; 1991.

The essence of the relevant chapters in the following books have also been numbered as references in this chapter. We recommend for further reading, the rich text in these books for greater integration and deeper understanding.

1. Goel KM, Gupta DK. Hutchinson's Pediatrics, 1st edn. Jaypee Brothers Medical Publishers (P) Ltd. 2009.
2. Marcdante K, Kliegman RM, Jenson HB, Behrman RE (Eds). Nelson's Essentials of Pediatrics, 6th edn. Saunders Elsevier, 2010.
3. Mason S, Swash M. Hutchinson's Clinical Methods, 17th edn. A BAILLLERE TINDALL book published by Cassell Ltd, 1980.
4. Milner AD, Hull D. Hospital Pediatrics. 3rd edn. ELBS with Churchill Livingstone. 1998.
5. Behrman RE (comps), Kliegman RM, Nelson WE, Vaughan VC III (Eds). Nelson's Textbook of Pediatrics, 14th edn. Philadelphia: WB Saunders; 1992.
6. Stephenson T, Wallace H (Eds). Clinical Pediatrics for Postgraduate Examinations. UK: Churchill Livingstone. 1991.

Chapter 3

Review of Systems

CORE OBJECTIVES

The review of systems (ROS)[1-28] is for the purposes of eliciting the following:
1. A list of questions focused on one organ system:
   a. Covers all important systems
   b. Covers all general symptoms of diseases[1-29]
   c. Utilizes a head-to-toe approach of organs in the body to clarify the history of present illness (HOPI) and all related symptoms

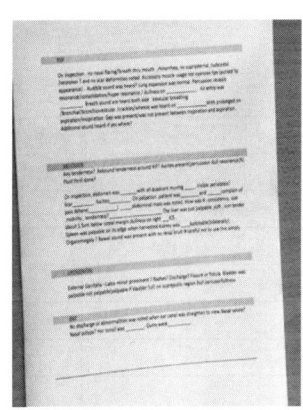

2. The collateral history of the mother pertaining to all related systems in the younger pediatric patient.
3. First-hand symptoms from the older patient himself or herself pertaining to all related systems.
4. Relevant negative symptoms of systems that will help exclude other diagnosis.

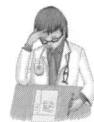

So the review of systems has a number of functions. Amongst the tasks are that it serves as a noninvasive tool that screens early symptoms of diseases. It also links and reviews symptoms that are relevant to the presenting problem. It is indeed a vital part of the pediatric history.

Features of the Review of Systems[5]

- Important health issues that involve systems other than the system in question, involved in the chief complaint are reviewed here
- These may be independently important or may contribute to making a diagnosis
- Strengthens the impressions or early differential diagnoses formed in the history of presenting illness (HOPI)
- Detailed questions of the systems with positive and negative answers which may allude to other differential diagnoses not already thought of after the HOPI may be asked here.
- Further defines the probable pathophysiological and etiological cause of the diagnosis
- Uncovers subtle symptoms of existing diseases
- Unmasks symptoms of early disease by direct questioning
- A history-taking tool to screen diseases.

SYMPTOMATIC ENQUIRY OF SYSTEMS

Examples to illustrate ROS in the gastrointestinal tract.

Take for example the importance of the systemic review in a child with abdominal symptoms:

Characteristics that may be linked to abdominal pain which are not already reviewed in the gastrointestinal system (i.e. the system in question).

1. **The importance of the review of system in a case of abdominal pain due to inflammatory bowel disease: elucidates disease etiology**

In the review of systems, you may gather information of weight loss or weight gain indicating how the

disease may have affected growth; you may ask about fever, joint complaints and rash.
- The occurrence of one or more of these indicates an inflammatory or infectious disease process.

2. **The importance of review of systems in vomiting due to gastroesophageal reflux: elucidates the influence of disease to other symptoms**

   In the review of systems, you may get information of the relationship of vomiting as a symptom in the HOPI to symptoms involving other systems.
   - Hyperactive airway disease, chronic cough and recurrent laryngitis may be more pronounced than the gastrointestinal symptomatology such as vomiting.

3. **The nondigestive tract causes of gastrointestinal symptoms: elucidates other causes of similar symptoms**

   In the review of systems, you get a chance to ask about similar symptoms that could occur in other systemic diseases.
   - Anorexia other than a sole symptom of gastrointestinal disease, could occur in many systemic diseases; vomiting can occur in gastrointestinal diseases, in urinary tract infections and increased intracranial pressure; diarrhea could be parenteral, constipation is seen in diverse simple etiologies and even in endocrine disorders like in hypothyroidism; dehydration can be due to many causes which can be individually asked in the ROS, abdominal pain can be a result of referred pain in many other etiologies, such as in renal diseases, pneumonias, some collagen vascular diseases and even as a psychogenic symptom. Hence, all other possible causes of the gastrointestinal symptom not reviewed in the HOPI can be thoroughly reviewed here.

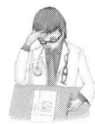

The ROS varies in its length and details in different ages. It is usually briefer in the infant. In the older child, the tendency is for the ROS to be longer.

REVIEW OF SYSTEMS SPREADSHEET[2,5,6,11,19,27,28]

Review of systems (ROS)	Symptoms	Yes or No
In general:	Fever	
	Chills and rigors	
	Change in activity	
	Weight loss or weight gain	
	Others	
Mouth:	Ulcers	
	Bleeding gums or swollen gums	
	Lesions of soft and hard palate	
	Soreness of tongue	
	Dental caries	
	Others	
Head, ear, nose and throat:	Mouth breathing	
	Snoring	
	Excessive salivation	
	Change in vision	
	Decreased hearing	
	Ringing sensation in the ears	
	Runny nose	

Contd...

Contd...

Review of systems (ROS)	Symptoms	Yes or No
	Thick white nasal discharge	
	Green nasal discharge	
	Ear pain	
	Ear discharge	
	Sore throat	
	Neck pain	
	Others	
Respiratory system:	Cough	
	Type of cough	
	Relieving and aggravating factors for cough	
	Wheezing and associated factors	
	Shortness of breath	
	Factors that reactivate breathlessness	
	Factors that relieve breathlessness	
	Recurrent chest infections	
	Other forms of noisy breathing	
	Change in color noted (e.g. pallor or cyanosis)	
	Others	
Cardiovascular system:	Shortness of breath	
	Sweating	
	Excessive sweating on scalp while feeding	
	Poor feeding	
	Unable to complete feeds	
	Color changes with feeding	
	Recent history of murmur detected	
	Chest pain	
	Palpitations	
	Fainting or dizziness	
	Exercise intolerance	
	Paroxysmal nocturnal dyspnea	
	Recurrent chest infections	
	Others	
Gastrointestinal system:	Stooling habits	
	Excessive regurgitation	
	Screaming episodes with legs drawn up	
	Abdominal pain	
	Nausea	
	Bloody vomitus or vomiting without blood	
	Bilious vomiting	
	Diarrhea	
	Constipation	
	Hematemesis	

Contd...

Contd...

Review of systems (ROS)	Symptoms	Yes or No
	Hematochezia	
	Melena	
	Symptoms indicative of gastroesophageal reflux disease (GERD)	
	Recurrent vomiting	
	Refusing to eat, gagging or even choking with feeding	
	Crying during feeding	
	Heartburn or "wind"	
	Symptom suggestive of abdominal pathology such as pain or discomfort	
	Others	
Genitourinary system:	Frequent unexplained fevers	
	Screaming episodes	
	Poor weight gain	
	Dysuria	
	Frequency	
	Urgency	
	Hematuria	
	History of sexual activity	
	Circumcision	
	Others	
Endocrine system:	Polyuria or polydipsia	
	Heat or cold intolerance	
	Precocious puberty	
	Delayed puberty	
	Feeding difficulties	
	Constipation	
	Growth pattern	
	Palpitations in teenage girl	
	Sweating excessively in teenage girl	
	Heat intolerance	
	Cold intolerance	
	Others	
Musculoskeletal system:	Myalgias	
	Arthralgias	
	Trauma	
	Limp	
	Muscle weakness	
	Others	
Neurological system:	Loud sounds are ignored	
	Does not follow objects with eyes	
	Head trauma	

Contd...

Contd...

Review of systems (ROS)	Symptoms	Yes or No
	Loss of consciousness (LOC)	
	Seizure activity	
	Developmental delays (later covered in detail under developmental history)	
	No eye contact	
	"Lazy eye"	
	Abnormal eye movements	
	Abnormalities involving chewing or swallowing	
	Constipation	
	Dysphagia	
	Recurrent chest infections (due to aspiration)	
	Pressure ulcers	
	Photophobia	
	Others	
Skin:	Rashes (with mother's description of site and nature)	
	Duration of rash	
	Exacerbating factors	
	Relieving factors	
	Noted petechiae	
	Noted bruising	
	Noted ecchymosis	
	Associated pruritis	
	Associated bruising	
	Associated petechiae	
	Associated nail problems	
	Associated hair problems	
	Others	
Infectious diseases:	Contact with adults with recent illnesses (later covered in detail under social history)	
	Contact with children in nursery with rashes (later covered in detail under social history)	
	Diarrhea	
	Cough	
	Fever	
	Recent travel to endemic areas (later covered in detail under travel history)	
	Immunizations (later covered in detail under immunization history)	
	Others	
Psychological or behavioral:	Decreased energy level	
	Extreme separation anxiety	
	Unusually obsessive	
	Cranky, temper tantrums (later covered in detail under behavioral history)	
	Others	

SYMPTOMATIC ENQUIRY USING THE CARDINAL TEN (HISTORICAL) AND THE HISTORICAL LINK

- First and foremost, for an accurate and meaningful history, it has been emphasized earlier that you must ensure that, in pediatric history-taking, you and the mother (or caretaker) are talking about the same thing. Once that is established, the points listed under each system may be useful in the symptomatic enquiry of patients. Each case must be considered individually and all related questions pertaining to the condition must be asked.
- In the symptomatic enquiry, consider asking **The Cardinal Ten (Historical)** and the historical link whenever relevant and related.

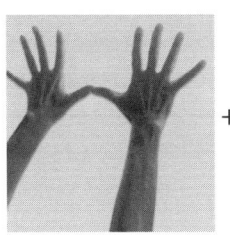 +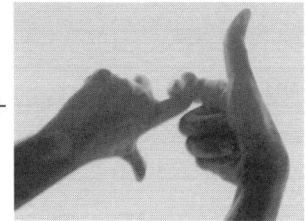

In the symptomatic enquiry of systems, use these tools, i.e. The Cardinal Ten (Historical) and historical links, whenever necessary

RESPIRATORY SYSTEM[2,6,11,19,27,28]

- This is the most common system that is affected by diseases in the pediatric age group
- This is because the caliber of the air passages is much smaller in infants than they are in adults. For this reason, minor degrees of obstruction caused by mucus plugging or bronchospasm can make significant differences in the ability of air to enter or to leave the lungs
- The developmental immaturity of immunological functions render children susceptible to many infections of the respiratory tract; mucosal secretory IgA is deficient in the young infant. This deficiency is compensated to an extent by exclusive breastfeeding
- Remember that pediatrics covers a spectrum of age groups with different susceptibilities to various diseases. In all diseases of children, due consideration must be given to the age in thinking of the differential diagnosis and etiology. The respiratory diagnosis, too, must be thought of with the age of the child in mind
- The influence of congenital anomalies on some respiratory diseases in childhood must not be forgotten. The younger the child, the more important this consideration is. It is good practice to think of and try to exclude congenital problems of the respiratory tract in all children under one year of age
- In congenital anomalies involving the respiratory tract, such as tracheoesophageal fistula, the pregnancy and birth history (e.g. history of polyhydramnios) can be used to give some clues to the type of congenital anomaly. Such historical links are important
- To make your history practical and clinically apt, go into the enquiry of necessary details on all activities of daily living (ADL) especially in children with chronic airway diseases
- Common respiratory symptoms such as coughing, mouth breathing, noisy breathing, breathlessness, exercise tolerance, sputum production and nasal congestion are typical respiratory symptoms that must be elucidated in detail.

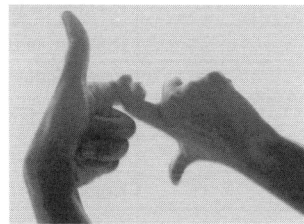

The history of polyhydramnios in pregnancy is a link to a possible diagnosis of a tracheoesophageal fistula with esophageal atresia

HISTORY OF COUGH AND ITS CHARACTERISTICS[2,6,11,19,27,28]

What do You Ask about Cough?

Expectoration

Remember that young children cannot effectively bring out their sputum and often swallow it, hence a productive cough is not routinely expected in young infants. If expectoration is present, ask about the color, quantity and nature. In the older child and adolescent ask about the color, where mucoid sputum occurs typically in chronic bronchitis when secondary infection is not present.

Tenacious sputum may be found in the older asthmatic child or the adolescent.

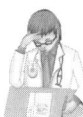

"I do remember the Charcot-Leyden crystals[22] and Curschmann spirals in the asthmatic sputum that I diligently learnt about in pathology. Such crystals may be seen in conditions associated with increased turnover of eosinophils and basophils"

Mucopurulent sputum is seen in upper respiratory infections and indicates secondary bacterial infection. The purulent sputum is thick and greenish yellow, often seen in bronchiectasis, bronchopneumonia or lung abscesses.

In lobar pneumonia the adolescent may bring forth viscid, rusty sputum. Hemoptysis may be due to tuberculosis or bronchiectasis. Hemoptysis may also have important extrapulmonary causes and systemic causes like bleeding disorders and systemic infections.

Characteristic Association of the Cough

This is useful to clarify. It may point towards the etiology or pathophysiology.
- A whoop may indicate pertussis or pertussis-like disease
- A brassy cough or one that is barking in nature may indicate acute inflammation of the larynx and is heard in croup
- A dry or hacking cough is of a viral infection
- A staccato cough is heard in chlamydial infections
- A cough that occurs in paroxysms may suggest pertussis, chlamydia, or foreign body
- A "honking" cough may suggest psychogenic cough
- A cough absent during sleep is suggestive of a habitual cough or even psychogenic in origin
- A "chesty" cough or a wet cough in bronchitis and in like lower respiratory infections like pneumonia
- A nocturnal cough is seen in asthma
- A recurrent cough worse on lying down in postnasal drip, bronchial asthma and in cardiac failure.

Associated Symptoms

When there are associated symptoms such as cyanosis and dyspnea, explain these pertaining to change of color, rapid breathing, struggling for air and in-drawing of chest.

If vomiting occurs, enquire about the nature of vomitus, color of phlegm in vomitus, how much vomitus, when it occurred and other relevant associated symptoms.

If the cough was associated with rapid breathing, the timing and association with cough or cyanosis or restlessness are important questions to ask. In the older child ask what activity brought it on. If breathlessness is sudden, explore the possibility of foreign body insertion into the nostrils or the choking associated with accidental aspiration of foreign bodies, such as peanuts. Here you must consider the age and development of the child.

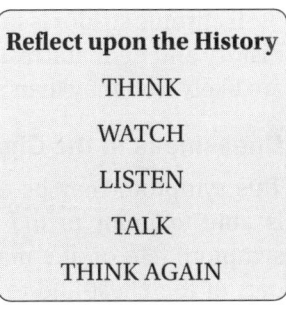

Reflect upon the History
THINK
WATCH
LISTEN
TALK
THINK AGAIN

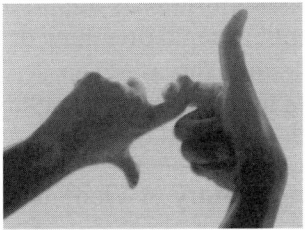

Link the age of the child and the development of a pincer as a fine motor milestone which enables the child to pick the peanut in the diagnosis of peanut aspiration

Accompanying Symptoms

If there are accompanying symptoms such as noisy breathing when crying, quiet or asleep and if these noises were not there prior to the cough, try to define this by asking mother how intense the noises are. Elucidate with **The Cardinal Ten (Historical)**.

In inspiratory or expiratory noise, ask on onset whether abrupt or slow or if associated with drooling of saliva. Ask on the ability to feed. Ask if there is any associated fever. The activity of the child prior to this, in the preceding days, and the presence of a runny nose prior to onset of the inspiratory noise can give a clue to the diagnosis.

Duration of cough[2,6,11,19,27,28]	Days, weeks and months[2,6,11,19,27,28]
Timing	Nocturnal or all through the day, during sleep or feeding
In older child, with or without expectoration	If expectoration present, what color is it?
Any precipitating factors?	Certain foods, colored drinks, or runny nose. Children swimming in cold water, exercise, cold weather or certain foods, colored drinks, flavors or odors
Characteristic association of the cough	Whoop, barking, paroxysmal, nocturnal and so on
Associated symptoms	Vomiting, cyanosis, or dyspnea
Accompanying symptoms	Noisy breathing when crying, quiet or asleep

If chronic stridor is suspected, ask briefly about birth history and neonatal history at this point. If such causes are likely, you may then proceed to indepth enquiry.

Uneasiness in the Chest or Chest Pain

This symptom may be elicited in the older child who is able to point to the chest when asked about this symptom. He or she may be able to point out to that part of the chest and to tell how painful it is, whether associated with symptoms suggestive of heart burn, when it occurs, during exercise, when playing at home or at school. In pleuritic pain, the chest pain is associated with deep breathing.

Feeding History

In infants a feeding history is important. This should be asked in depth as rapid breathing or tachypnea due to lower respiratory diseases can seriously interfere with the child's feeding. The feeding history is further elucidated under that section.

Hospitalization History or Visits to the Hospital

Information concerning hospitalization for respiratory illnesses, visits to the emergency department for treatment of respiratory illnesses and absence from school reflect the severity of the respiratory illness. Take note that missed school or inability to take part in school activities are vital components of the pediatric history. The past medical history is further clarified under that section.

Other History

If breathing difficulties are considered to be probably allergic in origin, ask of swellings of any part of the face suggesting urticaria. Angioneurotic edema can manifest as swellings involving the lips. The history of allergies are further dealt with in the section on allergies.

Immunization History

This is important (refer section on immunization history). Immunizations that are deemed immediately relevant to the presenting illness can be asked here. Remember that if the child is immunized against a disease, the likelihood of that disease is less than in an unimmunized child. A full immunization history can later be obtained under the section on immunization.

Family History

Concomitant occurrence of similar respiratory illness in the family is suggestive of an infective pathology, usually a viral etiology. The family history is important and should include questions about asthma, atopy, immune deficiencies and cystic fibrosis. Here too, relevant questions can be a clue to the differential diagnosis. Later, the family history can be explored under the appropriate section. In infections of the respiratory tract, a single virus may produce different illnesses in the family with typical flu-like symptoms in the parents, bronchiolitis in the infant, croup in the slightly older child, pharyngitis in another and a subclinical infection in yet another member of the family.

Environmental History

The link between the environment and many upper and lower respiratory illnesses are well known. The environmental history must include exposure to smoke, pets and pollutants. There is a recognized association between chronic pulmonary disease and air pollution. Air pollution also aggravates pre-existing pulmonary disease and impairs pulmonary function in children and teenagers. Smoking parents particularly whose children have chronic lung disease are subjecting their children's lungs to passive cigarette smoke at home. They should be educated in cessation of smoking.

Travel History

The History of Travel is Relevant

Remember that some respiratory diseases can be spread via travel including tuberculosis, influenza, SARS, meningococcal disease and measles. Visitors from endemic areas are also a source of infection. More details are stated under the appropriate section.

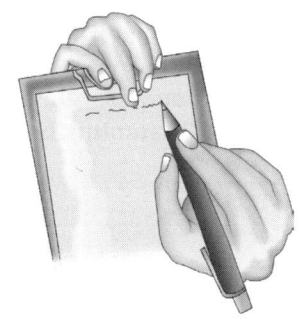

The History in Wheezing

Wheezing is both a common and an important symptom in respiratory diseases in children. Take the history of wheezing using **The Cardinal Ten (Historical)** and the historical link.

DISTINGUISHING FEATURES IN THE HISTORY OF WHEEZING[2,6,11,19,21,27,29]

History[2,6,11,19,21,27,29]	Interpretation of history[2,6,11,19,21,27,29]
	• When • What • How • How much • How long • How much less or how much more • What else • Worsened by • Lessened by • What was done
History[21]	**Interpretation of history[21]**
What is the child fed? Is there wheezing and chronic prolonged cough in the child fed cow's milk? Is there wheezing with rhinitis in the infant fed cow's milk? Is there recurrent wheezing, chronic cough, recurrent fever, tachypnea, failure to thrive or a family history of CMPA?	• Cow's milk allergy (CMPA) may be IgE mediated • CMPA may be IgE mediated • Non-IgE mediated respiratory reactions should be considered in infants with a form of chronic pulmonary disease (Heiner's syndrome)
At what age did the wheezing start?	• Differentiates congenital causes of wheezing from non-congenital causes
How did the wheezing start? Was it of acute or insidious onset?	• Foreign body aspiration is sudden or subacute in onset
Does the wheezing exhibit a particular trend or pattern?	• If it is intermittent wheezing, it suggests bronchial asthma • Wheezing that is persistent, suggests congenital or inherited genetic causes
Is the wheezing linked with a cough?	• Nocturnal cough and wheezing is suggestive of bronchial asthma
Is the wheezing precipitated by weather, cold air, smoke, chemicals, medications [e.g., aspirin and other nonsteroidal anti-inflammatory drugs (NSAIDs)], beta blockers, odors, exercise, bisulfite food additives and hormonal changes (menstrual cycle)?	• Varies triggers of bronchial asthma including drugs, food additives, emotion, activity, environment and pollutants
Is the wheezing linked to feeding?	• GERD (Gastro-esophageal reflux disease) or TOF (Tracheo-esophageal fistula) *Link wheezing to feeding and ask about recurrent vomiting, choking and gagging if suggested by history*
Is wheezing recurrent with multiple incidences of respiratory ailments in a child who has problems like loose stools and multiple unusual infections?	• Cystic fibrosis, immunodeficiency
In temperate climates, one may investigate as to whether the wheezing is linked to a specific season. Seasonal links are partly due to aeroallergens such seasonal pollen, mould, spores, dust mites and animal allergens In tropical or equatorial climates, it tends to occur all year round	• Croup: Occurs frequently from autumn to winter • Respiratory syncytial virus (RSV): Occurs frequently from autumn to spring • Allergic asthma: Sensitization to domestic mites[3] in the tropics
Is the wheezing affected by changes in position?	• Tracheomalacia, a pedunculated polyp of the lower respiratory tract and anomalies of the great vessels.
Are there any family members who suffer from wheezing?	• Infections, allergies
Does the child have an underlying cardiac problem such as a VSD or PDA or a cyanotic heart disease? Is the infant failing to thrive with feeding difficulties and excessive scalp sweating during feeding?	• Wheezing due to heart failure.

EAR, NOSE AND THROAT (ENT)[2,6,11,19,27,28]

- The nose is part of the upper respiratory system. The middle ear and throat are closely connected. Hence the history of the ENT is relevant independently and as a part of diseases of the respiratory tract and as part of some systemic diseases
- The ENT is commonly affected by viral and bacterial infection and may be the primary source of infection in children
- Infections of the middle ear are important to suspect in a febrile child and must be elucidated when there are historical clues
- Remember! While nose bleeds due to nose picking are common in children, a generalized hematological disorder may reveal itself by unilateral or bilateral epistaxis while epistaxis due to a foreign body is unilateral.

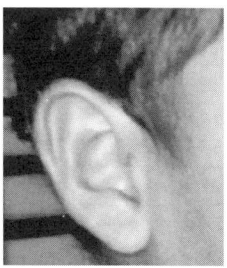 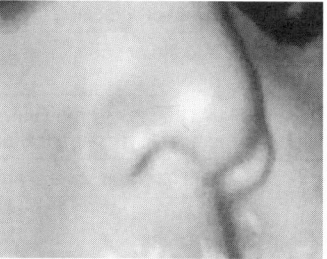

The history of problems of or related to the ear and nose are important in children (with kind permission from VRK)

Ears[2,6,11,19,27,28]	Nose[2,6,11,19,27,28]	Throat[2,6,11,19,27,28]
Ear pain	Watery nasal discharge (rhinorrhea) or thick or purulent nasal discharge (rhinitis)	Pain in the throat
Ear discharge	Nose block or obstruction	Difficulty swallowing (dysphagia)
Hearing loss or tinnitus	Noisy breathing	Painful swallowing (odynophagia)
Blocked sensation in ears	Nose bleeding, unilateral or bilateral	Neck swelling
History of insertion of foreign body	History of insertion of foreign body	Contact with persons with sore throat
Itching of the ear	Itching or discomfort of the nose	Itching of throat

Ears[23]

Ear Pain

The child may be pointing to the ears and crying or excessively rubbing the ears or may have difficulty going to sleep. Where foreign bodies are suspected, it may be useful to ask if the mother suspects that there is something in the ears; if so, ask her what she thinks it may be and for how long it has been in the ear.

Ear Discharge

Ask about the nature of discharge, color, amount, whether unilateral or bilateral, odor and nature whether mucoid, mucopurulent or blood stained. The carer may have seen the discharge or may have noticed staining of the child's pillow.

Remember that infections of the middle ear (otitis media) occur more frequently in the infant who has not been breastfed in children who habitually bottlefeed when sleeping, when there is a history of a sibling with ear infection, children taken care at day care centers and exposed to cigarette smoke. The symptoms of otitis media differ in the young infant compared to the older child. In the older child ear pain is an important symptom of acute otitis.

Symptoms of Otitis Media by Age[2,6,11,19,23,27,28]

Symptoms in infant	Fever, irritability, poor feeding (nonspecific symptoms)
Symptoms in the older child	Fever, ear pain (otalgia) (specific symptoms)

Otitis externa refers to a condition that involves inflammation of the external auditory canal. It is linked to swimming in pools or lakes. It is thus also called swimmer's ear. Ask about pain, tenderness and aural discharge. In otitis externa there is no fever. It is associated with pain on touch to the pinna or tragus of the ear.

Hearing

- Enquire about the child's response to sound from near and far. If there is difficulty in hearing, ask how parents noticed, enquire of recent flu. If sensorineural hearing loss is suspected, ask about parental concerns

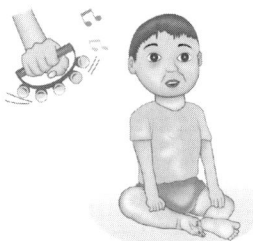

Enquire about the child's response to sound from near and far. When a history of suspected hearing loss is elicited hearing tests must be done

about learning, problems at school and language development.
- Ask about past hearing tests.

Tinnitus

- Does older child complain of buzzing in the ear?
- Ask for post-auricular swelling or tenderness (pain to touch) in association with history of upper respiratory illness.

Nose

Nasal discharge (Rhinorrhea) or Obstruction[23]

In a newborn, if the cyanosed child becomes pink on opening the mouth or when crying, think of the diagnosis of choanal atresia. Remember in the younger child, always exclude congenital anomalies. Ask if there is unilateral or bilateral discharge or obstruction seen. Also enquire if there is sneezing or a history suggestive of a post-nasal drip such as nocturnal cough or in an older child, a tickling sensation behind the throat.

Ask for history of a stuffy nose or frequent colds, if there is itching or a watery nose. Ask about the color and quantity of discharge (thick or light, mucous or blood stained). Enquire regarding disturbance of sleep due to breathing difficulty.

If there is a history of recent trauma, clear nasal discharge not associated with any symptom to suggest infection or allergy, must make you link the discharge to trauma and try to exclude this in the history and subsequent physical examination. If nasal discharge is offensive and unilateral enquire about possibility of foreign body in nose, like child playing with small toys or beads.

Sinusitis or paranasal sinuses infection may present with persistent mucopurulent bilateral or unilateral nasal discharge, nasal stuffiness and cough at night. This is a complication of the common cold or allergic rhinitis.

Pneumatization of the Sinuses in Children[23]

This information reminds the student of the age-related involvement of the paranasal sinuses. Hence frontal sinusitis is not a diagnosis made at birth!

Name of sinus[2,6,11,19,23,27,28]	Pneumatization of sinus[2,6,11,19,23,27,28]
Ethmoidal sinuses (formed at 3rd to 4th gestational month)	At birth
Maxillary sinuses (formed at 3rd to 4th gestational month)	At birth
Frontal sinus	7 years
Sphenoid sinus	5 years

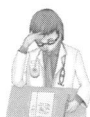
This is good to know......

Kartagener's syndrome is a syndrome of defective mucociliary clearance where patients are afflicted with chronic upper and lower airway disease. Recurrent chronic sinusitis is a feature. They present with persistent thick mucoid nasal discharge early on in life. It is associated with bronchiectasis and situs inversus. Other links include infertility due to immotile spermatozoa. An autosomal recessive pattern of inheritance is recognized. The enquiry of a family history of consanguinity is relevant.

Coughing

Enquire if child coughs when asleep.

Noisy Breathing

Ask for aggravating and relieving factors and whether the child breathes with mouth open. Ask if child snores.

Vomiting

Ask if there is vomiting at night or after feeding.

Nose Bleeds

If bleeding from nose is present, ask if it is unilateral or bilateral and whether the blood is fresh and enquire about the quantity of blood. Also ask for how long and how often it occurs. It may be associated with nose picking or may be spontaneous.

Throat

Enquire if there is any pain in the throat, inability to swallow or pain on swallowing, any contact with people with sore throat or associated vomiting or fever. Any noticed swellings of the throat or neck? Ask for any history of malaise or associated nasal congestion.

ENT symptoms of allergic rhinitis[2,6,11,19,23,27,28]
• Sneezing, often paroxysmal
• Rhinorrhea, often watery and profuse
• Nasal obstruction
• Itching of the nose, palate, ears
• Itching, redness, tearing of the eyes
• Complaints of periorbital swelling in severe conditions

GASTROINTESTINAL TRACT[2,6,11,19,27,28]

- There are many symptoms that begin in the gastrointestinal tract that may actually constitute important medical conditions within the gastrointestinal tract. Surgical causes of gastrointestinal symptoms must always be thought of and enquired into with **The Cardinal Ten (Historical)**.
- Remember that in children illnesses in other systems can cause abdominal pain. Therefore, ask about non-gastrointestinal symptoms like fever, headache, sore throat, cough, otalgia and dysuria.
- The influence of family illnesses on gastrointestinal symptoms of the index patient should not be forgotten. Hence, enquire about recent food ingestion with the family, members having similar symptoms help you with the diagnosis and the source of the infection. The history of gastrointestinal illnesses in the family, illnesses amongst classmates or in the nursery are factors that can help in making a diagnosis and to clarify etiology.
- Bear in mind that sometimes abdominal pain in children may not have an identifiable pathology with no specific diagnosis that can be made, hence a good and complete history and physical examination are important for clarification and appropriate management.
- The history (and examination) must focus at excluding life-threatening causes of abdominal pain and elucidate if a surgical cause must be considered. For example, bilious vomiting is always a sinister symptom in a child with abdominal pain.

Features that help in the characterization of abdominal pain in children[2,6,11,19,23,27,28]
• Severity
• Age of onset
• Location
• Timing of onset
• Character
• Associated features

ABDOMINAL PAIN[2,6,8,11,19,24,27,28]

Symptoms Suggestive of Abdominal Pathology such as Discomfort or Pain

Mother or caregiver will sometimes be able to tell if a child is having abdominal discomfort or not. Ask them what makes them think so; ask the details of 'when' and 'why'. The mother or caregiver may sometimes reveal their feelings about the cause of the pain (mothers may reveal important details about the time of day the child cries or the time the child is fussy or irritable or when the meal or milk feed was refused by the child.

Age of Onset

An important consideration in the history of abdominal pain is the age of the child.

The History of Pain

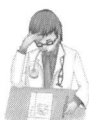

The causes of pain differ in etiology by the age of children. Pain is expressed in different ways by children. Abdominal pain in children is a symptom that challenges the diagnostic ability of the doctor.

- In a young infant, excessive inconsolable crying that is not relieved by the mother's touch or handling is indicative of pain. Many important points in the history (related to the child's age) can be asked
- Until children are much bigger they may not accurately express the onset or location of pain. The classic sequence of shifting pain from umbilicus to right iliac fossa usually occurs with acute appendicitis
- Young children who are unable to verbalize may present late. In such children, the history of vague nausea or periumbilical pain may be unnoticed. However, any child with pain that localizes to the right lower quadrant should be suspected of having appendicitis
- The pain of intussusception is intermittent and severe causing the child to draw up the legs in pain, a characteristic history to elicit
- In a child of school going age explore abdominal pain in relation to school, meals, eating of certain foods with each symptom detailed by **The Cardinal Ten (Historical)**
- Explore psychosocial stresses at school or at home, where applicable. Ask about teachers, homework, ability to cope, worsening and relieving factors of pain e.g. does the child experience similar pain during school holidays; do not forget to ask about friends at school, games and other activities
- However, in a child who is at an age where he or she is able to understand and give a reasonable history, the mnemonic acronym **SOCRATES**[7] is well-known and a tool in the history-taking of pain:

SOCRATES[7] is well-known and a tool in the history-taking of pain

Site	Ask where the pain is or the maximal site of the pain
Onset	Ask when the pain started, and if it was sudden or gradual. Did it get worse (progressive pain) or better (regressive pain)?
Character	What was the pain like? Burning, aching, stabbing are examples
Radiation	Ask if the pain radiates or moves systematically from one place to another
Associations	Ask if there was any other symptom or sign associated with the pain. Fever, weight loss and anorexia are important
Time course	Does the pain follow any pattern? Pain in children with colic is commonly in the evening or at similar times everyday
Exacerbating and improving factors	Ask if anything changes the intensity of pain
Severity	Ask about how severe the pain is. What the child does during the pain can give you a clue to its severity

Location

The child may use his or her finger or the whole hand to point towards the pain. Remember that it is important to consider seriously all locations of pain that a child indicates; however, periumbilical pain may also have a psychological cause.

Timing of Onset

The onset of pain is important. For example, if abdominal pain occurs at night or upon waking it indicates a likely peptic cause.

Character

This is useful if the older child can describe the pain. Involve the child in history-taking and give the child a chance to verbalize his or her pain if old enough to understand and to speak.

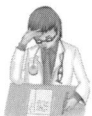

"The link between the nature of the pain and the diagnosis of the underlying condition is based on my knowledge of anatomy and pathophysiology."

Character of pain (in a child old enough to understand or express effectively) [2,6,8,11,19,24,27,28]	Possible cause [2,6,8,11,19,24,27,28]
Persistent, sharp pain in the periumbilical area later shifting to the right lower quadrant	Acute appendicitis
Burning pain in the substernal area radiating to the chest	Esophageal reflux
Severe burning, agonizing pain radiating to the back	Duodenal ulcer
Constant sharp, boring pain radiating to the back	Pancreatitis
Dull cramp like intermittent periumbilical pain	Functional irritable bowel syndrome
Cramping pain (+/- abdominal distension)	Lactose intolerance
Severe colicky pain often from loin to groin	Urolithiasis
Cramping pain with painless periods in between in the child who pulls his knees up intermittently and screams or cries and has red currant jelly stools	Intussusception

Surgical Causes of Abdominal Pain[2,6,8,11,19,24,27,28]

- It is important to have an index of suspicion of a surgical cause and exclude it, as many surgical causes require immediate intervention.
- It is always best to approach this by the age of the patient.
- Failure to pass meconium in the first 2 days of life with abdominal distension suggests Hirschsprung's disease, intestinal obstruction or imperforate anus. Enquire about constipation.
- In a child lesser than 2 months, ask if there is bilious vomiting as this suggests malrotation leading to volvulus. Exclude intestinal and extra-intestinal causes in neonates or young infants who present with vomiting.
- Ask for intermittent paroxysms of pain in a 4–10 month old with drawing of knees, vomiting (may be bilious) and 'red currant jelly' stool. These suggest intussusception.
- Bilious vomiting is an ominous history. In a preschool child with painful bilious vomiting in a boy, an incarcerated hernia must be excluded. Any cause of postampullary obstruction must also be thought of.
- If suspecting acute appendicitis, ask about central abdominal pain, sometimes systemically unwell, with poor feeding, nausea or vomiting, anorexia, pyrexia, diarrhea or constipation. The central abdominal pain, later localizes to the right iliac fossa. It is rare before the age of 12 months.
- In older children epigastric pain following trauma or viral illness requires that acute pancreatitis be excluded.

- A prior history of trauma in an older boy presenting with abdominal pain must make you consider a testicular pathology as well as to exclude splenic rupture or injury to any internal organ. A tubo-ovarian pathology must be thought of in a girl of similar age with a history of abdominal pain which occurs in the peri or post-menarchal period. The history of unprotected sex in the teenage girl with acute abdominal pain should raise the index of suspicion of tubo-ovarian pathology.

Functional Abdominal Pain[2,6,11,19,24,27,28]

- **Sometimes, abdominal pain may have a non-organic etiology.**
- Children with **functional abdominal pain** typically have pain almost daily. The pain is not associated with meals or relieved with defecation. Pain associated with anxiety and a personality that is obsessive in nature is seen in functional abdominal pain. It is often attributed to the adjustment to situations like parental separation or when starting school.
- The pain is often worse in the morning and that prevents them from attending school. Pain is commonly accompanied by school avoidance, lack of ability to cope and troubled relationships with friends at school. There can also be anxiety about imagined situations.
- In children with **irritable bowel syndrome**, the abdominal pain typically starts at the time of a change in stool frequency or consistency. They experience constipation which usually alternates with diarrhea. The pain is relieved by defecation. In irritable bowel syndrome some features overlap with functional abdominal pain. Pain is commonly accompanied by school avoidance, lack of the ability to cope and emotional problems with peers or teachers at school.

Severity or Intensity of Pain

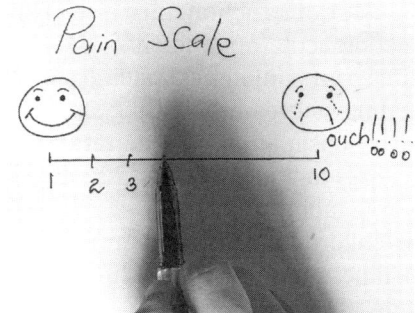

Clinical estimation of pain severity in a young child

This could be graded on a scale of 1 to 10; 1 being the least severe and 10 being the most severe. Younger children may exhibit facial expression which may range from a smile to frown or tears.

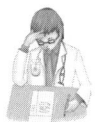

Come down to the child's level and use easily understandable analogies when asking the child about pain

Generally, children do not understand the exact description of pain so avoid terminology like "sharp pain" or "dull pain". Instead, you could ask if it hurts like a needle prick. Use easily understood analogies. Ask if it feels like butterflies in your stomach or if it helps to lie down or "poop"? Enquire if the pain improves on eating. Also enquire about the duration of pain and if it radiates.

History of Recent Trauma

A history of recent trauma may indicate the cause of pain.

Precipitating or Relieving Factors

Aggravation of Pain

Ask if any situation or position worsens the pain. A good example is parietal pain which is worsened by movement.

Relief of Pain

If there is pain relief after a bowel movement, that suggests a colonic source. When pain is better after vomiting it could suggest the involvement of the more proximal bowel. However, vomiting is a warning sign of underlying illness in children with recurrent abdominal pain. It is also a rather nonspecific sign in all illnesses in children.

Regurgitation

- Regurgitation is common in infants until 9–12 months of age and is accompanied by gastric contents that enter the pharynx or mouth and is expelled from the mouth. It is a nonspecific symptom in infants, and can be normal, or if excessive, can occur in gastroesophageal reflux disease (GERD)
- GERD can be part of the clinical picture of cow's milk protein allergy as well

- Ask how many times a day it occurs, whether it follows every feed. If significant, ask about growth and development.

Complications of severe regurgitation[2,6,8,11,19,24,27,28]
• Poor growth
• Aspiration
• Esophagitis

Nausea and Vomiting

Ask about frequency, contents, color and quantity of the vomitus; was it blood stained or not, whether it was forceful or projectile and was it associated with retching. Vomiting, is a nonspecific symptom with numerous causes. Vomiting is when contents of the stomach is expelled forcefully from the mouth with retrograde intestinal peristalsis. It is centrally controlled and often starts with salivation and is accompanied by nausea. The age of the patient in the history of vomiting is vital, as, the associated signs and symptoms and the temporal pattern of vomiting.

Rumination

It is abnormal regurgitation of recently swallowed food into the mouth followed by mastication and reswallowing. Commonly encountered in cerebral palsy, anorexia nervosa, and sometimes, in young children in cases of self-stimulation, or deprivation.

Posseting

Posseting is to be differentiated from vomiting. It peaks at around 1 to 4 months of age. It does not cause any pain or discomfort. The child is thriving normally and feeds appropriately.

Ask the mother if the baby brings out milk after feeding then enquire more specifically about this.

Flatulence

Ask if there is sensation of fullness or "bloatedness" in the older child, any noticeable abdominal distension and what the mother does during episodes of pain. Enquire about the relieving and aggravating factors.

Bowel Habits[2,6,11,19,24,27,28]

Compare with normal bowel habits as this puts the patient's symptoms into perspective and thus makes interpretation of symptoms more meaningful. Explore the pattern and frequency of any deviation from normal. Remember that the number, color and nature of the stools have a great degree of variation whether within the same infant at different times or between infants of similar age. The frequency of the stool may range from one to seven per day in normal babies.

Cause[2,6,11,19,24,27,28]	Nature of stool[2,6,11,19,24,27,28]
Earliest stool at birth	Meconium
Milk feeds begin 1–3 days of age	Green brown stools transition stools with curds
4–5 days	Yellow brown milk stools
Breastfed	Loose yellow stools sometimes with 'seeds'
Addition of complementary feeds	Carrot, corn and peas or worm-like threads of banana peel

Diarrhea[2,6,11,19,24,27,28]

Always compare to the normal bowel habits. Ask about quantity of fecal matter, whether stools seep through the nappies which indicate that the stools are very watery and the diarrhea is significant in quantity. Also ask of the odor and association with blood or with mucous. In a well thriving child, ask if the loose stool is associated with undigested vegetable-like matter, i.e. the "carrot and peas" stool of toddler's diarrhea.

If lactose intolerance is suspected, ask about association with abdominal "bloatiness", soreness or pain around anus or if child cries on changing nappies. Remember that lactose intolerance is often a secondary effect of prolonged, severe or explosive diarrheas in children. However, primary lactose intolerance is also a recognized entity.

If the child has chronic diarrhea, always ask about the growth of child; how growth percentiles have been affected since the onset of the diarrhea. Growth parameters plotted on appropriate growth charts give the clinician a clue on duration and severity, shedding light on pathology and etiology.

Enquire about the age of onset of diarrhea and the nature of stools. Was the child breastfed or formula fed? If the child was formula fed enquire about the type of milk fed to the child; was it cow's milk based, soy based or a pre-digested protein hydrolysate. If the child is on special milk formula, ask whether this was started by a medical practitioner and for what reason. Ask about bottle hygiene.

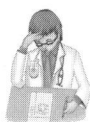

Cow's milk protein allergies (CMPA)—a diagnosis to consider in a symptomatic formula fed infant.

GASTROINTESTINAL MANIFESTATIONS OF ALLERGIES TO COW'S MILK PROTEIN[10,24,29]

Infants and toddlers[10,24,29]
Ask about the following
- Dysphagia, vomiting, frequent regurgitation, colic, abdominal pain
- Anorexia, refusal to feed, nausea
- Diarrhea, intestinal protein or blood loss
- Early satiety and growth failure are among the clinical features indicative of iron deficiency anemia
- Perianal rash and lip swelling

In older children[10,24,29]
- Ask about dysphagia, food impaction, regurgitation, nausea, vomiting, abdominal pain, constipation and symptoms suggestive of iron deficiency
- Ask about symptoms suggestive of gastroesophageal reflux disease (GERD). Vomiting may also be due to cricopharyngeal spasm, pyloric stenosis and in a recognized condition called allergic eosinophilic esophagitis (EoE)
- Vomiting and bloody diarrhea may be due to a recognized condition known as food protein induced enterocolitis syndrome (FPIES), proctocolitis, cow's milk protein induced enteropathy

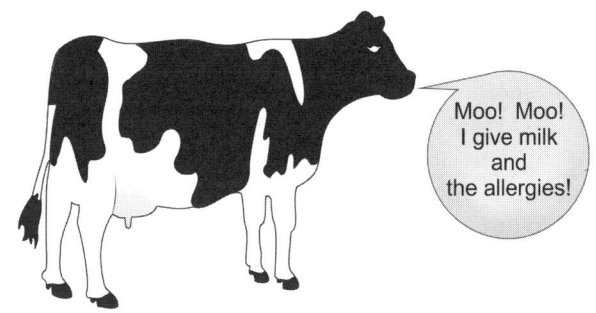

GASTROINTESTINAL LINKS

Dilution of Milk Feeds

The history obtained about the dilution of artificial milk feeds is important as concentrated feeds cause colic and constipation whereas diluted feeds for prolonged periods can interfere with the child's growth causing stagnation in growth parameters and even failure to thrive.

Make use of '**The Cardinal Ten (Historical)**' when necessary.

Constipation

Compare this with the normal bowel habits and the nature of stools. Attempt description such as if the stools were pellet-like or tooth paste like, the accompanying presence of or absence of blood, how much, whether staining pampers or fresh red or with streaks of mucus.

The history obtained about the dilution of artificial milk feeds is important. Concentrated feeds cause colic and constipation. An overzealous mother anxious about her child's weight may concentrate milk feeds. This may also be due to ignorance of mixing formula milk correctly.

Ask if the constipation has been present from birth and if severe, ask how fecal evacuation is done. If constipation has been present since birth, what historical link could you use? Hirschsprung's disease is a differential, so, besides other questions you would also ask about delayed passage of meconium, abdominal distension, the need for manual evacuation of feces, and so on. Remember also that delayed passage of meconium can be due to hypothyroidism, prematurity or anorectal malformations. If these differentials are considered link to appropriate questions.

Appetite

Explore if the child is choosy or fussy about food. Compare this to the child's appetite before the illness. Remember that appetites of children fluctuate enormously. During periods of rapid growth, appetite can be voracious, while during the intervening years some children may appear to eat very little but they grow and gain weight normally.

Loss of Weight

Ask the mother if she has noticed that the child has lost weight. Use practical daily living analogies like clothes that have become loose or whether others have commented on this. Ask if the mother can quantitate how much and how fast the weight was lost.

Difficulty in Swallowing (Dysphagia)

Ask why the mother thinks that there is dysphagia.
Ask if the child is refusing milk or is irritable. Differentiate from regurgitation. Elucidate further with **The Cardinal Ten (Historical)**.

In the older child or adolescent, ask if the dysphagia is specifically for solids or liquids or both.

Heartburn

In an older child, ask him to describe the nature of pain and explore using **The Cardinal Ten (Historical)**.

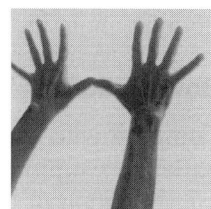

Use The Cardinal Ten (Historical)

Jaundice[2,6,11,19,24,27,28]

Jaundice is the visible yellow discoloration of skin and sclera.

History of Jaundice

- The cause of jaundice can be elucidated from history of presentation and age of the child. Ask when the yellow discoloration was first noticed and its duration and if there was any associated itching of the skin
- The age of the patient and history of presentation give important cues to the cause of the jaundice
- Causes in the infant of cholestasis and conjugated hyperbilirubinemia that present early in life include Alagille's syndrome, cystic fibrosis, alpha-1-antitrypsin deficiency and sepsis
- The history of poor feeding and vomiting is important to ask. Metabolic diseases or bilirubin encephalopathy can cause these symptoms
- Pale stools (or acholic stools) indicate an obstruction to the biliary tree such as biliary atresia, choledochal cyst, or gallstone disease
- The birth and perinatal histories, past medical and surgical histories, family history (including consanguinity), medication and dietary histories, social activity and school performance, and travel history should be recorded.

Appetite

Ask about the child's appetite; whether increased or decreased, association with growth and with activity.

Color of Stool and Urine

- Enquire about change of color of stool or urine
- Enquire about quantity of urine passed after diarrheal illness
- Ask about number of nappy changes and the color of urine on the nappy which can reflect the hydration status.

Other Relevant History

- Birth and perinatal histories
- Past medical and surgical histories
- Family history (including consanguinity)
- Medication and dietary histories
- Social activity and school performance histories
- Travel history.

Presentation[2,6,11,19,24,27,28]	Some probable causes[2,6,11,19,24,27,28]
Reflect on when and how the disease presents as this can give clues to diagnoses	Knowledge of childhood diseases that present with jaundice can help you link to diagnosis
Cholestasis and conjugated hyperbilirubinemia presenting in early childhood	Cystic fibrosis, biliary atresia, alpha-1-antitrypsin deficiency or Alagille's syndrome
History of poor feeding and vomiting	Metabolic diseases or bilirubin encephalopathy
Pale stools (or acholic stools)	Obstruction to the biliary tree such as choledochal cyst, biliary atresia, or gallstone disease as seen in children with hemolytic anemias

CARDIOVASCULAR SYSTEM[2,6,11,19,27,28]

- Both congenital and acquired heart diseases occur in children. Growth is a vital and sensitive indicator of cardiac function in children
- Enrich your questioning by a good theoretical knowledge of the basic pathophysiology of cardiac diseases in childhood
- Know about cyanotic and acyanotic heart diseases
- Know how cardiac conditions with increased pulmonary blood flow can give rise to frequent respiratory tract infections whereas conditions associated with decreased pulmonary blood flow usually manifest with symptomatology such as cyanotic spells
- The approach to the history-taking in heart failure would depend on the commonest causes that are age related

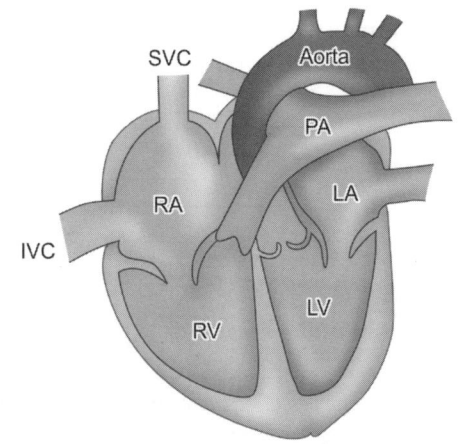

- Poor feeding, tachypnea, failure to thrive and difficulty during feeding are signs and symptoms of heart failure in infants whereas edema, shortness of breath and easy fatigability are signs and symptoms in older children.

Weight Gain

Ask for growth parameters and patterns. Ask to see previous plotted growth charts, if available. If weight gain is poor, enquire further on feeding or excessive vomiting; assess how much milk is consumed. Remember poor weight gain despite frequent feeding is an important sign of heart diseases in infancy.

Feeding History

- In a young infant this is very important.
- The infant in congestive cardiac failure takes less volume of milk per feeding or suckles for a short time on the mother's breast, becomes dyspneic while sucking, perspiring profusely.
- After the young infant falls into an exhausted sleep, the hungry infant will soon awaken for the next feeding. The child cries hungrily around the clock and this must be historically differentiated from colic or other feeding disorders which may have a cyclical or more predictable pattern.
- Ask about breathlessness during feeds, excessive scalp sweating during feeds in an infant, or diaphoresis, a clinical state due to sympathetic overdrive, inability to complete a feed due to exhaustion, excessive crying due to unsatisfied hunger and frequent feeding.
- While in the young infant, feeding difficulties may indicate fatigue, eliciting a history of fatigue in older children would require you to ask about specific activities like climbing up stairs, walking various distances, or riding bicycles. Ask about orthopnea and paroxysmal nocturnal dyspnea.

Change of Color

Cyanosis

- Congenital cardiac lesions may be cyanotic or acyanotic. The acyanotic lesions include ventricular septal defect (VSD), atrial septal defect (ASD) and patent ductus arteriosus (PDA).
- The cyanotic lesions include the 5Ts—tricuspid atresia (TA), total anomalous venous drainage (TAPVD), tetralogy of fallot (TOF), truncus arteriosus (TA) and transposition of the great arteries (TGA).
- Congenital cardiac lesions are more easily approached by rationalizing if it increases or decreases pulmonary blood flow as the change in pulmonary blood flow determines much of the child's symptoms.

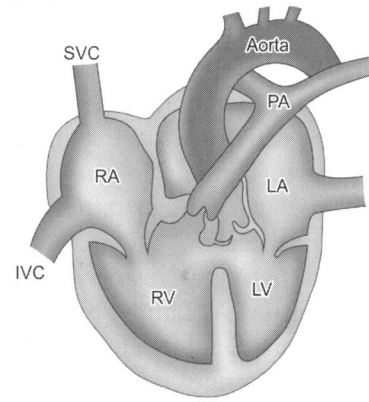

Tetralogy of Fallot

CONGENITAL CARDIAC LESIONS WITH INCREASE IN PULMONARY BLOOD FLOW[2,6,11,19,27,28]

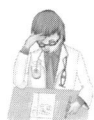

An increase in pulmonary blood flow will cause symptoms such as frequent chest infections that can worsen cardiac function and interfere with growth. That is why the history of chest infections is so important to ask.

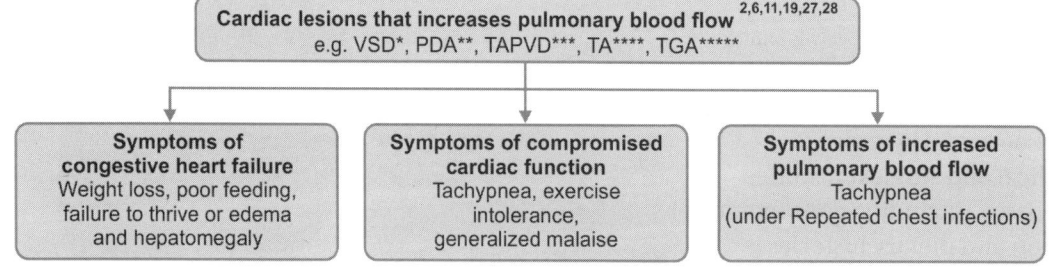

*ventricular septal defect, **patent ductus arteriosus, *** total anomalous pulmonary venous drainage, ****truncus arteriosus, ***** transposition of the great arteries

CONGENITAL CARDIAC LESIONS WITH DECREASE IN PULMONARY BLOOD FLOW [2,6,11,19,27,28]

Remember sometimes parents who are observing their child on a daily basis may not notice subtle changes that have occurred over days or weeks. Cyanosis may be recognized as a deep coloring. The cyanosis in TOF is usually intermittently severe. This occurs when there is pulmonary infundibular spasm. Ask when this occurs and what the child does when he or she turns cyanosed. Squatting to relieve the dyspnea of a hypercynotic spell in tetralogy of Fallot is well documented. Typically cyanotic spells occur early in the morning. The possible triggers are anxiety, anemia, fever, sepsis or even spontaneously without any cause. The spells may be initiated by the stress of feeding, crying or bowel movement, particularly after an infant awakens from a long sleep.

Possible Behavioral Differences in Infants with Cyanotic Spells Compared to Older Children[20]

Infant behavior during cyanotic spell[2,6,11,19,27,28]
• Appears fussy or irritable
• Inconsolable, progressing to increasing cyanosis
• Hyperpnea that is typical of a spell
The older child with cyanotic spell[2,6,11,19,27,28]
• Takes on a squatting position for recovery

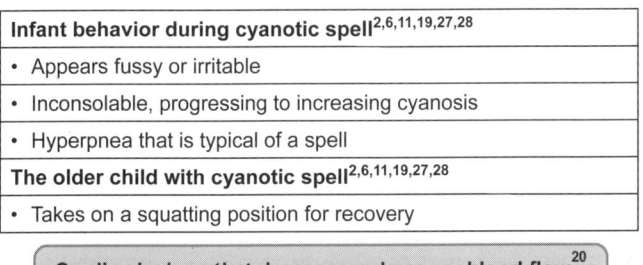

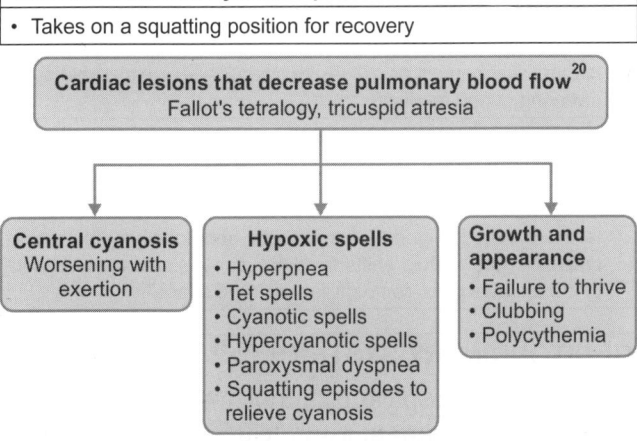

Cardiac causes that may present with cyanotic spells: [2,6,11,19,27,28]

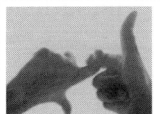

Think about a common factor in the cyanotic diseases that are associated with cyanotic spells. Reflect on why pulmonary stenosis is fundamental in such lesions. Rationalize your thoughts with the direction of the blood flow in the heart; discuss this by thinking aloud and think again!

- Tetralogy of Fallot
- Tricuspid atresia with pulmonary stenosis (PS)
- Transposition of great vessels with PS
- Single ventricle with PS or pulmonary atresia

LINKS TO CARDIAC FAILURE[2,6,11,19,27,28]

Pallor

When observed by the mother or caretaker and related in the history, it is a symptom. Ask details of this important clinical observation with the help of **The Cardinal Ten (Historical).**

Chest Pain

In a child who is older, ask if he or she complains of pain or points to any part of the chest due to pain. If so, make a detailed enquiry about when it happens; relationship to daily activity; can he or she play games in school or at home or can he or she climb up stairs.

Swelling of Ankles

If there is ankle swelling, ask how and when this was noticed. Also ask if it is increasing or decreasing. Enquire if the older child's shoes are getting too tight too fast. Ask for any diurnal variation.

Orthopnea

Orthopnea is a sign of left-sided heart failure. Can the child lie down without pillows? How many pillows does the child need? Does it disturb the child's sleep? Also ask what the child does when he or she wakes up.

Dyspnea

In an older child, enquire about the relation of dyspnea to daily activities. Ask if the dyspnea is sudden and worsened at night. Remember paroxysmal nocturnal dyspnea is a sign in cardiovascular diseases in older children and in adolescents but not seen in the younger child and is a historical feature to distinguish from the dyspnea of respiratory origin. Enquire about wheezing and orthopnea in left-sided heart failure.

Cough

In children, cough is a symptom of congestive heart failure. Enquire about distinctive features of the cough as a historical link to cardiac failure.

In infants feeding difficulties, irritability, a weak cry, noisy labored respiration with chest retractions which may be noticed by the mother indistinguishable from chest infections such as bronchiolitis may be present. Ask if cough is present. Productive cough occurs only in the older child.

Wheeze

Enquiry about the distinctive features of wheezing as a historical link to cardiac failure.

Use the historical link

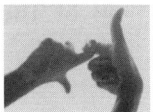

Link wheezing to the underlying pathophysiology of the disease.

Remember that the wheezing in cardiac failure is due to pulmonary edema whereas the wheezing in bronchial asthma has nothing to do with the accumulation of fluid in the lung. Explore when wheeze worsens and other associated features of the wheeze. Ask if it is sudden or chronic and recurrent. Explore where relevant, each of these symptoms using **The Cardinal Ten (Historical)**.

Syncope and Palpitations

In an older child, dizziness or fainting when standing may be indicative of certain valvular lesions like aortic stenosis. Syncope can be caused by cardiac abnormalities, circulatory anomalies with abnormal vascular volume or tone.

Palpitations or the awareness of one's own heart beat can occur in some dysrhythmias and valvular lesions. In the older child, ask if the child is aware of his or her own heartbeat. If so, ask when and how often this occurs and of associated symptoms.

Palpitations can occur in mitral valve prolapse. There are some associations of mitral valve prolapse to phenotypic features like tall stature and increased arm span in Marfan's syndrome. Though these are not common cardiac lesions, train your mind to link a historical fact with other possibilities as a way to arrive at or to exclude a possible clinical diagnosis.

Abdominal Distension

Explore when abdominal swelling was noticed; whether it is increasing or is it associated with decreased appetite or diarrhea. Hepatomegaly, edema and distended neck veins signify right sided heart failure. In children, the symptoms of congestive heart failure include fatigue, anorexia, effort intolerance, abdominal pain and cough.

The association of wheezing with feeding difficulties, failure to thrive and excessive sweating in a young infant is highly suggestive of heart failure.

Pain in Legs in Intermittent Claudication

This is rare in children and the commonest cause of pain in the legs in children is certainly not cardiac in origin! If it occurs in the older child, ask when the pain occurs; if it is on exertion, ask whether the child can play the games he or she used to in the past. Ask if the child is as active as before.

Summary of symptoms in the history indicative of congestive cardiac failure in children[2,6,11,19,27,28]
• Noted increased heart rate (the normal resting and active heart rate for "your" child—as this will vary with age)
• Noted increased respiratory rate, abnormalities of rate and depth of breathing, breathlessness (the normal resting respiratory rate varies with age)
• Have you noticed irritability, restlessness, or undue fussiness?
• Have you noticed sudden weight gain? (due to edema associated with heart failure)
• Do you think that there is puffiness or edema which is most noticeable at the hands, feet, or around the eyes?
• Is the child constantly crying of hunger due to difficulty to feed?
• Is there decrease in appetite or feeding due to loss of appetite?
• Is there poor weight gain? (due to a chronic progressive cardiac condition with failure to thrive)
• Have you noticed pale, mottled or greyish appearance in skin color?
• Is there diaphoresis or excessive sweating – or excessive scalp sweating during feeding?
• Is there frequent or persistent cough or wheezing?
• Have you noted a decrease in activity level (tiring more easily sleeping more often), fatigue and listlessness?
• Is there noted oliguria or in infants and toddlers, fewer wet diapers? (due to fluid shifts from the intravascular compartment to the extravascular compartment or "third space")

GENITOURINARY SYSTEM[2,6,11,19,27,28]

- An index of suspicion of problems pertaining to this system is important as protean symptomatology as nonspecific as poor weight gain and as specific as dysuria are symptoms referred to the genitourinary system.
- Urinary tract infections are the commonest cause of hematuria in children.
- Symptoms more specifically referred to the urinary tract are more frequent in older children while systemic symptoms related to sepsis are commoner in the young infant.

- Growth parameters must be enquired into if chronic or recurrent problems are suspected.
- The younger the child, the more important it is to consider congenital anomalies or hereditary problems of the urinary tract as cause(s) of the problem. In congenital anomalies, other parts of the history such as the history of pregnancy and the family history may give you clues to the underlying problem.

Urine Frequency

- Ask about the number of nappy changes in a day. In an older child, compare with normal urinary frequency.
- Decreased urine output (oliguria) as well as excessively increased urine output (polyuria) is abnormal. If polyuric, ask about increased thirst, weight loss, polyphagia and other symptoms to suggest diabetes mellitus.
- Remember that tubulointerstitial diseases of the kidney do not present with edema and hypertension; instead present with polyuria, polydipsia and growth failure.

NONSPECIFIC AND SPECIFIC SYMPTOMS

The predominant symptoms of urinary tract infections in children are different at different ages of presentations. The NICE guidelines[15] divides the ages as such: in infants less than 3 months and in infants more than 3 months. In infants less than 3 months, the most common symptoms are of a systemic septicemia like fever, vomiting, lethargy, irritability, poor feeding, failure to thrive and the least common are abdominal pain, jaundice, hematuria, and offensive urine.

The NICE guidelines indicate that in infants and children 3 months and older the commoner symptoms are fever, abdominal pain, loin tenderness, vomiting, while poor feeding, lethargy, hematuria, foul smelling urine and failure to thrive are less common than in the child less than 3 months. In the older child frequency, dysuria, dysfunctional voiding, changes to continence, abdominal pain and loin tenderness are the more common symptoms while fever, malaise, vomiting hematuria, offensive urine and turbid urine are less common.

Color of Urine[13]

- Ask if the urine is persistently frothy indicative of proteinuria; ask about any presence of blood and its odor. Ask if urine is dark in color indicative of hematuria; differentiate by history of painful or painless hematuria. Enquire the nature of the hematuria. Hematuria in the beginning of the urinary stream or initial hematuria suggests the source is from the urethra and that it is passed out by the initial passage of urine through the urethra; throughout the stream or total hematuria indicates that the bleeding occurs at the bladder or higher up in the urinary tract, so that the urine is completely mixed with blood, and the entire stream is bloody. This suggests that it is from the bladder, ureter, or kidneys; terminal hematuria can arise from the trigone, bladder neck or posterior urethra, and is noticed at the end of urination, when the bladder compresses these areas and occurs in some conditions including the parasitic infection, schistosomiasis.
- Previous episodes of gross hematuria and a history of trauma must be enquired. A family history of hematuria, proteinuria, renal disease, deafness or calculi may be relevant.
- Remember also that recent ingestion of certain foods like beetroot can make the urine red. Rifampicin and nitrofurantoin also make the urine red.
- If suspecting acute glomerulonephritis ask about preceding upper respiratory tract infection about 1 to 2 weeks prior to onset. The latent period between pyoderma and nephritis is variable. Ask about systemic symptoms like fever, malaise, anorexia and headaches.
- Extrarenal symptoms like arthritis and rash may be important in systemic lupus erythematosus (SLE) or SLE nephritis.

HISTORY IN HEMATURIA AND SUGGESTED DIAGNOSIS[11,13]

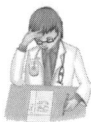

History of symptoms and preceding events in hematuria[2,6,11,13,19,27,28]	Suggested possible diagnosis[2,6,11,13,19,27,28]
Dysuria, frequency, hesitancy, urgency, flank or abdominal pain	Infection of the upper or lower urinary tract or nephrolithiasis
Recent trauma, severe exercise, menstruation, or bladder catheterization	Transient hematuria
A sore throat or skin infection within the past 4 weeks	Postinfectious glomerulonephritis

Drugs and toxins	Hematuria or hemoglobinuria
*Family history	Polycystic renal disease inherited bleeding disorders and Alport's syndrome
*A meticulous search in the family history on questions about hypertension, hearing loss, hematuria, nephrolithiasis, renal disease including renal cystic disease, coagulopathies, sickle cell trait, and dialysis or renal transplant.	

Pain During Urination (Dysuria)

- Does the child cry during micturition?
- Enquire if oliguria or polyuria is present. Both may be indicative of renal problems.

Urgency[4,11]

- Does the child who has been continent for some time, now pass urine before he or she reaches the toilet, suggesting urgency? Is there any hesitancy which is difficulty starting or maintaining the urine in the older child?
- Remember that nocturnal enuresis or bedwetting is wetting while asleep beyond 5 years Primary nocturnal enuresis means that the child has never achieved urinary continence for more than 6 months.
- Primary mono-symptomatic nocturnal enuresis (PMNE)[11] occurs in a patient who is otherwise well with normal voiding.
- Secondary nocturnal enuresis occurs when a child has gained urinary continence for at least 6 months (children are generally dry by day by two years and dry by night by three years) and then starts bedwetting. When children who have learnt to use the toilet without assistance suddenly begin to wet the bed at night, it is secondary enuresis. Urinary tract infection is a cause of this.
- Incontinence refers to absence of control over voiding. Such constant wetting may be due to urinary tract infection or a neuropathic bladder.
- Unstable bladder is frequent micturition associated with urgency and wetting. Certain postures like crossing legs or squatting may stop the urge in this type of bladder dysfunction.

Abdominal Pain

- In children, abdominal pain can occur quite frequently with urinary tract infection as well as in other specific and nonspecific conditions.
- Explore the site and nature with **The Cardinal Ten (Historical)**.

Fever

- Frequent and unexplained fevers without an obvious source of infection. In such fevers, one must exclude a urinary tract infection. The perianal area, the middle ear and the meninges are other reasons for fever without an obvious source.
- Ask about the pain or the passage of 'sand' or stones suggestive of calculi.

Weight Gain

Poor weight gain is recognized in recurrent urinary tract infections in children. In such cases, vesicoureteric reflux (VUR) and other congenital anomalies of the renal tract must be excluded.

Bowel Habits

- Establish normal bowel habits.
- Enquire about constipation, which has an association with urinary tract infections in children as constipation causes urinary stasis.
- Enquire about diarrhea.

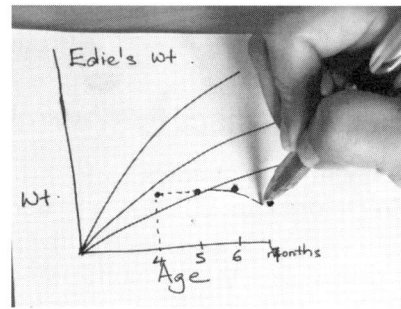

An infant with a urinary tract infection can fail to thrive

Periorbital Swelling or Edema

- Periorbital swelling is characteristic of kidney disease.
- Ask when it was first noticed. Is it more when the child wakes up in the morning? Ask if it interferes with the child's vision. Ask about noticeable weight gain. Are the clothes or shoes noticed to be tighter? Socks or a belt can leave an indentation in the skin that will persist and may have been noticed by the mother or caretaker.

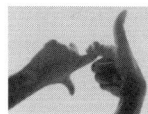

Link history of edema with activities of daily living such as indentations on the skin after taking the socks off in lower limb edema, for practical recall and a more meaningful history

Dyspnea

- Excessive accumulation of fluid in the lungs in renal disease causes dyspnea.
- Ask when it occurs and for how long. Are there any triggering or relieving factors? Ask if there is difficulty in lying flat in bed or orthopnea due to pulmonary edema.

Other Relevant History in Renal Diseases

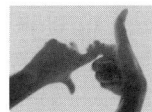

Often, you have to think "multidimensionally". Other components or subheadings of the history are very helpful in making a complete diagnosis. Hence, always take a complete history

- The historical link will subsequently link to appropriate questions.
- Ask for any loss of appetite, refusal of feeds or fussiness.
- Also ask for history of headaches from high blood pressure in kidney diseases (cause and effect), irritability and pain pointing to the head, inability to study or concentrate. Explore if the child had any recent illness in the past, any history of upper respiratory illness.
- Symptoms mistaken for 'gastric flu' such as nausea, vomiting, weakness, fatigue, loss of appetite can occur as symptoms are often non specific.
- Failure to thrive for the given age is a feature of chronic renal diseases. You may have to use historical comparison of growth with siblings.
- Difficulty concentrating and poor academic performance and easy fatigability is a noted feature in children with chronic renal diseases.
- Family history: Additionally, remember that in children, genetic diseases of the kidneys could manifest.
- The history of pregnancy is pertinent for many reasons in renal diseases. As mentioned, oligohydramnious occurs in congenital diseases of the kidneys.

CENTRAL NERVOUS SYSTEM[2,6,11,19,27,28]

- Diseases of the central nervous system have implications on the growth and development of the child.
- A clinical history suggestive of a neurological anomaly must localize to the neuraxis. Use 'the historical link' to try to discern this.
- The birth history, the history of developmental milestones achieved and the neurological history can be closely linked in some disorders and can give important clues to the areas to emphasize in the history.
- History must attempt to determine the pace at which a neurological abnormality develops. In pediatrics, this gives a reflection of the underlying nature of the disease. Symptoms of diseases of the nervous system may be gradual and progressive, static or episodic.
- Static or nonprogressive anomalies are usually due to congenital anomalies or due to brain insults in the prenatal or neonatal period.

LINKS OF ONSET TO NEUROLOGICAL EVENT[2,6,11,19,27,28]

The description of the onset of the neurological anomaly in history-taking can give you an idea of the etiological diagnosis. Some examples to illustrate this are:

Onset of neurological abnormalities[2,6,11,19,27,28]	Possible neurological event[2,6,11,19,27,28]
Sudden onset or hyperacute onset	A seizure or a stroke
Acute onset	Extradural hemorrhage
Sub-acute trigger	A brain tumor
Slowly progressive onset	Inherited conditions
Static	Cerebral palsy, hypoxia to brain in perinatal period
Intermittent attacks of similar abnormalities	Epilepsy or migraine
Episodic with exacerbations and remissions	Demyelinating diseases, autoimmune and vascular diseases

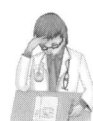

"There are many conditions that may closely resemble seizures in children and a good history will differentiate this; I must remember that an accurately described starting point in the chief complaint or the HOPI is vital for an accurate history thereon.... I simply must ensure that both the mother and I are talking about the same thing."

SYNCOPE[2,6,11,19,27,28]

Determine that it is a seizure and differentiate it from conditions that may resemble seizures like syncope, shock and coma.

Remember that a **vasovagal syncope** is precipitated by stress, emotions or can occur in confined spaces.

Syncope occurs when one temporarily loses consciousness and cannot maintain posture and that usually resolves spontaneously without medical or surgical intervention-differentiation from seizures is important.

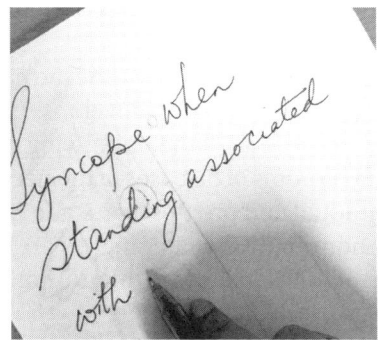

- The description of the syncope is important. There are many clinical conditions that can mimic a syncope
- Ask about the situation under which it occurs
- Ask if the episode of syncope was related to any change in posture
- Ask about prodromal symptoms like warmth, diaphoresis, or lightheadedness prior to or during the syncope
- In an older child, ask of feeling dizzy or fainting when standing
- Ask about association with chest pain, or the presence of palpitations in an older child
- Ask about pallor, clammy skin, sweating, nausea, lightheadedness, weakness or blurring of vision which indicate a neurogenic, vascular or cardiac cause of the syncope. Laryngeal syncope is linked to bouts of cough and unexplained sensations within the throat such as tickling in the throat followed by loss of consciousness
- Ask whether the child has ever turned pale, had nausea and visual changes suggesting a neurocardiogenic cause of syncope
- Vasovagal causes or post voiding micturition syncope must also be excluded if suspected
- Cough is usually paroxysmal for deglutition syncope
- Although rare in the pediatric age group, ask if the child was wearing a collar or had turned his or her head (i.e. carotid sinus cause of syncope) when the attack occurred
- Also enquire if the child was fasting or even feeding poorly if suspecting a hypoglycemia as a cause
- If the child suffers from diabetes mellitus, ask about the use of insulin and proceed enquiry with historical links
- Was there shortness of breath?

- Has the child ever suffered from phobias? Think of neuropsychiatric hyperventilation and psychological stresses in the older child or adolescent girl.

Reflex anoxic seizures are seen in toddlers after trauma, orthostatic hypotension is sometimes seen in adolescents after standing for long periods, and cardiac syncope can result from the hemodynamic effect of cyanotic heart diseases that decrease blood flow to the lungs, arrhythmias, valvular prolapse or severe aortic stenosis in the adolescent.

Breath holding spells are recognized in children from six months to three years. The child holds the breath in expiration usually at the peak of anger. This causes cyanosis, limpness and can lead to unconsciousness. If this is severe, there is tonic stiffness of the limbs. The child will recover rapidly. This is a behavioral problem seen in some children.

From two years of age to seven years, children may partially wake up from deep sleep and may be very restless. This agitation is difficult to calm and is described as night terrors.

Benign positional vertigo occurs between one and five years. It is of sudden onset, associated with pallor, nystagmus and vomiting. The child remains conscious. This may be related to migraine.

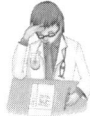

"Attentive listening to the historian followed by open and closed ended questions making use of historical links will help me decide on the clinical episode and differentiate a syncope from a seizure".

SEIZURES[2,6,11,19,27,28]

History of Fits

- **A fit may be an important clinical manifestation of intracranial and extracranial disease**.
- Make use of **The Cardinal Ten (Historical)** and the 'historical link' to ascertain its true nature.

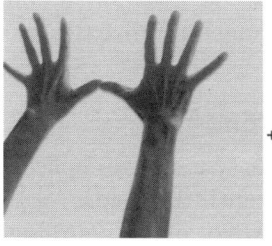 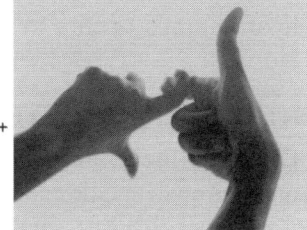

- Clarify the origin of the seizures; whether intracranial or extracranial. Remember that neurocardiogenic causes, vasovagal causes, micturition and breath holding spells can cause or mimic seizures. All associated features can give you a hint to its etiology.[2,6,11,19,27,28]

- When did it occur?
- How often did the fit occur within 24 hours of the initial fit (to assess severity) or fever (for febrile fits) did it repeatedly occur?
- Ask what the child was doing when it occurred or before it occurred and the nature of the fit
- What were the postictal events?
- Describe the post fit period
- Were there abnormal or unusual behaviors?
- Was there a period of postictal drowsiness?
- Was there associated loss of consciousness or was the child arousable? Was it associated with tonic and clonic movements, up-rolling of eyeballs, incontinence of urine and passage of feces—'**The Cardinal Ten (Historical)**'.
- Ask questions about the mental state, e.g. drowsiness before or after the fit
- Ask about response to instructions given at that time
- Ask for symptoms to suggest headache in the past. Does the child point to the head and cry or is the child unusually irritable?
- Is there blurring of vision or associated vomiting? If so make use of **The Cardinal Ten (Historical)** to enquire about such symptoms in detail
- Ask about recent school performance

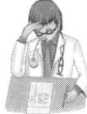

Neurodevelopmental delay can be the cause or the effect of seizures.

Growth and Developmental History

The neurodevelopment of the child including birth history and developmental history are vital. Realise that an intracranial lesion causing neurodevelopmental delay can cause a seizure and likewise repeated seizures can also lead to neurodevelopmental delay.

Fever

Was the child having a fever? How high was it? How many times did the fit occur during the first 24 hours of fever?

There are many important causes of seizures that occur in children with fever that must be excluded. Simple febrile seizures occur in neurodevelopmentally normal children. Certain criteria have to be fulfilled to make the diagnosis of a simple febrile seizure. It is wrong to assume that all seizures in a febrile child is a febrile seizure.

Causes of seizures in children with fever[2,6,11,19,27,28]
• Central nervous system infections like meningitis, encephalitis or brain abscess
• Unrecognized epilepsy triggered by fever
• Simple febrile convulsions
• Complex or atypical febrile convulsions

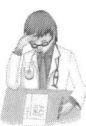

"I must exclude preventable and treatable causes first"

Factors to fulfill for the diagnosis of simple febrile convulsions[2,6,11,19,27,28]
• Occurs in children from 6 months to 6 years; the mean age is 22 months
• Precipitated by rapid increases in temperature
• Occurs in the first day or two of fever
• Occurs in 2–4% of all children
• They are generalized motor seizures
• Lasts less than 15 minutes
• Occurs once in a 24 hour period
• The child is neurologically and developmentally normal
• A cause for the fever is usually found
• If no obvious source is found, a viral infection, viral exanthem or a urinary tract infection may be the cause

If the child is febrile and there are focal features to the seizure, if the seizure lasts more than 15 minutes, or the seizures occur many times within one febrile event or if followed by Todd's palsy (transient focal weakness) the seizure is called a complex febrile seizure. In such cases, it is mandatory to exclude an underlying treatable cause of seizures such as meningitis.

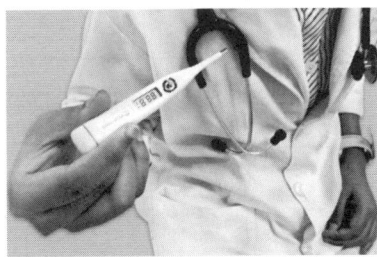

The recording of temperature is a vital assessment in a child with seizures

History Suggestive of Aura or Migraine or Nausea

There may be a preceding aura described by the family as a change in behavior. There may be migraine or nausea.

Enquiry of Limb Paresis or Paralysis

Require regarding weakness or paralysis of limbs or muscles. How much this interferes with activities of daily living must be gauged by questioning. Ask about change in gait or if there is reduced movement of the limbs. Also ask if there is numbness in limbs or elsewhere.

Enquiry of Giddiness or Staggering

Enquire about frequent falls prior to the fit. Changes in gait or unsteady gait can occur in intracranial lesions, neoplasms and drug toxicity.

Enquire about Visual Disturbance

If suspecting visual problems, you may ask if the child holds objects close to him, sits in the front row of the classroom, is showing declining school performance or skews eyes on watching television.

Directly ask about parental concerns about vision.

Enquiry about Deafness

If indicated, ask about parental worries about hearing. Ask if child responds to call of his or her name, ask if child startles to loud noise. Ask if child has recently started to speak in a loud tone when he or she talks (conductive deafness).

History Suggestive of Tinnitus

A buzzing sensation in the ear described by an older child may indicate tinnitus. Try to link its causes to medications or ear infections; then follow-up with **The Cardinal Ten (Historical)** and historical links.

Speech Disturbance

Can the child speak? Does the child respond to sound normally? Deafness interferes and delays speech.

Ask if child says any word with meaning and relate this to his or her age.

Environmental Stimulation or Siblings or Nursery[1]

Ask how many siblings there are and how they interact.

Ask if child is sent to the nursery. How many children are there? The first child in a family may not be exposed to as stimulating an environment as the second or third child. However, parental attention is usually, but not always, more intense in the only child.

Has the caregiver or mother noticed that the child cannot say the things he or she used to before. This indicates developmental regression which is suspected when a child who has been normal in development and has met milestones appropriate for age starts to regress, unable to perform milestones that he or she has already achieved. This is an extremely worrying symptom.

After determining that the episode is a seizure and not a condition mimicking a seizure, determine the seizure type from history.

Seizures[2,4,6,11,19,27,28]

Seizure Type

If it is a partial seizure, determine if consciousness was impaired, lost or maintained. In simple partial seizures, consciousness is not affected. In complex partial seizures consciousness is impaired. Such

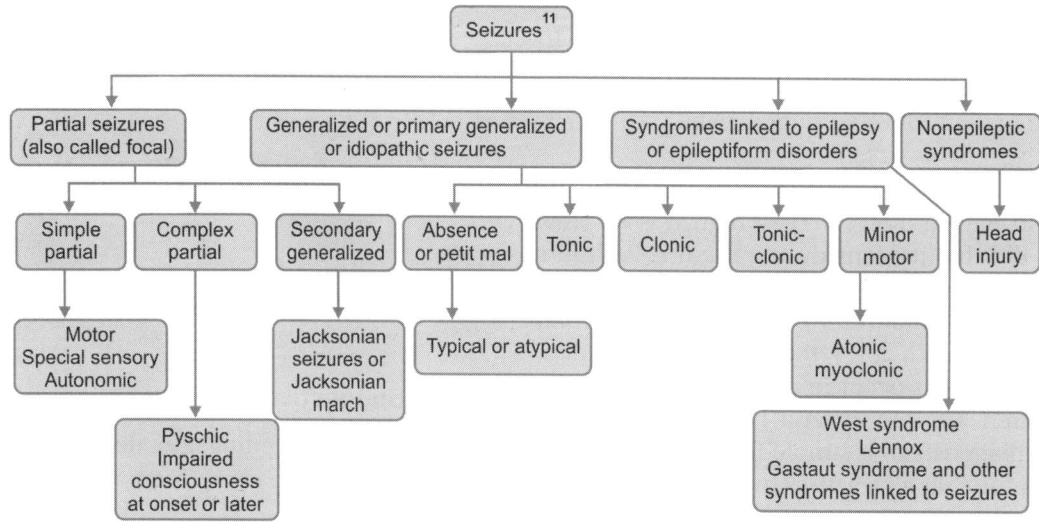

impairment in consciousness may be either at onset or it may affect the patient more gradually during the course of the seizure.
- Did the child exhibit any injury?
- Was the child noticeably pale before falling?
- In the older child, ask if the child was able to respond to questions?
- Was the patient in an unconscious state or was there just a mild impairment in his or her awareness?
- Was it the whole body or part of the body involved?
- Which part of the body was involved?
- Briefly describe the manner in which the child fell to the ground. Did the patient have a stiff fall or did he or she gradually droop to the floor?
- What was the time period for the tonic stiffening or clonic jerking?
- Which part of the body exhibited clonic activity?

Determine postictal states and postictal events

Postictal sleep
- Such changes occur after complex partial and generalized convulsive seizures.

Postictal changes
- Are not observed after the occurrence of generalized absence seizures.
- Loss of speech postictally (indicative of left temporal lobe seizure).
- Enquire if lateralized motor activity-like-movement of the child's eyes to one particular side or dystonic positioning of a limb was observed by the parents.
- The diagnosis of **simple partial seizures** is supported by motor activity without impaired awareness.
- Impaired awareness and automatisms are suggestive of a **complex partial seizure**.

Important Points to Note in Seizures

- Paroxysmal events are not necessarily always epileptic seizures hence these two conditions must be differentiated.
- Seizure onset that might be localized best explains a partial or focal seizure. An aura may occur before the clinically apparent seizure. An aura is usually observed by the family as changes in behavior prior to the onset of the seizure.
- In the history, ask about the details of events before, during and after the seizure.
- The patient or parent may provide a description of a feeling that they have perceived in the child (e.g. feeling of fear, or tingling sensation felt in the fingers, or bright lights in one visual field). These specific symptoms might enable you to identify the possible location of seizure onset. A well-known example in the older child or adolescent is déjà vu which indicates involvement of the temporal lobe.

MUSCULOSKELETAL SYSTEM[2,4,6,9,11,14,19,27,28]

- In pediatrics, all ages can be affected by musculoskeletal problems.
- Some normal developmental changes in children must be known before pathological diagnosis of the musculoskeletal system is made.
- Most cases of musculoskeletal problems in children are self-limiting hence the differentiation of benign musculoskeletal disorders of children from pathological ones is important.
- Remember, however, symptoms of the musculoskeletal system can be the initial feature of severe and even life-threatening systemic illnesses such as leukemia or osteomyelitis or social problems such as non-accidental injury.
- Specific problems of muscles and bones, if present, must be asked in detail using the historical link.
- The history is a tool to anatomical, etiological and pathological diagnosis. The history identifies symptoms that reflect the root or cause of the problem which could be inflammatory, infectious, traumatic or malignant.
- Delay in the diagnosis of some important musculoskeletal problems in children can adversely affect the prognosis and even lead to musculoskeletal deformities.

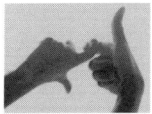

In the musculoskeletal history, link the chronological and developmental age to the history obtained. Determine true pathology. Differentiate this from normal physiological variation in children

MUSCULOSKELETAL PAIN[2,9,11,14]

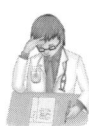

"In the musculoskeletal system, I find that I have to link many questions in the history to activities of daily living". In diseases affecting this system, the historian also expresses concerns about the inability to conduct these activities. These difficulties essentially affect the quality of the child's life."

Inflammation of the joints (arthritis) or inflammation of the synovium (synovitis) causes:[2,9,11,14]
• Joint pain
• Joint swelling
• Morning stiffness
• Gelling or stiffness of joints after inactivity
• Difficulty in using the affected joint and this makes daily activities difficult
• Difficulty in playing games or conducting usual activities
• Absenteeism from school

Enthesitis is when the insertion of a ligament or tendon to bone is inflamed. Pain and swelling commonly involves the Achilles tendon but can also involve toes and fingers, elbows, pelvis and chest wall.

Inflammation of the muscle (myositis) causes[2,9,11,14]
• Muscle pain
• Weakness
• Difficulty in performing activities of daily living

- Ask "Is the pain consistently localized?"
- Ask if the pain is triggered by movement of that particular joint if possible joint pathology.
- Is the pain initiated by rest or upon bearing weight on the limb which could be associated with underlying pathology? If so, this is suggestive of disease of the bone.
- Is the child able to move normally despite having pain at rest? i.e. pain in the limb after physical activity? This is often linked to an innocuous cause.
- Self-limiting musculoskeletal conditions must be differentiated from more innocuous ones. The following are historical clues.

The following are suggestive of a benign cause of a musculoskeletal problem[2,9,11,14]
• Pain that is better during rest
• Worsened by activity
• Pain towards late evening
• Nocturnal pain with improvement after simple analgesics
• No history to suggest evidence of arthritis
• No history to suggest muscle weakness
• A normal physical examination
• Normal laboratory tests

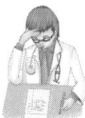

"How will I choose the least number of investigations with the most yield?"

The following indicate musculoskeletal conditions that require investigation[2,9,11,14]
• Pain better by activity and present at rest
• Morning stiffness
• Pain at night which does not improve with simple analgesics
• The presence of gait abnormality such as a limp
• History indicative of arthritis
• History indicative of muscle weakness
• Abnormal physical examination
• Abnormal laboratory tests
• Systemic symptoms

In children, benign musculoskeletal pain or growing pains peaks between three to seven years of age and may have a family history. It is described as deep, cramp-like pain in the thighs typically occurring in the evening or at night. Growing pains are commoner in boys, in children who are very active and may be exacerbated by increased physical activity. The typical history and a normal physical examination is elicited when one diagnoses growing pains.

Remember that persistent nocturnal leg pain, especially if associated with fever, needs to be investigated. Leukemia is a cause that must not be forgotten in children.

Trauma[2,4,6,9,11,14,19,27,28]

- In musculoskeletal symptoms you must always ask about the preceding history of trauma.
- Traumatic fractures potentially occur anywhere in the body depending on the type of trauma and severity.
- When would you consider non-accidental injuries (NAI)? You must think of NAI whenever there are inconsistencies in the pediatric history with fractures at sites that do not tally with the mobility in keeping with the developmental age of the child.

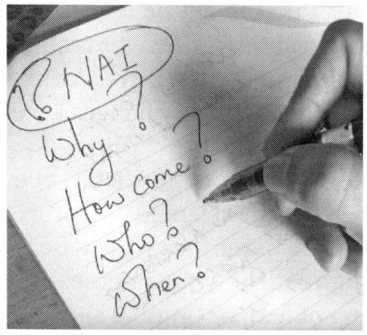

Review of Systems

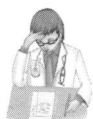

"Why can't I make sense of the history and what I see? Is there something more in pediatrics that I must think of?"

NAI should be suspected when: [2,4,6,9,11,14,19,27,28]

• The caretakers do not allow you to ask the child the history or seem to resist when you want to interview a child who is at an age to understand
• An injury is unexplained, the severity of the injury is incompatible with the history
• The history keeps changing
• The injury is not in keeping with the developmental age of the child
• There are multiple fractures at various stages of healing in a child
• There are rib fracture which are rare in children as the rib cage is flexible
• There are skull fractures as skull fractures are uncommon in young children below 18 months and are a consequence of direct force on the skull
• There are sternum, scapula, or spinous processes involved in fractures

LIMB ABNORMALITIES OR DEFORMITIES[2,4,6,9,11,14,19,27,28]

- Ask if affected joints are swollen, hot or tender; explore systemic symptoms like fever and bleeding gums which point to a systemic cause.
- Ask also of associated symptoms like rash, fever, malaise or weight loss.
- Ask if there is a family history of bleeding tendencies, or excessive bleeding after circumcision in child or in family member(s), at birth or later in life.
- If limb deformity is present, is the deformity unilateral or bilateral? Was the deformity present from birth? Is the deformity static or is it resolving or progressing? A progressing deformity indicates that the mechanism of growth is affected and intervention should be started early.
- Genu valgum and varum must be interpreted in the light of a child's normal development.
- Usually if these conditions occur at ages other than that associated with normal developmental changes and if associated with short stature, think of a possible pathological cause like skeletal dysplasia. Ask for other associated features of renal diseases, trauma or fever.

Physiological genu varum [2,4,6,11,19,27,28]	Pathological genu varum [2,4,6,11,19,27,28]
• Most common in children older than 18 months	• Blounts disease, trauma, rickets
• Improves by 2 years	• Osteogenesis imperfecta, benign tumors

Physiological genu valgum [2,4,6,11,19,27,28]	Pathological genu valgum [2,4,6,11,19,27,28]
• Between 3 and 4 years of age children	• Unilateral renal rickets, skeletal dysplasias
• Improves and resolves by age 7	• Bilateral trauma, infection, benign tumors

Pathological genu varum (bow legs) and genu valgum (knock knees) should be suspected in the following circumstances: [2,4,6,11,19,27,28]

- Ages are not inkeeping with physiological variations
- Asymmetrical genu varum or genu valgum
- Family history of skeletal deformities
- Poor dietary history
- Absence to sun exposure
- Short stature
- A history of pathological fractures
- Angular deformities of skeleton—suspect skeletal dysplasia
- Systemic diseases such as renal or, hepatic or other systemic manifestations such as abnormalities of the eye, deafness and so on

Limb Weakness[14]

The child may have difficulty in standing up or combing hair. If pain is present, decide if it is bone pain, joint pain or muscle cramps. Use **The Cardinal Ten (Historical)** to further inquire about the joint pain or swelling.

As mentioned earlier, 'growing pains' are benign nocturnal limb pains of childhood. It is a diagnosis of exclusion that is characterized by cramping pains of the thigh, shin, and calf. It usually occurs at night and may arouse the child from sleep but disappears by morning and is without a limp or a change in gait.

Limb Pain[14]

- Ask if any particular posture or position relieves the pain. Explore if the pain is experienced on waking up. Is it migratory or constant in nature? Is the pain radiating in nature? Is there any associated rash; if so, ask for details of the rash. Ask for other associations. Ask about swelling, limited range of movement and loss of use of a limb.
- Enquire about early morning stiffness and improvement with activity which is typical of inflammatory arthritis.

- Preceding upper respiratory illness, vaccinations, chickenpox and rubella may link to post infectious arthritis.
- Ask if any particular posture or position relieves the pain.

CHILD WITH A LIMP
(Refer to Chapter 14)[2,6,11,19,27,28]

Gait Abnormalities[2,4,6,9,11,14,19,27,28]

- Is there any noticeable change in gait? If so, give details using 'The Cardinal Ten (Historical)'.
- Is the abnormality preceded by a sore throat?
- Was it preceded by a possible tick bite?
- Are there any triggering or relieving factors for pain?
- Are there any associations of pain with fever, eye symptoms, weight loss, bleeding or bruising, or bloody stools?
- Ask about associated systemic symptoms such as fever, bowel symptoms, urinary symptoms, and symptoms suggestive of liver disease or renal disease where relevant. Ask about weight loss, swellings in lymph nodes and easy fatigability.
- Explore the possibility of trauma where relevant.
- Ask about related symptoms, make use of 'the historical link' to describe the pathophysiological connection.

The age of the child and whether it is painful or painless is important in determining the differential diagnosis. An acute course makes infections or trauma more likely whereas a chronic course makes a rheumatic, inflammatory or neurological course more likely. A bone pain worse at night is seen in neoplastic causes whereas a limp worse in the morning may be suggestive of an inflammatory cause.

Questionnaire in a Child with a Limp[2,6,11,14,19,27,28]

• Age of child.
• Duration of limp.
• Has it improved or worsened since onset?
• When is the limp worst? Morning or night?
• Is it painful?
• Where is the pain mostly felt?
• How severe is the pain? What does the child do when in pain?
• Duration of pain.
• What relieves the pain?
• Is there any radiation of pain?
• Is there a history of trauma?
• Are there associated systemic symptoms?

• Is there weight loss or anorexia?
• Is there a history of fever?
• Is there any rash?
• Is back pain present?
• Are there arthralgias involving the joints of the affected limb or are other joints involved?
• Are there problems of voiding or passing stools?
• Is there any recent history of illness including viral or streptococcal infection?
• Has the child been exposed to antibiotics? (may change course of illness)
• Is there any history of sports activity?

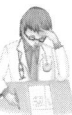 A history of recent or strenuous sports activity can indicate an overuse injury such as a stress fracture or Osgood-Schlatter disease, as would a history of worsening pain with activity.

Family history
- This could suggest a collagen vascular disorder, irritable bowel syndrome (IBD) in an older child or adolescent, a hemoglobinopathy or bleeding disorder.
- Is there a known neuromuscular disorder?

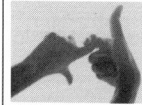 The presence of fever would link to an infectious, inflammatory or malignant cause.

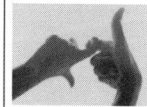 A history of upper respiratory illness (URI) or sore throat may make post-infectious arthritis or myositis to be considered in the differential diagnosis

ENDOCRINE SYSTEM[2,6,11,12,19,27,28]

- There are many causes of growth disorders. Congenital anomalies, chronic diseases, chromosomal and endocrine disorders must be considered.
- Growth and metabolism are closely related and is regulated by the endocrine system which is an important body function managed by hormonal messengers.
- Many different syndromes are linked to the endocrine system or are also associated with endocrine abnormalities. Disorders of growth due to deficiencies of GHRH, GH and IGF-1 are recognized.
- The clinical expressions of an endocrine disorder could be related to the response of the peripheral tissue to excessive or deficient hormones.
- Endocrine disorders thus may manifest due to excessive hormone, deficient hormone, abnormal end organ response, and absence, dysgenesis, atrophy or enlargement of the endocrine gland.

Pattern of Growth[2,6,11,12,19,27,28]

- Review all previous heights and weights recorded on suitable age and gender appropriate charts. This will give you an idea of the questions that are relevant to ask in the history.
- Remember that familial causes of short stature and of tall stature are common so observe parental height as you take the history.
- Ask about birth weight, growth and weight gain in infancy. Ask whether the child has always been short or has not increased in height as expected.
- Also ask about any chronic ingestion or administration of medications that could have influenced growth like systemic steroids, antimetabolites or even some quinolones which should not be chronically prescribed in the young child.
- Do not forget to ask about symptoms suggestive of chronic diseases that could have impacted growth.

ENQUIRY AND LINKS[2,6,11,12,19,22,28]

Remember the causes of a child with short stature when enquiry is made: (Refer to chapter 14)
• Familial short statute and constitutional delay in growth and puberty (CDGP) are common causes that must be considered
• Short stature due to chronic childhood diseases
• Short stature due to inadequate intake or malnutrition
With the causes in mind, ask about symptoms that reveal the possible etiology of short stature:
• Typical features of familial short stature and CDGP (Refer to Chapter 14)
• Chronic diarrheas suggest inflammatory bowel diseases or food allergies
• Lethargy, constipation, hair loss, poor school performance suggest hypothyroidism
• Sometimes, infants who are small for gestational infants (SGA), do not catch up and reach optimal adult height

General questions that indicate possible endocrine causes of underlying problems[2,6,11,12,19,27,28]

- What is the known duration of the problem?
- Has the child been experiencing abnormal weight gain or loss?
- Explore for history of heat or cold intolerance, alterations in bowel habits, hair loss, irritability and inability to focus or palpitations in the older child or teenager.
- Ask about factors that relieve and exacerbate fatigue.

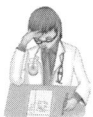

"These are nice to know."

"When I think of endocrine dysfunction in the differential diagnosis, I must categorize my knowledge of pathophysiology into hormone excess, hormone deficiency and end organ dysfunction. Then I make use of the historical links to think about it in depth."

Enquire regarding peculiar eating habits, unusual behavior, visual problems and headaches. In suspected or suggestive cases of diabetes mellitus, enquire also on the age of onset of the disease.

The commonest type of diabetes mellitus in childhood is type 1 diabetes mellitus. Other types are neonatal diabetes, an underlying disease with diabetes like cystic fibrosis. Type 2 diabetes mellitus, maturity onset diabetes mellitus (MODY), drugs like steroids can cause diabetes mellitus (*Refer to Chapter 14*). Certain syndromes are linked to diabetes mellitus.

Pediatric diabetes mellitus with genetic syndromes[2,11,17]
• Turner syndrome (TS)
• Prader-Willi syndrome (PWS)
• Friedreich ataxia (FA)
• Down syndrome (DS)
• Klinefelter syndrome (KS)
• Bardet-Biedl syndrome (BBS)
• Berardinelli-Seip syndrome (BSS)
• Alström syndrome (AS)

Food and Water Intake[2,6,11,12,19,27,28]

- Hypoglycemia in infancy and childhood can be a consequence of many metabolic and endocrine causes (*Refer to Chapter 14*). Hypoglycemia is commonly transient in the immediate newborn period but when it occurs after 48 to 72 hours it can also be due to endocrine or metabolic disorders.
- The diagnosis of hypoglycemia is made on the basis of a low serum glucose concentration. The symptoms of hypoglycemia are mainly the result of the release of adrenaline or cerebral glycopenia.
- In infants, nonspecific symptoms are common. Symptoms such as hunger, confusion, headaches, visual changes and tremors can be present.
- The etiological diagnosis of hypoglycemia requires a detailed history including birth, family and drug history.

50 The Link: Pediatric History-Taking and Physical Examination

Symptoms of hypoglycemia[2,6,11,12,19,27,28]	Signs of hypoglycemia[2,6,11,12,19,27,28]
• Anxiety	• Perspiration
• Nausea	• Vomiting
• Weakness	• Pallor
• Headache	• Paresthesia
• Inability to concentrate	• Trembling
• Hunger	• Mental confusion
• Somnolence	• Difficulties in concentration
• Personality changes	• Staring
	• Palpitations
	• Trembling
	• Convulsions
	• Diplopia
	• Ataxia
	• Coma
	• Stroke

When suspecting diabetes mellitus, ask about excessive fluid intake, loss in weight or increased urine output.

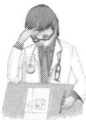

That is why diabetes mellitus is referred to as a condition where there is 'starvation in the midst of plenty' where the excess glucose extracellularly cannot enter the intracellular environment for optimal function due to the lack of insulin.

Ask for the presence of polyphagia (excessive hunger) and the onset and correlations like weight gain. Polyphagia, polydypsia and weight loss is recognized in Type 1 diabetes mellitus.

Drug and Food History in Diabetes Mellitus[2,4,6,9,11,14,19,27,28]

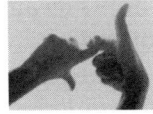

Breastfeeding probably has a protective effect against IDDM.

The drug history could be helpful as some forms of secondary diabetes is associated with certain drugs. Ask for history of maternal drug ingestion-medicines linked to diabetes mellitus such as Danazol and steroids. Remember that some traditional medicines and herbs may contain steroids. Iatrogenic steroid therapy is a known cause. Also enquire on cow's milk feeding prior to the age of 2 years. Preceding history of viral infections is associated with the destruction of the islet cells and is a cause of childhood diabetes mellitus.

NEONATAL HISTORY IN THYROID DISORDERS[2,6,11,19,26-28]

Thyroid hormones are vital for early brain development. During pregnancy, both maternal and fetal thyroid hormones contribute to fetal brain development. The early influence of maternal hormones explains why most newborns who are born with thyroid agenesis or hypofunction seem asymptomatic at birth.

Fetal or neonatal hypothyroidism is a rare disorder. Its incidence, by neonatal screening, is about 1:4000.

Enquire about the history of prolonged jaundice. This is due to delayed maturation of the glucuronide transferase enzyme. This may be the earliest sign of hypothyroidism. Feeding difficulties, respiratory difficulties, sluggish development, bowel habits, a coarse cry and somnolence are typical clinical features of hypothyroidism.

In the history you could try to differentiate congenital hypothyroidism and acquired hypothyroidism which present with different symptoms.

Symptoms like neonatal jaundice, poor feeding, hypothermia and protuberant abdomen present early in congenital hypothyroidism. Failure to gain weight, decreased stool frequency and poor sucking are also symptoms of congenital hypothyroidism. Symptoms that occur later are umbilical hernia, dry skin with carotenemia and a hoarse cry. Also recognized are symptoms that may be present after 3 months of life.

In acquired hypothyroidism, short stature, delay in the eruption and shedding of teeth, myxedema, precocious sexual development, delayed onset of puberty and galactorrhea in girls are recognized symptoms. Also recognized are symptoms of muscle weakness and pseudohypertrophy.

Permanent Congenital Hypothyroidism (Refer to Chapter 14)

- Primary thyroid dysgenesis: Thyroid ectopy, agenesis and thyroid hypoplasia (most common)—TSH high, T3, T4 low.
- Inborn errors of biosynthesis of thyroid hormone are also causes of permanent congenital hypothyroidism.

- Mutations involving Thyroid Transcription Factors (TTF)[26] influence altered fetal thyroid development.
- Fetomaternal deficiency of transcription factor (Pit-1, Prop-1, LHX-3)[26] is also a rare cause of fetal hypothyroidism.
- Secondary (central) part of syndrome with midline defects (e.g. septooptic dysplasia) or inherited—TSH low; TRH and other hormones may be affected.

Transient Congenital Hypothyroidism

- Discovered at birth.
- TSH high, T3, T4 low with thyroid hormone levels returning to normal in weeks to years.

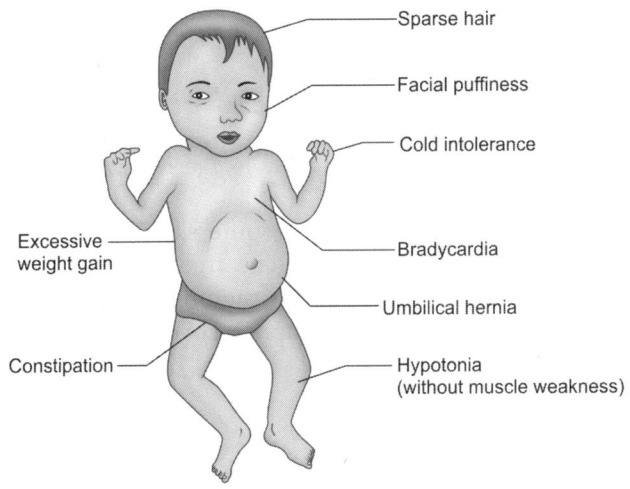

Features of hypothyroidism

Goiter and Thyroid Disease

- Take the history in a chronological manner. Clinical symptoms may be nonspecific. Certain genetic disorders like Turner's syndrome and Down syndrome have a higher incidence of acquired hypothyroidism (Hashimoto thyroiditis).
- Infants born to mothers with Graves' disease may develop neonatal thyrotoxicosis. The passage of transplacental thyrotrophin receptor stimulating antibodies (TRAb) cause neonatal thyrotoxicosis. Neonatal Graves' disease usually improves and resolves on its own within less than 12 weeks as maternal thyroid stimulating immunoglobulins are cleared from the circulation.
- Thyrotoxic fetuses may develop tachycardia, a goiter on physical examination, craniosynostosis and even accelerated bone maturation. Excessive fetal movement and the retardation of growth are other possible features. Fetal thyrotoxicosis can cause hydrops due to cardiac failure.
- In infant's premature birth, poor feeding and failure to thrive must be asked. Sometimes abnormalities of cranial bone fusion or craniosynostosis may be seen.
- In older children and teenage girls, ask about weight loss, palpitations, tremors, heat intolerance, diarrheas, polyphagia, hair loss and proximal muscle weakness.

CHILD WITH AMBIGUOUS GENITALIA[2,6,11,19,27,28]

This is not a common condition. Nevertheless, when suspected a detailed history must be taken. Ask about history of consanguinity of marriage. Enquire about a possible family history of similar problems particularly among the siblings as **congenital adrenal hyperplasia (CAH), 46XY gonadal dysgenesis and 5-alpha reductase** are autosomal recessive or familial conditions.

In infants, ask about maternal drugs during pregnancy as drugs containing androgens taken at that time, especially early in pregnancy, cause virilization of the female external genitalia. Ask about history of unexplained neonatal death. Find out the time and pattern of pubescence in precocious puberty. Correlate other clinical symptoms with 'the historical link' and ask details with **The Cardinal Ten (Historical)**.

Family History[2,6,11,19,25,28]

Enquire about the growth history of siblings, parents and relatives. Enquire about the social background (if relevant) in the family history of similar or associated diseases. Enquire if there is a history of sudden and unexplained infant death in the family which is suggestive of **salt losing CAH**.

Precocious Puberty

- The urgency of referral depends on the age of onset and the clinical signs.
- Early puberty in boys is worrying and any boy who develops signs of puberty before nine years of age requires referral to an endocrinologist to be investigated.
- Early puberty in a girl, is more likely to be benign, unless occurring at a very young age.
- A frequent cause of early development of axillary or pubic hair in childhood is premature adrenarche.
- The main physical changes of adrenarche are the effects of androgens and the appearance of pubic hair (pubarche).

- In a child with precocious puberty investigations and referral to an expert are necessary. Yet in these cases, although challenging, you could try to exclude pathology, thinking about the causes.
- The clinical manifestation of hyperandrogenism includes the complaint of premature development of pubic and axillary hair, the development of body odors due to increased sweat glands and accelerated growth. It is important to try to clinically distinguish from **central precocious puberty, congenital adrenal hyperplasia** and from **androgen secreting tumors** of the adrenal glands and the gonads.
- Although not always easy, try to elicit and exclude in the history, symptoms that suggest tumors of the adrenal gland and pituitary gland which can cause precocious puberty in boys and girls. Ovarian tumors are known to cause precocious puberty in girls.
- Ask about rarer causes that are linked to bone and skin lesions. You may have to refer further to remember examples such as McCune Albright's syndrome which cause precocious puberty in both boys and girls.
- The intake of medications containing estrogen or testosterone or even the regular application of topical creams or ointments containing estrogen or testosterone over altered or abraded skin can be simply obtained from the history.

School Going Age

Remember that a recognized common cause of delayed puberty in boys is due to constitutional delay in growth and puberty (CDGP). These children are healthy and have no underlying organic cause for the delay in growth. However, in these children, a careful history to exclude systemic illness is important to exclude other causes. You may enquire as to how the child is faring in school when trying to exclude central causes of precocious puberty. Has the teacher observed poor school performance recently?

SKIN[2,6,11,19,27,28]

- The skin is the largest organ in the body and its protective function against noxious external agents is important.
- There are differences in the child's skin as compared to the adult skin which contribute to the difference in susceptibility and spectrum of skin diseases in children.
- Rashes of the skin may be ailments of the skin per se or may be part of a systemic illness
- Rashes with fever indicate a local or systemic infection.

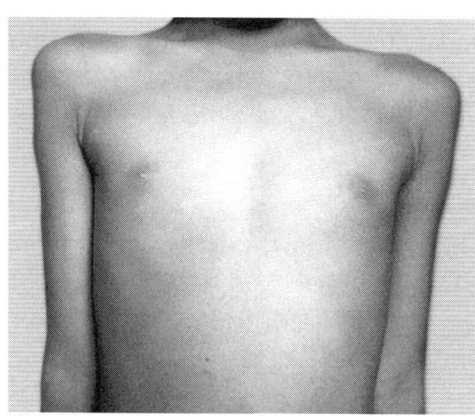

5-year-old boy with fever and maculopapular rash due to measles. (Courtesy: Associate Professor, Dr Loh Keng Yin, reprint with permission)

- The typical morphology of some skin lesions may warrant the need for urgent treatment as seen in palpable petechiae in meningococcemia or exfoliation of the skin in staphylococcal scalded skin syndrome (SSS).

Age[2,6,11,19,27,28]

- The skin of the child has less well-developed sebaceous glands and hair follicles. The amount of subcutaneous fat and the regulation of temperature are different in the child's skin as compared to adults. These differences are important to realize as topical medication applied on the skin can have different responses in this age group. As an example, the sensitive skin of an infant can be affected by irritant damage to the skin.
- The age of the child also influences the differential diagnosis considered as certain conditions are more common in certain age groups. The distribution can differ in the different ages, e.g. atopic eczema in infancy is seen on the cheeks, in the toddler in the extensors and a flexural distribution in the older child and adult.
- Seasonal predilections of skin conditions are linked to allergic diseases. Environmental influences and genetic predispositions pertaining to skin diseases are recognized and are important.
- Remember that enquiry must always be made into previous treatment of skin conditions whether topical or oral.

Historical clues to the diagnosis of skin lesions[2,6,11,16,19,27,28]

• The age of patient
• Onset of lesion
• Where and how did it start?
• Duration of lesion, i.e. how long has it been present?
• Progression of lesion, i.e. does it come and go or is it persistent?
• Has it changed and if so, in what aspect?
• Exacerbating factors, i.e. are there any factors that make it worse?
• Relieving factors, i.e. are there any factors that make it better or make you feel more comfortable?
• Associated cutaneous symptoms, i.e. is it itchy, painful or burning?
• Associated systemic symptoms like fever, malaise or weight loss
• Is there any use of over the counter remedies (OTC)? OTC remedies can significantly alter the appearance of a rash and this may confuse the clinical picture, making it more difficult to make a diagnosis.

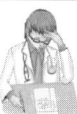

Probe this history in depth by asking closed ended questions related to possible medications as patients may not consider topical creams as important enough to relate to you.

• History of allergies
• Any significant environmental exposure
• Other aspects of history including history of travel and previous treatment
• Other family member(s) who has a similar rash or lesion

Questionnaire on site and descriptive morphology of skin rash
• When did the rash start?
• Which area of the body did it affect?
• What was the pattern of spread?
• If it did spread, did it spread rapidly?
• Did it spread from the center of the body to the peripheries or from the peripheries to the central areas? (centrifugal or centripetal)
• Is it fluid filled? If so, probe into the nature of the fluid contained
• Is it pustular?
• Is it papular?
• Is it red?
• Is it red and scaly?
• Is it itchy?
• What are the borders like? Are they raised or serpiginous?

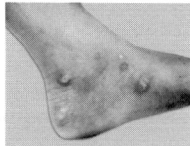

Leg of school boy with intensely itchy lesions due to Sarcoptes scabiei (Courtesy: Associate Professor Dr. Loh Keng Yin, reprint with permission)

Contd...

Contd...

• How would you describe the rash?
• Is it generalized, intensely pruritic papulovesicular, crusted rash of scabies in a child?
• Is it red and eczematous?
• Is it red and pruritic?

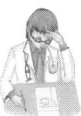

"How would an infant manifest pruritis? Would he or she wiggle?"

• Is it red and nonpruritic?
• Is it painful?
• Is it persistent or intermittent?
• Is it impetiginized?
• Is it oozing?
• What brings it on?
• What makes it worse?

DERMATOLOGICAL LINKS TO THE DIAGNOSIS OF ALLERGY TO COW'S MILK PROTEIN[2,6,10,11,19,24,27-29]

- The enquiry into the history of ingestion of cow's milk as a cause of skin lesions is important as CMPA is a common condition in children. They usually outgrow this between the ages of 2–4 years. Remember that breastfeeding mothers on large amounts of cow's milk may also transmit this allergy via breastfeeding.
- The skin manifestations of CMPA can occur in infants, toddlers and even children.
- CMPA can manifest as urticaria that may be unrelated to infections, drug intake or atopic eczema.
- Angioedema as a result of CMPA may be manifested by swelling of lips or eyelids. This can pose as management emergencies. It may manifest as atopic eczema.
- Sometimes CMPA causes a chronic relapsing pruritic inflammatory disease of the skin.

In atopic eczema you must ask about:
- The feeding history including:
  - The history of introduction to artificial formula
  - The age of introduction of the weaning diet.
- The family history of atopy such as:
  - Bronchial asthma
  - Hay fever
  - Urticaria.

Clinical Spectrum on the Skin of Cow's Milk Protein Allergy (CMPA) in Children[2,6,10,11,19,24,27-29]

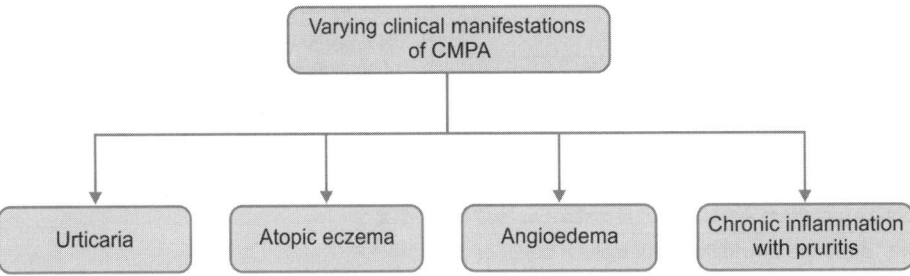

HEMATOLOGICAL SYSTEM[2,6,11,19,27,28]

- The hematological system may be primarily or secondarily involved in childhood diseases.
- The age related normal variations are important to know before pathology is thought of. For example, the normal newborn has a relatively increased hemoglobin and hematocrit levels than the older children. Physiological adjustment to extrauterine life contributes to the physiological 'anemia' of infancy. In the term infant the mean Hb levels are about 9–11 g/dL and in the preterm infant about 7–9 g/dL at 2–3 months of age.
- Anemias linked to nutritional deficiencies can occur in children especially in chronic diseases.
- In the hematological system, ethnicity and race are important considerations as certain hematological conditions are common in specific races.
- The clinical features of sickle cell anemia and β-thalassemia appear as fetal hemoglobin disappears by about 6 months.
  The presence of anemia should heighten the index of suspicion of underlying pathology. Childhood anemia results primarily from decreased production of red cells or hemoglobin from increased destruction of red cells or loss of red blood cells.

Symptoms of severe anemia regardless of cause[2,6,11,18,19,27,28]
• Weakness
• Dyspnea on exertion
• Poor concentration in school or deteriorating school performance
• Exercise intolerance
• Palpitations
• Failure to thrive if chronic
• Symptoms of congestive cardiac failure

- Ask about the family history of bleeding disorders or of unusually prolonged bleeding such as autosomal recessive conditions (e.g. Fanconi anemia) and autosomal dominant conditions (e.g. hereditary spherocytosis) and X-linked conditions (e.g. G6PD deficiency).

In evaluating a possible bleeding disorder ask yourself:[2,6,11,19,27,28]
• Is it likely to be a bleeding disorder? If so, why?
• Is it an inherited bleeding disorder?
• If it is likely to be a congenital bleeding disorder, what is the main clinical expression of the bleeding site? – If mucosal bleeding consider platelet defects, von Willebrand disease (sometimes both mucosal and deep tissue bleeding) or blood vessel disorder – If deep tissue bleeding consider a coagulopathy
• Is it an acquired bleeding disorder?
• Is there an underlying disease causing the bleeding? If so, what could the underlying disease be and why?
• Is there an underlying drug causing or exacerbating the bleeding?

LINK HISTORY TO HEMATOLOGICAL ABNORMALITY[2,6,11,16,18,19,27,28]

The age of bleeding, gender of the patient and nature of bleeding can shed light onto the diagnosis of hematological disorders.

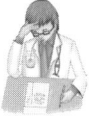

The historical links must lead you to think of the type of blood disorder; hence a detailed history of the presenting complaint, the onset and site of bleeding, the past history and the family history as well as factual knowledge on blood disorders are useful tools for diagnosis.

Blood disease[2,6,11,18,19,27,28]	History suggestive of disorder[2,6,11,18,19,27,28]
Suspect any severe inherited bleeding disorder. *Early bleeding is the link to explore further in history-taking, physical examination and investigations.*	• Bleeding in early childhood • Circumcision bleeding • Umbilical cord bleeding • Cephalohematomas following delivery • Intracranial or subdural hemorrhages following delivery
Factor XIII deficiency *Early, intracranial bleeding are links to diagnosis.*	• A 10-day-old term infant with a normal delivery and postpartum period is found to have an intracranial hemorrhage
Vitamin K deficiency *A home delivery is the link to diagnosis as vitamin K may not have been given in the home delivery*	• A 12-day-old male infant delivered at home is circumsized and develops severe hemorrhage following the circumcision
Hemophilia *The age of onset, the gender and the family history are clues to explore further in the history and physical examination*	• A male infant just starts to walk and presents with a painful swollen knee joint after a fall • A young boy goes to school, has a minor injury during a game of football and develops a huge swelling of his knee. His maternal uncle has a bleeding disorder
von Willebrand disease (vWD) *The site and age are clues that suggest the need for further investigation.*	• A teenage girl presents with menorrhagia, recurrent nose bleeds • A history of prolonged and excessive bleeding after a minor surgery in the past
Acute ITP *Age, preceding viral infection, site and a well-child give clues to possible diagnosis.*	• A well young child of 3 years presents with petechiae in the lower limbs and a recent viral infection
Chronic ITP *Age and family history provide clues to explore further in history and examination.*	• A teenage girl with fatigue and easy bruising with a family history of autoimmune disorders, e.g. systemic lupus erythematosus

56 The Link: Pediatric History-Taking and Physical Examination

Blood disease[2,6,11,18,19,27,28]	History suggestive of disorder[2,6,11,18,19,27,28]
Acute leukemia *Fever, bone pain, bleeding and toxicity are vital links to warrant urgent investigations.*	• A nine-year-old girl with high fever and bone pain, ecchymosis and gum bleeding of 2 weeks' duration

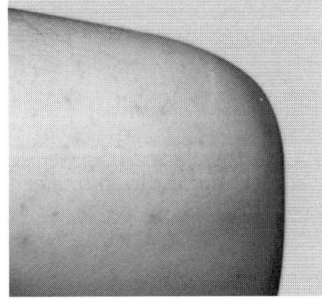

A 10-year-old boy with fever and petechiae on the thigh (Courtesy: Associate Professor, Dr Loh Keng Yin, reprint with permission)

Important Links in the Nutritional History and the Hematological System[2,6,11,16,18,27,28]

- Cow's milk diet may be associated with iron deficiency anemia. Goat's milk diet is linked to folate deficiency. Pica is associated with iron deficiency. Cholestasis and malabsorption are associated with vitamin A, D, E or K deficiency. The presence of diarrhea can be linked to vitamin B_{12}, iron or vitamin E deficiency.

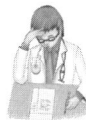

"How does diarrhea link to these deficiencies? Where does absorption of these vitamins take place? Where is intrinsic factor produced?"

Intestinal infections with *Giardia lambia* are associated with iron malabsorption; *Diphyllobothrium latum* **infections are linked** to vitamin B_{12} deficiency and hookworm infestations to iron deficiency anemia.

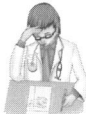

Parvovirus causes erythema infectiosum or "slapped cheek" disease and aplastic anemia is an uncommon but important condition to bear in mind.

Some viruses can suppress the bone marrow or cause anemia via hemophagocytosis such as parvovirus infections; Epstein-Barr and cytomegalovirus can suppress the bone marrow. *Mycoplasma* infections can cause hemolytic anemia.

The drug history is important as oxidants cause hemolysis in G6PD. Immune-mediated hemolysis is linked to penicillins. Phenytoin increases the requirement for folate and bone marrow suppression occurs in chemotherapeutic drugs.

Appetite

How is the appetite? What type of diet is the child on?

General questions, hematological problems and bleeding diasthesis[2,6,11,18,19,27,28]
• Has the patient had blood loss?
• Have you noticed petechial or purpuric spots on the child's skin?
• Have these spots appeared without fever?
• Does the child bruise easily?
• Does the child have bleeding gums?
• Are the stools ever black?
• Any dyspnea noticed? 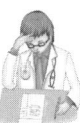 *"What has dyspnea to do with bleeding? What is the clinical link?"*
• Any lethargy noted or does the child tire easily?
• After intramuscular vaccination or following a minor trauma has the child developed a large swelling at the site?
• After a small cut or minor trauma does the child hemorrhage excessively?
• Did the child hemorrhage excessively after a circumcision?
• Is there a known family history of bleeding problems? If so, who are the members of the family involved? Is any particular gender involved exclusively?
• Are the parents consanguineous? 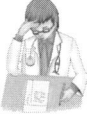 *"What is the main mode of inheritance enhanced by consanguinity?"*

REFERENCES

1. Autistic Spectrum Disorders: A Guide for Paediatricians in India. Available at: http://autism-India.org/AFA%20 Paediatrician%20booklet.pdf.
2. Richard E. Behrman (comps). Robert M Kliegman, Waldo E Nelson, Victor C Vaughan III. (eds). Nelson's textbook of pediatrics (14th ed). Philadelphia: WB Saunders; 1992.
3. Caraballo L, Puerta L, Fernández-Caldas E, Lockey RF, Martínez B. Sensitization to mite allergens and acute asthma in a tropical environment. J Investig Allergol Clin Immunol. 1998;8(5):281-4.
4. Elizabeth KE. Clinical Pediatrics for Undergraduates. India: Jaypee Brothers Medical Publishers (P) Ltd, 2009.
5. Elston DM. Avoid downcoding by documenting a review of systems. Dermatology world. 2001;12:6–7.
6. Goel KM, Gupta DK. Hutchinson's Pediatrics (1st edn). Jaypee Brothers Medical Publishers (P) Ltd, 2009.
7. HA Clayton. "SOCRATES on Pain Assessment". Med Surg Nursg 2000. Retrieved. 2008-03-31.
8. Hammond P, Curry J. Pediatric acute abdomen. Br J Hosp Med. 2004;65(11):686-9.
9. Junnila JL, Cartwright VW. Chronic Musculoskeletal Pain in Children: Part I. Initial Evaluation. Am Fam Physician. 2006;74(1):115-22.
10. Koletzko S, Niggemann B, Arato A, et al. Diagnostic approach and management of cow's milk protein allergy in infants and children: ESPGHAN GI Committee practical guidelines. J Pediatr Gastroenterol Nutr. 2012;55(2):221-9.
11. Marcdante K, Kliegman RM, Jenson HB, Behrman RE (Eds). Nelson's Essentials of Pediatrics (6th edn). Saunders Elsevier, 2010.
12. Massoud A. Endocrine disorders. In: Bannon M, Carter Y (Eds). Practical Pediatric Problems in Primary Care, Oxford University Press, 2007:281–304.
13. Meyers KEC. Evaluation of hematuria in children. Urol Clin North Am. 2004;31(3):559–73.
14. Myers A, McDonagh JE, Gupta K, et al. More 'cries from the joints': Assessment of the musculoskeletal system is poorly documented routine pediatric clerking. Rheumatology. 2004;43:1045–49.
15. National Institute for Health and Care Excellence. Urinary tract infection in children: diagnosis, treatment and long-term management 2007.
16. Robinson MJ, Lam LE. Pediatric problems in tropical countries. Pelanduk Publications (M) Sdn Bhd.1994.
17. Schmidt F, Kapellen TM, Wiegand S, et al. Diabetes mellitus in children and adolescents with genetic syndrome. Exp Clin Endocrinol Diabe. 2012;120(10):579-85.
18. Sharathkumar AA, Pipe SW. Bleeding disorders Pediatr Rev. 2008;29;121-30.
19. Stephenson T, Wallace H (Eds). Clinical pediatrics for postgraduate examinations. UK: Churchill Livingstone, 1991.
20. Taksande A, Gautami V, Padhi S, Bakshi K. Hypercyanotic spells. J MGIMS, 2009;14 (ii):7-9.
21. Weiss LN. The Diagnosis of Wheezing in Children. Am Fam Physician. 2008;77(8):1109-14.
22. Sakula A. Charcot-Leyden crystals and Curschmann spirals in asthmatic sputum.Thorax. 1986;41(7):503–507.
23. American Academy of Pediatrics Clinical Practice Guideline: Management of Sinusitis Subcommittee on Management of Sinusitis and Committee on Quality Improvement PEDIATRIC. 2001;108(3):798-808
24. Venter C, Brown T, Shah N, et al. Diagnosis and management of non-IgE-mediated cow's milk allergy in infancy - a UK primary care practical guide. Journal of Clinical and Translational Allergy. Available at http://www.ctajournal.com/content/3/1/23.
25. Robertson M. Manifestations of Gastrointestinal Disease in the ChildWith sections authored by: JD Butzner, H Machida, SR Martin, HG Parsons and SA Zamora. https://www.cag-acg.org/uploads/firstprinciples/z_pdf/EN_GAST_14B.pdf.
26. Radetti G1, Zavallone A, Gentili L, Beck-Peccoz P, Bona G. Foetal and neonatal thyroid disorders. Minerva Pediatr. 2002 Oct;54(5):383-400.
27. Mason S, Swash M (Eds). Hutchinson's Clinical Methods, 17th edn. A Bailllere Tindall book published by Cassell Ltd; 1980.
28. Milner AD, Hull D. Hospital Pediatrics, 3rd edn. ELBS with Churchill Livingstone. 1998.
29. Guidelines for the management of cow's milk protein allergy in children 2012 (CMPA in children). Available at http://www.allergymsai.org/file_dir/6296706325048109343baa.pdf. Accessed in April 2015.

The essence of the relevant chapters in the following books have also been numbered as references in this chapter. We recommend for further reading, the rich text in these books for greater integration and deeper understanding.

1. Goel KM, Gupta DK. Hutchinson's Pediatrics, 1st edn. Jaypee Brothers Medical Publishers (P) Ltd, 2009.
2. Marcdante K, Kliegman RM, Jenson HB, Behrman RE (Eds). Nelson's Essentials of Pediatrics, 6th edn. Saunders Elsevier, 2010.
3. Mason S, Swash M (Eds). Hutchinson's Clinical Methods, 17th edn. A Baillere Tindall book published by Cassell Ltd; 1980.
4. Milner AD, Hull D. Hospital Pediatrics, 3rd edn. ELBS with Churchill Livingstone. 1998.
5. Behrman RE (comps), Kliegman RM, Nelson WE, Vaughan VC III. (Eds). Nelson's Textbook of Pediatrics, 14th edn. Philadelphia: WB Saunders. 1992.
6. Robinson MJ, Lam LE. Pediatric problems in tropical countries. Pelanduk Publications (M) Sdn Bhd. 1994.
7. Stephenson T, Wallace H (Eds). Clinical pediatrics for postgraduate examinations. UK: Churchill Livingstone, 1991.

Chapter 4

History of Pregnancy, Delivery, and the Neonatal Period

- The history of the pregnancy and birth can have a significant influence on the health of the infant and young child. This part of the history is important in pediatrics especially during these periods.
- The diagnosis of the case may be dependent on historical features that are elicited in this part of the history; hence, this must be done wisely.
- As children get older, this part of the history may be less significant in the normal child.
- In the child with chronic illnesses, whatever the age, this part of the history is important as it may give clues to the pathophysiological and etiological diagnosis.

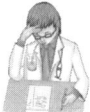

Do all these historical events affect the newborn child?

HISTORY OF EVENTS RELEVANT TO BIRTH AND DELIVERY[1-11]

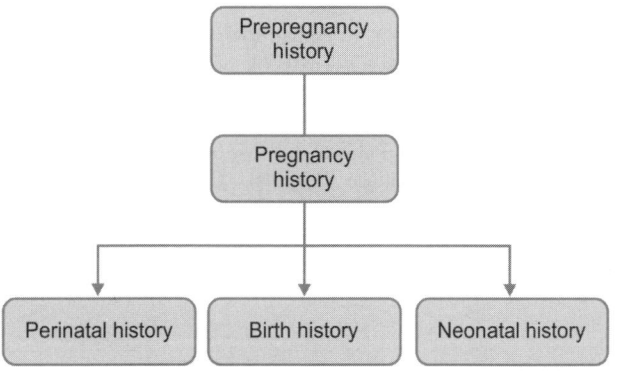

RELEVANT PREPREGNANCY HISTORY[1,4,8,10,11]

The details of important social and demographic features include:
- Age
- Ethnic origin
- Sexually transmitted diseases including hepatitis and AIDS
- Use of unlicensed drugs, alcohol abuse, cigarette smoking and cocaine
- Immune status including blood group, syphilis, rubella (German measles) and hepatitis B
- Exposure at work.

Bear in mind that the prepregnancy nutrition and health status can influence the health of the young infant.

Brief questions indicative of the mother's overall health status before conception are sufficient. This involves enquiry of the following details:
- Number of children
- Spacing of pregnancies
- Maternal nutrition
- Maternal vaccination
- Other maternal illnesses of relevance to her pregnancy and delivery
- Related surgeries
- Medication(s) before conception.

History on the following is also important:
- Abortions
- Intrauterine fetal death
- Congenital anomalies
- Birth weight
- Incompetent cervix
- Multiple pregnancies
- Preterm deliveries
- Blood group sensitization
- Neonatal jaundice

- ABO or Rh incompatibility
- Fetal hydrops
- Infertility.

HISTORY OF PREGNANCY AND DELIVERY[1,4,8,10,11]

This history influences the immediate postnatal period. The subsequent health status of the child pertaining to development as well as some acute and chronic infections and disorders is linked to the events that occur during pregnancy and delivery. Complications of pregnancy that result in poor fetomaternal outcome can be due to the following causes:
- Causes attributable to the mother
- Causes attributable to the fetus
- Both maternal and fetal causes.

Pregnancy

Age

Enquire about the mother's age when the child was conceived. Some anomalies and syndromes are associated with advanced maternal age.

Nutrition and Social Habits

Ask about nutrition during pregnancy, habits during pregnancy, i.e. if mother consumes only certain types of foods which do not have nutritious value or which may interfere with the absorption of nutrients (e.g. chappati and iron absorption). Smoking and alcohol consumption can affect the fetus.

Antenatal Check-ups

Ask whether antenatal check-ups are regular or not and if any medications were consumed during pregnancy. History of abnormal fetal presentations detected later on in pregnancy should be enquired. Ask if the mother who was on regular antenatal check-up was compliant with the hematinics and multivitamins given. The incidence of neural tube defects are significantly reduced with maternal folate supplementation.

Antenatal problems can lead to congenital malformations, hypoxia or transient diseases in the newborn, including some forms of neonatal hypothyroidism, neonatal myasthenia and immune thrombocytopenia. These diseases are due to transfer of preformed maternal antibodies.

Ask also about antenatal complications, such as preeclampsia and gestational diabetes mellitus. Ask about the quantity of amniotic fluid. Oligohydramnios refers to a reduction in amniotic fluid. Rupture of the membranes is a recognized common cause of oligohydramnios. In the mid and late trimesters of pregnancy, the amniotic fluid is derived mainly from fetal urine. Decreased fetal urine production or urinary tract obstruction can then cause oligohydramnios.

Polyhydramnios is a condition where there is increased amounts of amniotic fluid for a stipulated period of gestation. Physiologically, the act of swallowing by the fetus reduces the quantity of amniotic fluid, hence the absence of swallowing or an obstruction to the fetal gastrointestinal tract causes polyhydramnios which is also called hydramnios.

Ask if fetal ultrasounds were all normal

Abnormal fetal ultrasound findings such as **oligohydramnios** are associated with intrauterine growth restriction (IUGR) and chromosomal syndromes as well as significant renal anomalies. Historically, oligohydramnios may be sometimes elicited by the mother telling you about decreased fetal movements during that pregnancy. Although a subjective sensation, this is particularly helpful if she has had previous pregnancies as she may have been able to compare fetal movements to her other pregnancies.

Polyhydramnios is linked to maternal diabetes mellitus, both immunological and nonimmunological causes of fetal hydrops, fetal chromosomal abnormalities and multiple pregnancies. Esophageal and duodenal atresia, cleft palate and neural tube defects decrease fetal swallowing resulting in polyhydramnios. During the pregnancy the mother may have felt excessive fetal movements, again more easily observed by the mother who has had previous pregnancies.

Causes of polyhydramnios[1,4,8,10,11]

• Idiopathic
• Defects in the diaphragm such as hernias
• Cleft lip and cleft palate
• Tracheoesophageal fistula
• Intestinal obstruction due volvulus, ileal atresia or duodenal atresia
• Gastroschisis
• Omphalocele
• Neural tube defects: meningomyelocele, anencephaly, spina bifida
• Rhesus isoimmunization
• TORCHES
• Beckwith-Wiedemann syndrome
• Multiple congenital anomalies
• Maternal diabetes mellitus (preexisting or gestational)
• Twin pregnancies

Causes of oligohydramnios[1,4,8,10,11]

• Unilateral renal agenesis (Potter syndrome)
• Pulmonary hypoplasia
• Severe placental insufficiency
• Fetal polycystic kidneys
• Preterm premature rupture of membranes
• Maternal dehydration
• Maternal drugs like angiotensin converting enzyme inhibitor usage

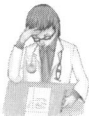

"How do I utilize my knowledge of the causes of polyhydramnios and oligohydramnios?"

Use your knowledge of the cause of abnormalities in the amniotic liquor and try to link specific problems that may have emerged in the history. As an example, in a history of abnormally delayed walking in a child and if there is an elicited history suggestive of polyhydramnios during pregnancy, together with other clinical symptoms, would you consider a neural tube defect in your differential diagnosis? What links in the history can you use? In history-taking, apply all that you already know. You may then discover new things that can help make a good diagnosis.

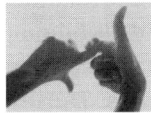

Link your knowledge of associations of the history of the pregnancy to the patient's story to help you make a good clinical diagnosis

Placental Anomalies[1,4,8,10,11]

- Enquire about complications like placenta previa which could be indicated by painless vaginal discharge unrelated to labor. Painful vaginal discharge is indicative of abruptio placentae.
- **Placental causes of fetal hypoxia**[5] can be due to placental insufficiency, abruptio placentae, and prolapsed cord.
- Maternal hypertension with its undesirable hemodynamic effects can result in placental insufficiency leading to placental hypoxia and its growth implications on the fetus.
- Maternal anemia and its complications can cause fetal hypoxia. Fetomaternal hemorrhage and erythroblastosis fetalis are fetomaternal causes of hypoxia.

Effects of Maternal Infections of the Genitourinary Tract[1,4,8,10,11]

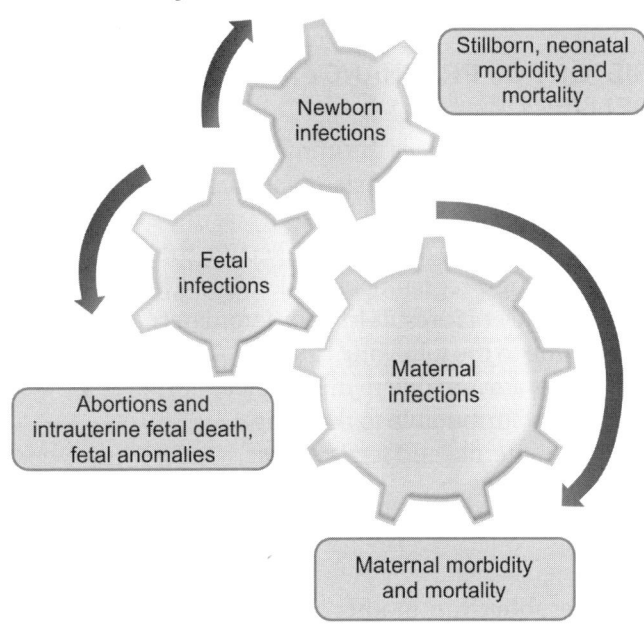

Impact of Infections of the Mother, the Fetus, and the Newborn

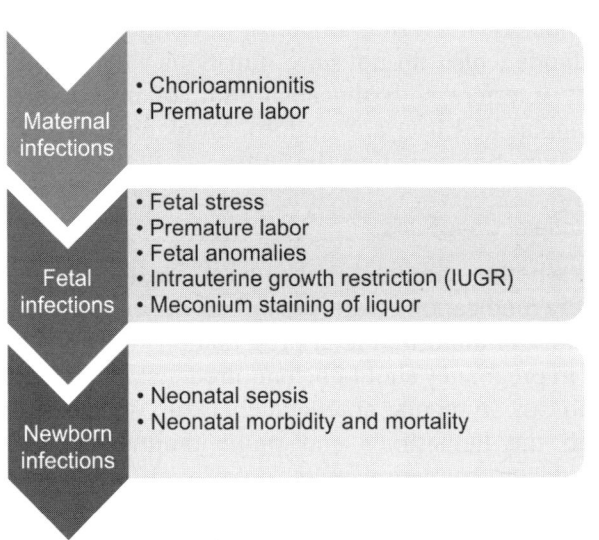

Ask about vaginal infections and vaginosis. Ask about yellow malodorous vaginal discharge. Ask about a known or suggestive history of urinary tract infection in the mother. Enquiry on the administration of antibiotics intrapartum or postpartum is important. Remember infections of the birth canal can affect the newborn leading to dire sequelae if untreated.

Maternal infections affecting the fetus[1,4,7-10]

Bacterial
• Group B streptococci • *Escherichia coli K1* • Enteroviruses • *Chlamydia trachomatis* • Genital mycoplasma • Ureaplasma • *Neisseria gonorrhoea* • Mycobacterium
Viral
• Rubella • Cytomegalovirus • Hepatitis B • Hepatitis C • Epstein-Barr • Varicella zoster • Coxsackievirus B • Poliomyelitis • Herpes simplex 2 • Parvovirus • Human immunodeficiency virus
Parasitic
• Toxoplasmosis • Trypanosomiasis • Malaria
Fungal
• Candida

Vaginal Bleeding

Vaginal bleeding in the first trimester is important to ask as this can be linked to birth defects and various chromosomal anomalies.

Maternal Medical Complications[10]

Enquiry must include morbid conditions in the mother associated with fetal wastage and abnormalities. Some maternal complications include the following.[1,4,5,8-11]

• Metabolic and hemodynamic maternal problems such as diabetes mellitus, hypertension and significant heart disease
• Collagen vascular diseases
• Severe anemia, idiopathic thrombocytopenic purpura
• Hyperthyroidism
• Myasthenia gravis
• Inborn errors of metabolism like maternal phenylketonuria
• Malignant melanoma and other malignancies
• Drug addiction
• Hyperparathyroidism
• Rh or blood group sensitization
• Systemic lupus erythematosus
• Hepatitis B, tuberculosis
• Sickle cell anemia
• Phenylketonuria

Maternal diseases like cyanotic heart diseases, hypertension, and preeclampsia can cause intrauterine growth restriction (IUGR), diabetes mellitus can cause fetal macrosomia, fetal hypoglycemia and even IUGR due to placental vasculosclerosis. Endemic goiter can produce fetal hypothyroidism. Sickle cell anemia can cause preterm labor as well as or IUGR. Maternal phenylketonuria is associated with microcephaly and mental retardation. Maternal Graves' disease is linked to transient neonatal thyrotoxicosis.

Maternal medications and exposures that can affect the fetus[1,8,10]

• Alcohol
• Aminopterin
• Coumarin
• Isotretinoin
• Lithium
• Misoprostol
• Penicillamine
• Phenytoin
• Radioactive iodine
• Radiation
• Diethylstilbesterol
• Tetracycline
• Testosterone-like drugs
• Thalidomide
• Vitamin D
• Streptomycin
• Sodium valproate
• Nicotine
• Cyclophosphamide
• 6-Mercaptopurine
• Primaquine
• Progesterone
• Quinine

Maternal Surgery or Trauma

Enquire on maternal trauma or surgery during or prior to pregnancy.

Maternal Immunization Status

Confirm the mother's immunization status; also enquire specifically if the mother has taken the rubella vaccine.

Laboratory Investigations in the Mother[2]

- **Pregnancy-associated plasma protein screening (PAPP-A)** is a placental protein in early pregnancy. Abnormal levels are linked to a heightened risk for chromosome anomalies.
- Quantitative abnormalities of estriols, chorionic gonadotropin or alpha-fetoprotein detected during antenatal visits are important if such information is obtained.
- **Alpha-fetoprotein (AFP),** the origin of which is from the yolk sac and fetal liver, can be tested in maternal blood. In open neural tube defects, greater concentrations of AFP is measured in maternal blood as fetal skin is not complete or intact. In Trisomy 21, the AFP is notably decreased in the mother's blood. Abnormal levels of AFP may also indicate the following:
  - Other chromosomal abnormalities
  - Congenital openings in the abdominal wall of the fetus, such as omphalocele and gastroschisis
  - Twins
  - A wrongly calculated due date, because of fluctuations in pregnancy.
- **Estriol** is a placental hormone, utilizing constituents from the fetal liver and adrenal gland. Estriol levels are decreased in pregnancy with Trisomy 21.
- **Human chorionic gonadotropin (hCG)** hormone is a placental hormone and is used to test for pregnancy. A precise subunit, the **beta subunit**, is elevated in pregnancies with Down syndrome.
- **Others maternal tests include:**
  - Nuchal translucency on ultrasound testing (early pregnancy)
  - Inhibin (from placenta)
  - Amniocentesis.
  - Chorionic villus sampling.

HISTORY OF EVENTS RELATED TO LABOR AND DELIVERY[1,4,8,10,11]

Consequences of Maternal Infections

The following history should be included in this section:
- Duration of labor
- Presentation, i.e. vertex or breech
- Mode of delivery, i.e. vaginal or cesarean section
- Spontaneous, induced labor or instrumental delivery
- Term or preterm birth, i.e. the gestational age
- Enquire on weight, length or circumference of head (COH). You may ask to see the birth card and vaccination card. If the child was born premature, enquire on gestational age and weight
- Place of delivery, i.e. at home or in the hospital and unusual cultural or traditional practices especially in villages or home deliveries
- Mode of delivery, i.e. spontaneous vaginal delivery (SVD) or forceps or cesarean section. If it was a cesarean section, explore indication, fetal or maternal
- Presentation at birth, i.e. vertex or breech
- Presence of meconium stained fluid.

Components of meconium: Mucus, bile salts, epithelial cells, enzymes. In some cases, due to fetal distress, the liquor is stained by meconium, which is passed by the fetus *in utero*. This is due to the fetal anal sphincter becoming lax, significant dark green or black, thick, tenacious meconium is passed. The bile salts and enzymes in meconium are potentially dangerous if inhaled by the fetus during labor.

It can cause meconium aspiration syndrome (MAS) causing severe lung pathology, including:
- Obstruction of the airways and the ball-valve effect of meconium that causes air trapping
- Meconium-induced chemical pneumonitis
- Respiratory distress with loss of surfactant
- Pulmonary hypertension.

Causes of birth asphyxia[5,6]

Intrapartum causes
• Birth trauma: Insufficient or inadequate fetal monitoring, instrumental deliveries, abnormal presentations, shoulder dystocia, cephalopelvic disproportion (CPD), none or inadequate resuscitation of the newborn
• Spinal cord transaction
• Hypoxia: Compression or prolapse of the umbilical cord, abruptio placentae

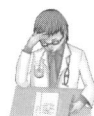

A large number of causes of intrapartum birth asphyxia are preventable. Better feto-maternal monitoring, birth care and effective resuscitation at birth will reduce neonatal morbidity and mortality.

APGAR SCORE[1,8]

- Ask about gestation and leaking liquor. Premature rupture of membranes at term (PROM) and premature preterm rupture of membranes (PPROM)

History of Pregnancy, Delivery, and the Neonatal Period

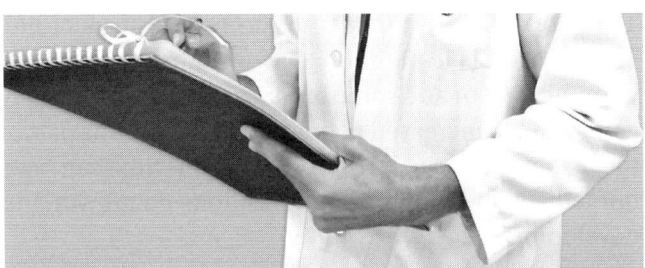

Write the history down with a sense of purpose, reassuring the mother that you too are interested in her story

before term are both linked to fetal infection. Enquire about intrapartum antibiotics which are given to decrease the risk of sepsis in the neonate.
- Other important history is cephalopelvic disproportion (CPD), prolapsed cord or fetal distress.
- Ask about clamping of cord. Delayed clamping may lead to polycythemia, raised pulmonary vascular resistance, hypoxia and jaundice. Early clamping may lead to anemia, a cardiac murmur and poor peripheral perfusion.
- Was there history of maternal fever (suggestive of maternal sepsis)?
- Ask the Apgar score if known. If it is not available ask if the child cried immediately after birth, moved all four limbs vigorously and was put to the breast soon after delivery. Did the infant require any form of resuscitation?
- The Apgar score is used to assess the need for resuscitation of the newborn. At 1 minute and 5 minutes after birth, each of the five physiological parameters are observed or elicited by a trained examiner. Some mothers may have the Apgar score in the birth card that they keep, so do request for it.

Apgar score[1,8]

Signs	Points		
	0	1	2
Heart rate	0	<100/min	>100/min
Respiration	None	Weak cry	Vigorous cry
Muscle tone	None	Some extremity flexion	Arms, legs move well
Reflex irritability	None	Some movement	Cry, withdrawal
Color of body	Blue	Pink body, blue extremities	Pink all over

Interpretation of the Apgar score[1,8]

At 1 minute	At 5 minutes	Indication of status
8	9	Normal cardiopulmonary adaptation
4–7	4–7	Close monitoring and further intervention if not improved
0–3	0–3	Cardiopulmonary arrest or severe bradycardia, hypoventilation, central nervous system depression

Often the Apgar score as such is not known. If it was a home delivery, there will be no documentation of the Apgar score. Therefore, during history-taking indirect questions to see if all was well at the time of birth and soon after will give a clue to the APGAR score.

Some questions to be asked if the Apgar score is not known[1,4,8,10,11]

• Did the baby cry?
• Was it a lusty cry?
• Was the baby active?
• Was the baby put to mother's breast as soon as or shortly after birth? Healthy babies are put on mother's chest soon or shortly after birth for skin-to-skin contact.
• Was the baby pink?
• Did the baby need help from the nurse?
• Did the baby need to be resuscitated?
• Was the baby taken away for medical intervention?

Causes of birth asphyxia[1-8,10]

Postpartum causes
• Infections—congenital pneumonia
• Central nervous system—maternal medications, episodes of fetal hypoxia or acidosis, trauma
• Congenital neuromuscular disease—congenital myasthenia gravis, myopathy, myotonic dystrophy
• Airway problems: choanal atresia, laryngeal webs, large obstructive goiter
• Pulmonary disorder: prematurity, pulmonary hypoplasia, pneumothorax, pleural effusion, diaphragmatic hernia
• Renal disorders: renal agenesis, pulmonary hypoplasia
• Congenital cardiac defects: severe congenital cardiac anomalies

Questionnaire guide if life-threatening congenital anomalies are suspected[1-8,10]

• What was the duration of gestation? Preterm, term or post-term?
• Was the mother on any medication?
• Was there a history of maternal gestational diabetes?
• Was there a history of preeclampsia or eclampsia?
• Was there a history of maternal infection?

Contd...

Contd...

- Is there a family history of congenital anomalies?
- Was there polyhydramnios or oligohydramnios?
- What was the mode of delivery?
- If vaginal delivery, was there instrumentation like forceps or vacuum?
- If cesarean section, what was the indication? Was it a maternal or fetal indication?
- Was there fetal distress?
- Was the liquor meconium stained?
- Did the infant cry, grimace, move after birth?
- Was it a lusty cry? Any resuscitation required?
- Was the infant ventilated?
- If ventilated, for how long?
- Did the doctor tell you of the diagnosis?
- Was there respiratory distress in the delivery room?
- Was the abdomen scaphoid?
- Was there cyanosis?
- Was it difficult to pass a nasogastric tube?
- Did the newborn look abnormal?
- Was there bile stained vomiting?
- Any family history of abortions, stillbirth, neonatal death?
- Is there a history of parental consanguinity?

Postnatal Events[1,4,8,10,11]

- Ask when the child was discharged from hospital. If the child was discharged home soon after delivery with the mother, it usually is an indicator that the child had no immediate problems of concern.
- Determine if this period was eventful or uneventful.
- Ask if the child stayed in the hospital. Ask about the duration of hospitalization. Did baby "room in" with mother; ask for how long the child was in an incubator and enquire on the requirement for oxygen. Was the baby in a special care nursery.
- Enquire specifically about initial and early feeding.
- If the child was ventilated, ask for the duration of ventilation and indication for ventilation. Also ask if the parents were told of any complications; if so, the details of the complications must be asked.

NEONATAL HISTORY[1,4,7,8,10,11]

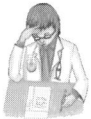

"Nonspecific symptoms and signs of diseases in this age group make this part of the history challenging. I must have a high index of suspicion of the suggestive history and signs on physical examination and link to the diseases that I will read about"

The neonatal period refers to the first 28 days of life. This is a crucial period. Relative immaturity of the immune system and some unforeseen birth events may contribute to increased neonatal morbidity. This part of the history is crucial. Any problem at this time can have immediate and long-term implications on growth and development.

Events to note in the postnatal and neonatal period include the following:
- Presence of respiratory distress
- History of cyanosis
- History suggestive of pallor
- History of convulsions
- History of feeding difficulties
- Jaundice
- History of known or suspected infections
- History of interventions, e.g. transfusions, lumbar puncture, umbilical vein catheterization.

During the neonatal period respiratory distress is important as a sign of disease that refers to both the respiratory system and as a symptom of systemic disease.

Respiratory distress can be due to congenital pneumonias, aspiration pneumonias at or soon after birth. Important historical links to aspiration in the newborn are prematurity, fetal distress and meconium-stained liquor. Postnatal aspiration can occur in infants with cleft palate. Aspiration at this time is also seen in neonatal sepsis and in tracheoesophageal fistula. Maternal pyrexia, foul smelling liquor, birth asphyxia, and premature rupture of membranes are links to congenital pneumonias, and these must be actively sought for in the history.

Hyaline membrane disease occurs in premature infants and in infants of the diabetic mother and constitute an important cause of both morbidity and mortality during this period.

Transient tachypnea of the newborn (TTN) occurs in a term baby delivered by cesarean section.

Congenital malformations of the lungs and diaphragm such as diaphragmatic hernia and congenital lobar emphysema can cause early respiratory distress.

Different from other age groups, distinct nonrespiratory problems can contribute to respiratory distress in the neonatal period.

Malformations of the central nervous system, birth injuries affecting the CNS as for example asphyxia in a preterm neonate due to a difficult delivery is an example of a central CNS cause of respiratory distress in a neonate. Traumatic breech deliveries can cause palsy of the respiratory muscles or diaphragmatic paralysis and be a reason for respiratory distress. Congenital myopathies and myasthenia gravis are other causes.

During the newborn period hypoglycemia, organic acidemias, and hyperammonemias are inborn errors of metabolism that could present early with respiratory distress. The family history of sudden unexplained neonatal death or parental consanguinity which propagates autosomal recessive genes (as many metabolic disorders have autosomal recessive inheritance) are supportive of the diagnosis.

Sepsis in the newborn of early onset can have a similar presentation. Antenatal history, birth history and neonatal history about the risks associated with sepsis must be sought for as pathological and etiological diagnoses depend, to an extent, on these histories.

As in other age groups one must not forget the cardiac causes of respiratory distress such as congestive cardiac failure and anomalous pulmonary venous drainage and pulmonary hypertension. Link historical questions to your knowledge of inheritance patterns, antenatal history and neonatal history. Ask about maternal immunization status for rubella. Also enquire about maternal health and other related events mentioned in this chapter.

Neonatal Conditions Linked to Medications[1,4,7,8,10,11]

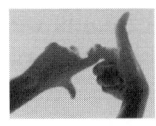

• Gray baby syndrome	Chloramphenicol
• Staining of teeth	Tetracycline
• Deafness	Streptomycin
• Hyperbilirubinemia	Salicylates, sulfonamides

HISTORY OF NEONATAL JAUNDICE[1,4,7,8,10,11]

Ask when it was first noticed and for how long; ask about phototherapy, for how long it was used. Ask if the mother was told why the baby was jaundiced. Enquire about the highest bilirubin reading and when. If jaundice was high, was exchange transfusion done? Was the child breastfed? If prolonged jaundice is suspected, ask for how long? Enquire about the color of the stools and the general activity of the child.

Infants with high-risk factors for neonatal jaundice include the following:[1,8]

Jaundice in the first 24 hours
Prematurity
Glucose -6- phosphate dehydrogenase (G6PD) deficiency
Jaundice persisting beyond the first week of life
Significant cephalhematoma or bruising
Incompatibility of blood group antigens with a positive direct Coombs' test
Increasing serum bilirubin levels at a rate greater than 5 mg/dL/24 hours
A reading of serum bilirubin that is more than 12 mg/dL in full term infants or 14 mg/dL in preterm infants
At any time, a reading of greater than 1 mg/dL of direct reacting bilirubin

When you take a history of neonatal jaundice, some knowledge on the time of the appearance of the jaundice will help you make sense of the history and will guide you in thinking of relevant historical links.

Neonatal jaundice occurring in the first 24 hours is ominous and is due to conditions like Rh isoimmunization, ABO incompatibility and occasionally minor blood group incompatibilities. Intrauterine infections, maternal drugs like salicylates, vitamin K, and sulfisoxazole are also causes of such early onset jaundice.

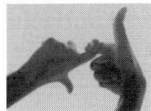

Link the time of onset of jaundice to clarify your differential diagnosis of jaundice

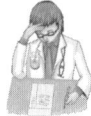

"These syndromes are good to know. In the far more common type of neonatal jaundice such as physiological jaundice, I see the importance of the negative history. The history of the absence of birth trauma or a hemolytic blood disorder are important to first exclude."

Hemolytic anemias like Crigler-Najjar syndrome and Lucy-Driscoll syndrome are other rarer causes. Here, the enquiry of relevant details of siblings with jaundice in the family history is relevant.

Jaundice appearing between 24 and 72 hours could be physiological in an active term baby. Due to the many causes of jaundice you must ensure that there is no risk of sepsis, be informed about the mother's and baby's blood group and G6PD status. Instrumental deliveries

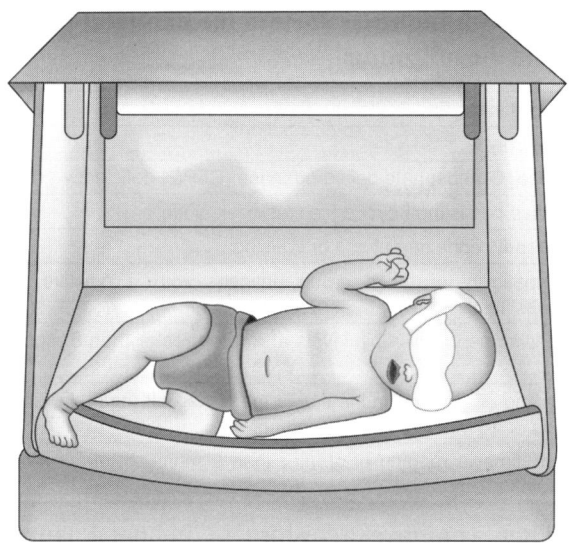

Phototherapy: *An effective method of reducing indirect hyperbilirubinemia. Light with maximal irradiance in the 425–475 nm wavelength band converts bilirubin to isomers that are water-soluble and easily excreted.*

must be asked for in the history as cephalhematomas can sometimes cause very high levels of jaundice. The family history of jaundice and whether siblings required phototherapy or exchange transfusion can also be asked. Essentially, a diagnosis of exclusion, the pertinent negative history obtained pertaining to these factors, in an active, term baby who feeds well and who is mild-to-moderately jaundiced then fulfills the criteria of physiological jaundice.

The preterm baby manifests physiological jaundice a little later and it lasts a little longer. It warrants close observation in the preterm baby who also has a cephalhematoma, polycythemia, hypoxia or acidosis as there is a risk of kernicterus with moderate or high bilirubin levels. The history must determine the age of gestation, must exclude any prenatal or birth factors that increase the risk of infections and the mode of delivery, whether instrumental or not.

Hypothyroidism also causes unconjugated hyperbilirubinemia at about this time. Besides factors in the history (as has been mentioned in Chapter 3), a screening test is universally done and a guide to early diagnosis.

Jaundice appearing after 72 hours could be due to causes like neonatal sepsis, neonatal hepatitis, neonatal cholestasis and biliary atresia.

Jaundice in breastfed babies can manifest during this time (Cases Discussed in Chapter 13). It must be determined from the history which actively excludes other important causes. Decreased breast milk production and poor sucking or ineffective latching on the breast, causes dehydration and is a cause of early breastfeeding jaundice in the breastfed child.

Metabolic causes of jaundice during this period are galactosemia and tyrosinemia. Remember that some causes of early breastfeeding jaundice due to hypothyroidism can still be first noticed at this time.

Intrauterine infections also contribute to jaundice after 72 hours of life. Gilbert's syndrome and Dubin-Johnson syndrome are other causes that may be clarified by the family history.

Surgical causes like intestinal obstruction and pyloric stenosis are not to be forgotten as causes of jaundice at this time. Here, historical links to the time and nature of vomiting as well as suggestive physical findings must be sought to support the clinical impression.

Monitoring an Infant under Phototherapy[1,8]

Remember that when a child is receiving phototherapy, the doctor looks for the signs and symptoms:
- To suggest improvement in jaundice (by regular serum bilirubin levels) as visual checks for the level of jaundice are unreliable.
- Of bilirubin encephalopathy which must be regularly checked for by asking about activity, movement, sucking, cry (refer below)
- To prevent complications like dehydration and diarrhea, retinal damage, ileus especially in preterm infants, skin rashes, overheating or overcooling (due to exposure) by constantly checking the body temperature.

Additionally, 'bronzing' of infants or greenish brown skin color of infants occurs when infants with conjugated hyperbilirubinemia are incorrectly put under phototherapy.

Remember that parental anxiety due to jaundice and separation distress must be allayed. Vigorous, exclusive breastfeeding must continue.

Bilirubin Encephalopathy: Early and Late Symptoms and Signs[1,4,5,8-11]

Early symptoms and signs
• Feeding problems
• Inactivity or even lethargy
• Excessive irritability
• Sleep disturbances
• The infant's activity—initially inactive, later lethargic

Contd...

Contd...

• The infant's muscle tone—initially hypotonic, later becomes hypertonic
• The infant's cry which is weak, later shrill
Advanced symptoms and signs
• Poor feeding
• Cycling movements
• Inconsolable cry or extreme irritability
• High pitched cry
• Fever
• Convulsions
• Coma
• High tone sensorineural deafness
• Paresis of gaze
• Cerebral palsy of the choreoathetoid type
• Dental hypoplasia
• Learning difficulties and psychomotor retardation

Neonatal Sepsis[1,3,8,10]

Onset and sources of neonatal sepsis is showing in following Flowchart.

Antenatal risk factors that are importantly associated with an increased incidence of neonatal sepsis including:[1,4,5,8-11]

Prolonged rupture of membranes
Maternal pyrexia
Maternal colonization with Group B Streptococcus
Chorioamnionitis or suggestive history
Male gender
Birth asphyxia
Preterm
Urinary tract infection in the mother

Sepsis is an important cause of morbidity and mortality in the neonatal period. The signs are nonspecific. A high index of suspicion is needed.

Common signs:[1,4,5,8-11]
Reduced spontaneous activity or lethargy
Hypotonia
Poor sucking
Apnea or cessation of respiration for more than 20 seconds often associated with bradycardia and cyanosis
Bradycardia
Usually hypothermia, sometimes hyperthermia
Respiratory distress
Vomiting, especially if persistent and bilious
Diarrhea
Abdominal distention
Jitteriness
Seizures
Jaundice
Umbilical cord sepsis
Bleeding
Pallor
Central cyanosis
Absence of the passage of meconium in the first 24 hours
Significant congenital anomalies

Remember that other than sepsis, neonatal seizures can also be caused by hypoglycemia, hypocalcemia, hypomagnesemia, electrolyte imbalance, intracranial hemorrhage and birth asphyxia. Additionally, these can either be caused by or be the result of sepsis.

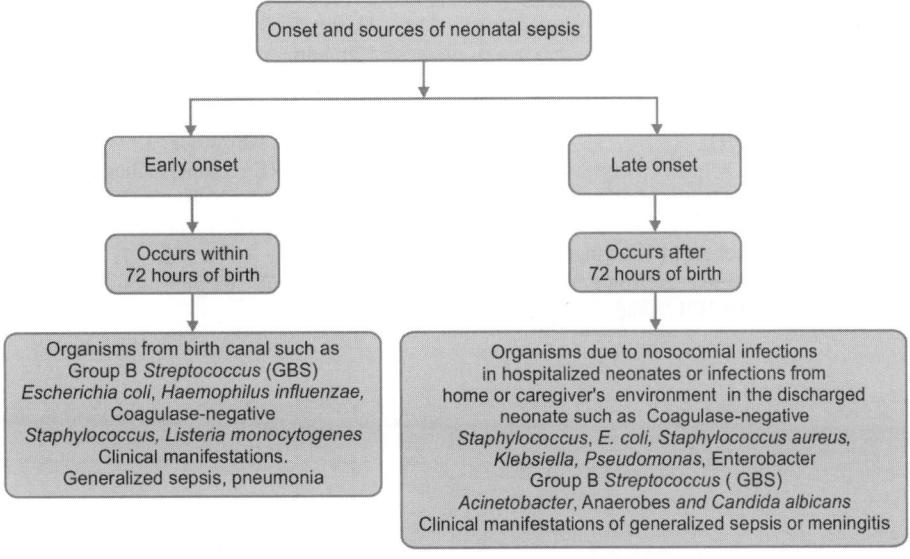

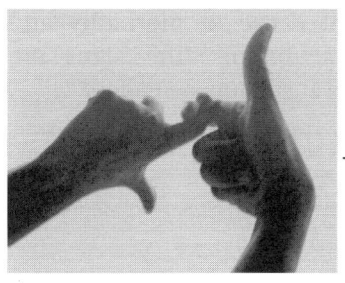
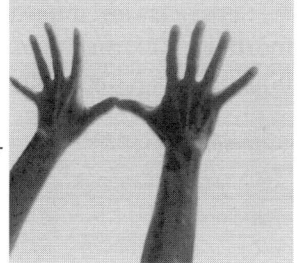

Neonatal sepsis: *Linked to high morbidity and mortality rates. The maternal history of pregnancy and delivery are important.*

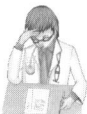

"Why does cytomegalovirus produce microcephaly, periventricular calcification and chorioretinitis and toxoplasmosis produce hydrocephalus and diffuse calcification in the affected infant? Would knowing the pathology of these infections help me remember this?"

Intrauterine Infections (TORCHES)[1,8]

These infections result in a clinical spectrum of intrauterine growth restriction (IUGR), microcephaly or hydrocephalus, cataracts, glaucoma, pigmentary retinopathy, keratoconjunctivitis, congenital heart defects, bone changes, skin rashes, mucocutaneous scarring, pseudoparalysis and persistent rhinitis. These symptoms and signs in the newborn make TORCHES a possible diagnosis. The maternal history must also be taken in detail:

- Toxoplasmosis
- Others, e.g. human immunodeficiency virus, enteroviruses, coxsackievirus, varicella zoster virus, Parvovirus B19, chlamydia, human T-lymphotropic virus and hepatitis B virus
- Rubella
- Cytomegalovirus
- Herpes simplex
- Syphilis (*Treponena pallidum*).

REFERENCES

1. Richard E. Behrman (comps). Robert M Kliegman, Waldo E Nelson, Victor C Vaughan III (Eds). Nelson's Textbook of Pediatrics (14th ed). Philadelphia: WB Saunders; 1992.
2. Common Tests During Pregnancy. Available at http://www.hopkinsmedicine.org. Accessed in January 2015.
3. Elizabeth KE. Clinical Pediatrics for Undergraduates. India: Jaypee Brothers Medical Publishers (P) Ltd, 2009.
4. Goel KM, Gupta DK. Hutchinson's Pediatrics, 1st edn. India: Jaypee Brothers Medical Publishers (P) Ltd; 2009
5. Havdial J, Jekyll AM (ed). Learn pediatrics: The basics of cerebral palsy. Learn pediatrics. 2010; July.
6. Lawn J, Shibuya K, Stein C. No cry at birth: global estimates of intrapartum stillbirths and intrapartum-related neonatal deaths. Bulletin of the World Health Organization 2005;83(6):409-17.
7. Levene MI, Tudehope DI, Thearle MJ; Essential Neonatal Medicine, Third edition. Blackwell Science, 2000
8. Marcdante K, Kliegman RM, Jenson HB, Behrman RE (Eds). Nelson's Essentials of Pediatrics (6th ed). Saunders Elsevier, 2010.
9. Mason S, Swash M (Eds). Hutchinson's Clinical Methods (17th edn). A Bailllere Tindall book published by Cassell Ltd; 1980.
10. Milner AD, Hull D. Hospital Pediatrics. 3rd edn. ELBS with Churchill Livingstone. 1998.
11. Stephenson T, Wallace H (Eds). Clinical Paediatrics for Postgraduate Examinations. UK: Churchill Livingstone; 1991.

The essence of the relevant chapters in the following books have also been numbered as references in this chapter. We recommend for further reading, the rich text in these books for greater integration and deeper understanding.

1. Goel KM, Gupta DK. Hutchinson's Pediatrics, 1st edn. Jaypee Brothers Medical Publishers (P) Ltd, India 2009.
2. Havdial J, Jekyll AM (Eds). Learn pediatrics: The basics of cerebral palsy. Learn pediatrics. 2010.
3. Levene MI, Tudehope DI, Thearle MJ; Essential Neonatal Medicine, 3rd edn. Blackwell Science. 2000.
4. Marcdante K, Kliegman RM, Jenson HB, Behrman RE (Eds). Nelson's Essentials of Pediatrics, 6th edn. Saunders Elsevier, 2010.
5. Mason S, Swash M (Eds). Hutchinson's Clinical Methods, 17th edn. A Bailllere Tindall book published by Cassell Ltd; 1980.
6. Milner AD, Hull D. Hospital Pediatrics, 3rd edn. ELBS with Churchill Livingstone. 1998.
7. Behrman RE (comps). Kliegman RM, Nelson WE, Vaughan VC III (Eds). Nelson's Textbook of Pediatrics, 14th edn. Philadelphia: WB Saunders. 1992.
8. Stephenson T, Wallace H (Eds). Clinical Paediatrics for Postgraduate Examinations. UK: Churchill Livingstone. 1991.

Chapter 5

Other Components of the Pediatric History

DEVELOPMENTAL HISTORY[1,10]

- Distinctive to the pediatric history, this enquiry looks into four categories of development.
  The four categories of development are the following:
  a. Movement and posture or "gross motor"
  b. Vision and manipulation or "fine motor"
  c. Hearing and speech (language)
  d. Personal, social and psychosocial.
- The activities of daily living are also a component that encompasses all aspects of development.
- The normal cephalocaudal progression of human development is unique and important.
- A craniocaudal developmental sequence is appreciated when a child learns to control his head first before sitting, sits before standing, and stands before walking.
- Developmental disorders[1-3] may specifically affect one realm of development or may affect at least two areas of development or more and may be linked to significant cognitive impairment.
- History of all four categories of development must be asked. Wherever necessary, a comparison with other siblings should be made.
- When more than two areas of development are abnormally slow and are outside the normally accepted limits and associated with cognitive impairment, it is termed "global developmental delay."
- Delay in speech alone as may occur in a hearing defect is termed "isolated developmental delay."
- Omitting a single milestone may be quite normal, provided the rest of the milestones appear normally.
- In prematurity, allowance for the prematurity is given and correction of post gestational age is done for up to 2 years.

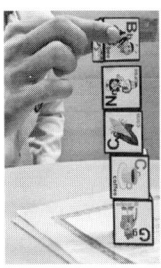
Development

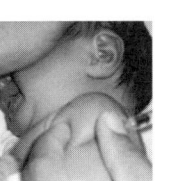
Immunization

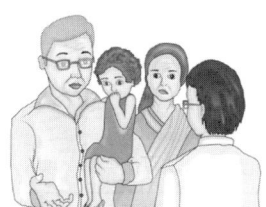
Family

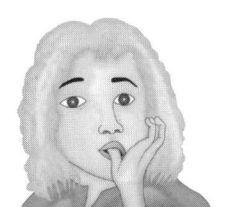
Behavioral

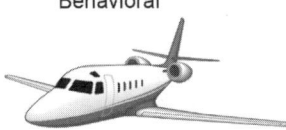
Travel

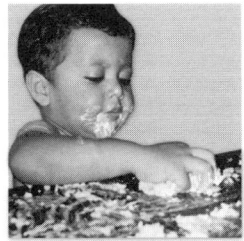
Dietary

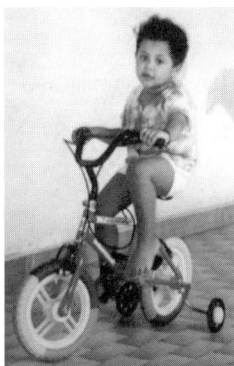
Social

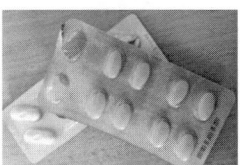
Drugs

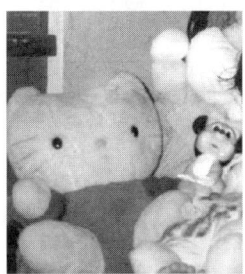
Allergy

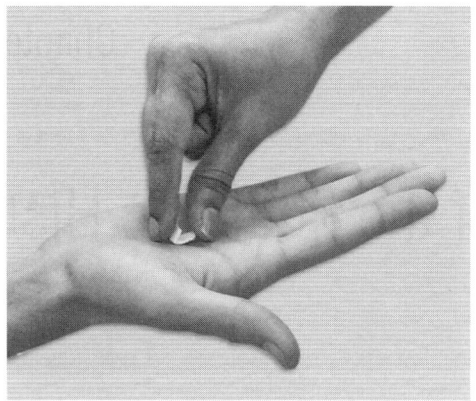

Demonstration of a pincer grip.

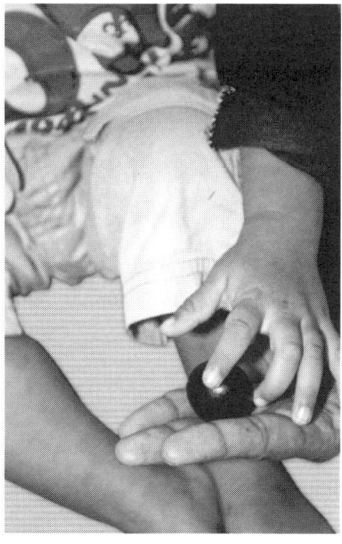

Index finger approach. The pincer grip-requires fine motor skills and intact vision. It is a fine motor development that is seen between 7 and 11 months. Before the use of a thumb-finger pincer grasp, the infant typically picks things up with a more immature palmar grasp.

- In the developmental history, ask whether the child has achieved a milestone
- If so, ask when the milestone was achieved
- You may want to know with what maturity or how well the milestone is carried out
- You must know that one developmental milestone can depend on another

AN APPROACH TO THE DEVELOPMENTAL HISTORY[1-3,8-10,15]

- Ask when the parents first noted a meaningful or responsive smile, vocalization, and response to sound, if the child is approximately 6 weeks old. Enquire when the child could hold a rattle placed in his or her hand, turned his or her head to sound and reached out and achieved an object if the child is approximately 6 months old or less. If the child is aged between 6 and 12 months, ask of the age of onset of sitting, crawling, creeping, and standing. Ask also when the child pulled himself or herself to sit and stand.
- Ask when the child waved goodbye or said any meaningful word. If the child is approximately 12–18 months, enquire when the child was able to join words together to make a sentence.
- Ask if the child is dry by day and/or night and is able to walk alone. Also ask if the child is able to dress and feed himself or herself. How many meaningful words can the child say?
- If the child is approximately 2 years old, is the child able to understand things said to him or her? Does the child come when called from another room? Observe and note parental worries about development. Ask about differences in development in comparison with other siblings, and ask if there have been parental concerns with development in the other siblings.

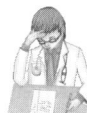

"Is this a disorder of development or a normal variation in development?"

Suspected developmental disorders: Checklist and historical links[4-10]
What are the parents' immediate concerns?
At what level is the child currently functioning?
Is it a behavioral problem or a problem of developmental delay?
Consider prenatal factors—maternal illnesses, drugs and substance abuse
Consider perinatal history—gestational age, birth weight, labor, delivery and Apgar score
Consider neonatal history—illnesses, seizures, hyperbilirubinemia, and congenital malformations
Are there illnesses in the child outside the neonatal period like recurrent otitis media, seizures, and developmental delay?
Is there a history suggestive of chronic illnesses?[4,11]
Is there a history that suggests a possibility of head injury?[12]
Is the nutritional history suggestive of poor nutrition or indicating possible nutritional imbalances?
Is there a possibility of toxic exposure?[13,14]
Are there possible visual problems?
Do you suspect hearing problems?

Contd...

Contd...

From the history, is there reason to suspect nonaccidental injury?[12,15-17]
Are there significant emotional stresses?[15-17]
Consider family history[15-17]—consanguinity, sudden unexplained deaths among the young, ask if there were members requiring special school
Consider social history[12]—parental education, extended family support and parental behaviors that are risky such as alcoholism or substance abuse

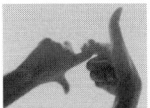

Other Historical Components that Influence the Developmental History[10,15,17,18] and the Developmental Diagnosis

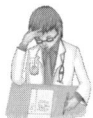

Development evolves from the interaction of intrinsic and extrinsic factors[10,19-25]

Components of the developmental history[10]

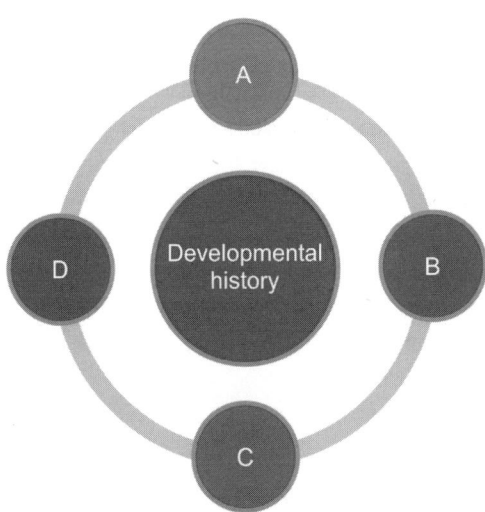

Development: *Some historical factors of importance.*

Appreciate how the events around pregnancy, birth and the neonatal period, as well as the family history, the past medical history and socioenvironmental history have a role in influencing the rate at which a child attains his or her developmental milestones.

Other Components of the Pediatric History

A. Pregnancy history, birth history, and neonatal history[10,29]

Prenatal factors—Potential teratogens including maternal drugs, alcohol, medications, maternal infection (cytomegalovirus, rubella, toxoplasmosis) and chicken pox, maternal diabetes mellitus and phenylketonuria in the mother. Tests done during pregnancy like special maternal blood tests (Refer to Chapter 4), amniocentesis and ultrasounds that may reveal important fetal anomalies
Birth factors like low birth weight and preterm delivery; prematurity and appropriate for gestational age (AGA) is different from intrauterine growth restriction (IUGR). Try to differentiate this in the history and by asking for its documentation in the birth card, where possible
Remember that a premature baby has not successfully completed a period of development in the uterus and correction must be made for this period until the age of 2 years. The corrected age, which is the chronological age minus the period of prematurity, is used for developmental assessment. This is the adjusted age based on the due date
Enquire about the Apgar score. Also ask if any resuscitation, birth asphyxia, feeding difficulties, history of hypotonia, admission to special care nursery (SCN), neonatal intensive care unit (NICU), ventilation or infections had occurred
Birth injuries that primarily affect the motor aspects of development include shoulder dystocia, subluxation of the hip, and fetal hypoxia leading to a nonprogressive brain condition, such as cerebral palsy

B. Family history is important in the developmental history[10]

How does the family history influence development?
A detailed family history of three generations is important. A pedigree must be drawn.
Normal developmental milestones fall in a range so that in some families walking may be faster than in others or talking may be earlier or later than in others. Hence, the mother may compare development of her children; the comparison will give her an opportunity to remember events and will give you a chance to understand some aspects of normal development in the family

Contd...

Contd...

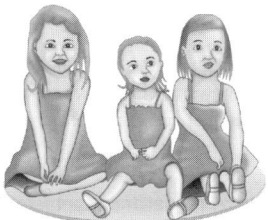

Comparison—an opportunity to recall events.

It is known that mothers and fathers appear to influence children in different ways
Language development of children raised by parents with a high level of education may be different from that of children raised by parents with a low level of education (Hoff E Naigles L)[9]
Family illnesses can influence development • A family history of deafness and blindness • Family history of degenerative diseases of the nervous system • The family history of genetic conditions and genetically related conditions
Familial risk factors that can affect a child's development • Maternal depression • Mental illness in the family • Parental substance abuse • Family violence • Poverty
• Other forms of family stresses involving parents or siblings or any member of the nuclear or extended family
• Lack of extended family support
• Living in isolation

C. Past medical or surgical history influences the developmental history[10]

Chronic diseases can potentially affect gross and fine motor movement, muscular strength, motor function, coordination and sensation. Otitis media, meningitis, chronic helminthic infections, malaria, HIV, diarrheal diseases especially severe or reccurent diarrhea in the first two years of life can affect cognition and child development.[26] There is a link between neurological and cognitive impairments associated with cerebral malaria.[26]
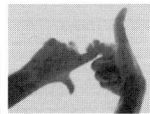 *Nutrition contributes to the overall health of a child and this links to the achievement of all aspects of development. Micronutrients such as iron, iodine and zinc are important in normal cognitive and other developmental achievements. Developmental milestones are often interlinked.*
Neurological and neuromuscular disorders can be a cause for motor delay. Any cause of a global developmental delay can cause motor delay. Other child risk factors include malnutrition, blindness, deafness, recurrent or chronic illness. Chronic illnesses can cause global developmental delays. A physical anomaly or neuromuscular disorder can be responsible for a defect in articulation and affect speech.

Contd...

Contd...

Long-term medications-chronic illnesses that require long-term medications with potential side effects[27] if therapeutic levels are not adequately monitored (e.g. antiepileptics in cases of epilepsy) can make a child less alert and influence cognitive development
After the developmental history, developmental testing must take into account that the performance of developmental tests may be affected by physical diseases; hence, developmental testing in a child who is obviously ill would be inaccurate

D. Social, environmental, and child factors affect development[3,10,21]

Environmental and child factors affect the development of social and emotional milestones. These influencing factors include the following:

Environmental risk factors[3,10,13,21,29]
Living in unsafe communities with environmental pollutants such as contaminated drinking water
Poverty
Receiving care within a low-quality child care setting
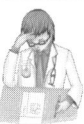 *Education is vital for both individuals and a community to emerge from poverty. Poverty can adversely affect the development of a growing child directly and indirectly.*
Lack of resources available in the community
Lack of motivation or stimulation can result in delays in communication
Genetic factors can cause "global developmental delay"
Pyschological stresses can also be a cause of global developmental delay
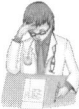 *Is there anything in the present or past upsetting the child?*
The influence of past experiences and opportunities on the child's development
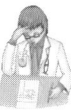 *Has the child ever been given a chance to have done this at home?*
Has the child been given the opportunity to stack up bricks at home? Interpret the child's ability for these tests in the light of the past experience of the child. If the child has never learnt to stack up cubes but has been putting toys into round and square pegs then test him on familiar tasks of putting toys into pegs instead of stacking up cubes
If suspecting problems involving mother–child relationships, the social history is of importance.

Contd...

Contd...

Some behavioral patterns may be influenced by cultural and environmental factors. In some eastern countries, looking at adults directly in the eye may be disrespectful. 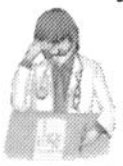 *Is there a cultural reason influencing the milestones in this child different from what I understand to be the norm?*

Contd...

Contd...

In certain cultures, the norm is to speak only when spoken to. The saying "speak only when spoken to" or "children should be seen and not heard" still holds true in some cultures. The child is expected to answer questions using respectful titles like aunty, uncle, sir or ma'am. The upbringing of some children may be to ask permission from an adult before starting an activity

An Approach to the Developmental History[10]

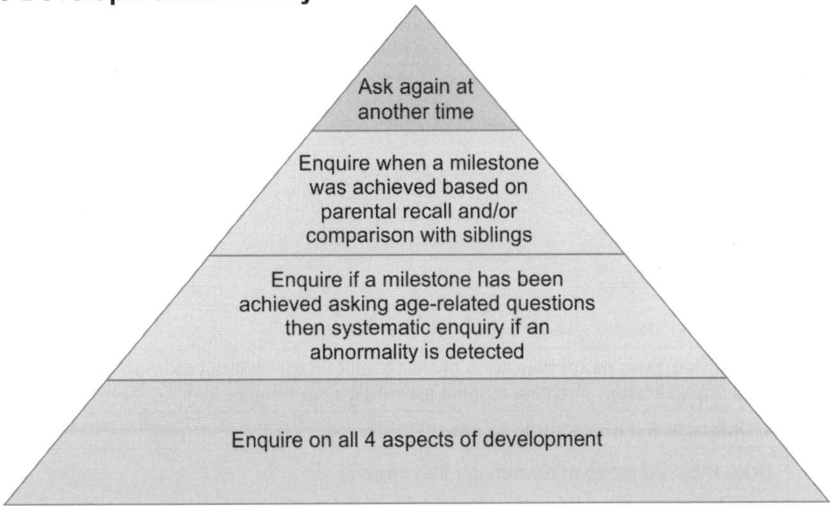
Ask again at another time
Enquire when a milestone was achieved based on parental recall and/or comparison with siblings
Enquire if a milestone has been achieved asking age-related questions then systematic enquiry if an abnormality is detected
Enquire on all 4 aspects of development

Enquiries Pertaining to the Developmental History[1,10,15,17]

The enquiry into a child's developmental milestones: The developmental history deals with the achievement and timing of all milestones involving the four areas of development. It uses comparison of events with siblings or close relatives as a means of reminding the parents of distant events.

Questions in the Developmental History[1,10,15,17]

Gross motor milestones[1,10,15,17] Rationale—enquiries on locomotion, physical activities of daily living covers many gross motor milestones	**Some gross motor enquiries**—remember that the motor development of a child starts in a craniocaudal manner. **At 2 months an infant lifts his or her shoulder while prone.** **At 4 months an infant lifts the body up when prone using arms; rolls from front to back and has no head lag when pulled to sit from supine.** Rolling over, sitting, creeping, cruising and walking are gross motor milestones. When lying with face down, can the child lift the head from a lying position? 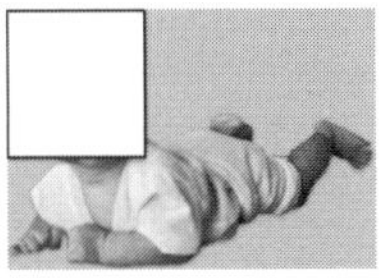 *Child supports body with forearm on prone position.*
	Can the child roll over?
	Can the child support himself or herself in the prone position with forearm?
	The child at six months supports himself steadily with forearm and head well above the horizontal when prone. If a child has not been able to do this at six to nine months, enquire in greater depth using **the Cardinal Ten (Historical)** and historical link. 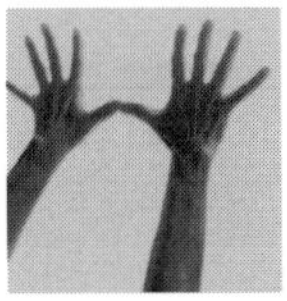 The Cardinal Ten enquires with greater depth into a milestone that is delayed or not achieved.

Contd...

74 *The Link*: Pediatric History-Taking and Physical Examination

Contd...

	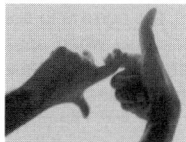
	The historical link asks about the possible causes of the delay.
	Ask details of birth history, history of delivery, and postnatal period to look for events likely to cause hypoxia.
	Ask about other parts of the history like family history, parental consanguinity and so on to look for familial patterns of development and inherited or familial causes of developmental delay.
	Can the child pull himself or herself to a standing position?
	Does the child sit with or without support? When did the child first sit without any support?
	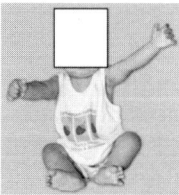 *Child sitting steadily without support at 6–7 months*
	The normal gross motor milestone of sitting supported, at about six months of age in a normal infant is referred to as "tripod sitting", or sitting leaning forward on the hands.
	An infant at 9 months pulls to stand
	Does the child creep and when did that begin? 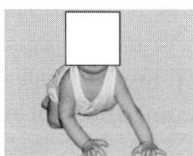 *When did the child start to do this?*
	Does the child walk holding on to furniture? (cruise).
	A child walks, stoops and stands at around 12 months.
	Does the child walk without any help or independently?
	A child walks backwards at 15 months, runs and kicks a ball at 18 months, walks up and down stairs at 2 years.
	Can the child climb up one leg at a time, or with alternate feet?
	Can the child climb down stairs? How does he or she do so?
	Can the child ride a tricycle?
	A child rides a tricycle at 3 years, walks steps with alternating feet and can jump with a broad base at the same age.
	At 4, the child balances with each foot quite well and can even hop on one foot.
	The 5-year-old child is able to skip and heel-to-toe walk and at 6 years he or she balances on each foot for 6 seconds.
	In pediatrics, always link developmental achievements with age to avoid erroneous neurological diagnosis.

Contd...

Contd...

	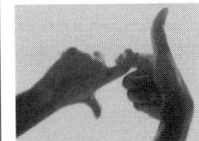 The link to the age of the child. The developmental history must link achievements of milestones to age to understand the physiology of growth; hence, any pathology must be interpreted in the light of such aberrant physiology.	
	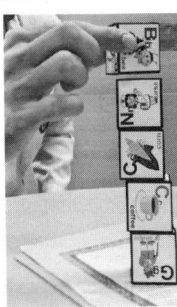 Building a tower of cubes on a flat, hard surface is fine motor development. A child stacks 3 to 4 blocks at 18 months, 5 to 6 blocks at 2 years, and 8 blocks at 3 years.	
Fine motor milestones[1,10,15,17] Rationale—enquiries on intricate movement of hands and fingers related to activities of daily living	**Some fine motor enquiries: Reaching out, transferring and the pincer.** 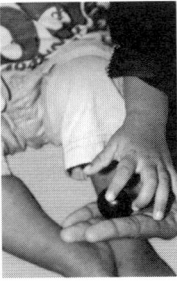 *The pincer grip is an example of fine motor development.* Does the infant hold a rattle or toy when you place it in his or her hand? **An infant tracks past the midline at 2 months, reaches for objects with a raking grasp at 4 months.** Does the infant engage in play with the toes? The playful infant is aware of his or her feet at 4–6 months. Will the child reach out for a toy? When did he or she begin holding toys? Does the infant pass a toy from one hand to the other? An infant is able to transfer objects from one hand to another at 6 months, starts to pincer grasp at 9 months, bangs two blocks together at 9 months. When did the child pass objects from one hand to the other? Does the child hold his or her own cup or bottle? Does the child point towards things with the index finger? Does the child pick up little objects?	
	A child puts a block in a cup at 12 months, scribbles at 15 months, stacks 3 to 4 blocks at 18 months, 6 blocks at 2 years, and 8 blocks at 3 years. He or she copies a circle and draws a person with 3 parts at 4 years, copies a square at 5 years, a triangle at 6 years. At 6 years, he or she can draw a person with 6 parts.	
	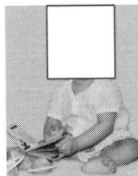 *When did the child turn pages? How many pages at a time?*	

Contd...

Contd...

Personal, social and psychosocial[1,10,15,17] Rationale— Integration and coping with others and environment	Some enquiries on social interaction: Enquire about bonding or feelings of affection of the parent towards the newborn which occurs soon after birth. 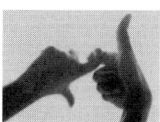 *A link between the feeding history and psychosocial development is that breastfeeding enhances bonding.* Attachment is the feeling between the infant and parent and is a gradual developmental event. 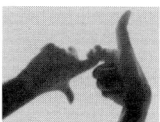 *The link between one psychosocial milestone and another is that efficient bonding during the early postpartum period strengthens the development of attachment.* Does the infant pay attention to you when you talk to him or her?
	Has the infant started to smile at you when you interact with him or her? When did you first notice the social smile? 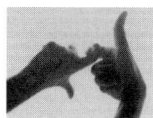 A link in this history is that a social smile appearing at the right time is an early sign that vision is normal. It is also indicative that the concerned neurological pathways are intact. Does the infant make noises and smile when you talk to him or her? **An infant smiles responsively at 6–8 weeks, holds a bottle at 6 months, waves bye-bye at 9 months.** Does the child show any interest when the child sees a feed being prepared? *Imitation* At what age did the infant start to imitate your actions? **A child drinks from a cup and imitates others at 12 months and uses a spoon and a fork at 15 months.** Does the child imitate you doing things in the house like sweeping, dusting or washing up? (domestic mimicry). **Domestric mimicry starts at 15 months, the child washes and dries hands at 2 years.** *Early social interaction* Does the child wave bye? When did the child begin to do that? Does the child clap hands? When did the child begin? Does the child help when you are dressing him or her?
	Can the child dress himself or herself fully? **A child can put on his/her own T-shirt at 3 years.** How does the child compare in understanding of simple instructions with his or her brothers or sisters? **At 2 years the child can brush teeth without help and dress without much help.** 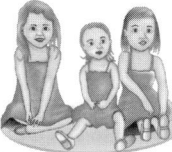 *Comparison to siblings is a tool to use in the developmental history.*

Contd...

Contd...

	Does the infant become insecure when the mother or the father is away? **Separation anxiety develops as early as 9 months and as late as 18 months. Stranger anxiety develops and abates around the same time.** Micturation and bowel competencies. 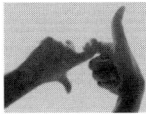 *Link questions to age and ask logically.* Does he or she tell you when he or she wants to use the potty? Is the child generally dry throughout the day? When did the child become reasonably dry by day? Is the child normally dry by night?
	When did he or she become dry by night? 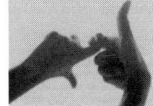 If sphincter control has not been achieved at an age when it should, determine whether it is primary or secondary enuresis. Make use of the historical links of the causes when proceeding to ask further questions.
Hearing[1,10,15,17] Rationale Responses to near and distant sounds	*Some enquiries on hearing* 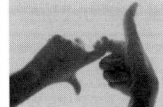 Remember that an isolated delay of development can happen when there is delay in speech in a child with a hearing defect. Response to loud sound, music and familiar sounds. Does the child turn the head in response to sounds when hearing sounds? When did that begin? Do you think that the child can hear? Why do you think that the child can hear? Does the child respond to music?
	What does the child do when there is music? 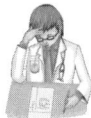 *"Appreciation of music tells me that the child can hear. That is a straightforward deduction. Yet, what more can I infer from this? Are there conditions where a child hears but does not respond appropriately? I do not think that I need to know every such condition, but I would like to also think of other reasons to explain this when I am told of these historical details by the busy mother. Yet I must not lose sight of the common things first".*
	Does the child sing along his or her favorite nursery rhymes? Does the child like being sung to? 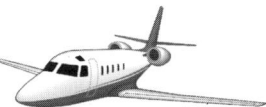 Children may respond by excitement to hear a plane if they are familiar with the sound. Others may be frightened by the loud sound. What does the child do when he hears a plane? Does the child respond to the ring of the telephone? Does the child respond to the father's footsteps?

Contd...

	"In a case of a child with speech delay, if a child can indicate the ability to hear footsteps or the call from another room it tells me that the child has no hearing impairment. That is what I infer. Yet I keep my mind open to all possibilities and make a scientific conclusion only after the entire history and physical examination is complete." Will the child come from another room when you call him or her without him or her seeing you? *"Many questions in the developmental history can be put in different ways to the historian. I must remain focused as to why I ask these questions and obtain maximum information from the responses."*
Speech[1,10,15,17]	**Some enquiries on speech**
The formation of words, sentences and development of language	Realize the link that normal speech requires normal hearing.
	Meaningful words and sentences.
	An infant coos at 2 months, laughs and squeals at 4 months, and babbles at 6 months.
	Does the child say any word which has a particular meaning?
	At 9 months an infant says Dada and Mama, at 12 months says 2 other words.
	At 15 months the child says 3–6 words, at 18 months at least 6 words, puts two words together at 2 years, at which time the child knows body parts. At 3 years the child names pictures and says 3 word sentences. At 4 years, the child is able to name colors and understand adjectives. At 5 years, the child understands opposites and counts. At 6 years, he delineates and defines words.
	What does the child say?
	How much does the child understand of what you say to him or her?
	Does the child join words together to make short sentences?
	A child shows understanding of the concept of today at 2 years, tomorrow and yesterday at 3 years.
	At 6 years, a child begins to comprehend right and left.

When should you be concerned?[1,10,15,17,21]

Developmental milestones amongst children have an age range that is considered normal. As there are such age ranges for the normal achievement of developmental milestones, allowances must be made for apparent delays within such reasonable limits. However, there are recognized developmental alerts, warning signs or 'red flags' that should raise your concern.

The following conditions indicate a delay or deviation from the normal development that requires medical intervention.

Red flags that should raise concerns over developmental delay[1,15]
Absence of visual fixation after 8 weeks
Persistent fisting beyond 3 months
Uncoordinated eye movements with unusual head turning movements after 3 months
Inability to control head by 6 months
Not able to sit independently by 10 months
Unable to walk independently by 18 months
Absence of pointing to show demand or interest by 14 months
No words with proper meaning by 18 months
Not able to combine two words by 30 months
Hand preference less than 1 year (this usually develops at 18–24 months)
Unusual or pervasive development

Developmental Abnormalities[1,5,10,15,17]

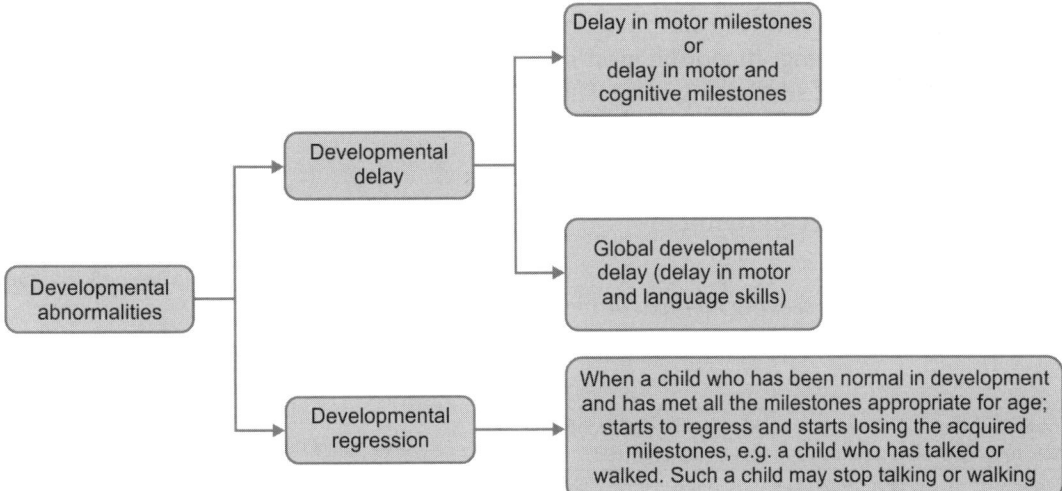

A hypothesis as to a reason why regression occurs in some metabolic or neurological diseases is that the toxic insult or an abnormal metabolite or cerebral event reaches critical levels to damage sufficient neuronal pathways or interfere with neuronal activity or conduction, such that clinical manifestations are apparent.

Some causes of developmental regression:[1,5,10,15,17]
Metabolic neurodegenerative disorders
Ceroid lipofuscinosis
Mitochondrial diseases
Mucopolysaccharidosis
Autism
Cerebral tumors
Certain types of epilepsy
Subdural hematomas
Hydrocephalus

Dietary or Feeding History[1,5,10,15,17]

- This history is important in assessing present and future growth and health. It also gives an idea of parental knowledge and attitudes towards feeding methods and infant nutrition.
- The history of breastfeeding must be explored. Remember that some proteins if consumed in large quantities by the mother, can pass through breast milk so the diet of the breastfeeding mother can influence the breastfed child.
- Cow's milk allergies and food allergies are important to discover by history taking.
- Marasmus refers to severe protein-energy malnutrition and wasting. Primary nutritional factors and many secondary factors can cause this.
- Kwashiorkor is malnutrition as a result of protein deficiency with significant edema due to inadequate protein intake or excessive protein losses in the presence of fairly good caloric intake. Primary nutritional factors and many secondary factors can cause this.

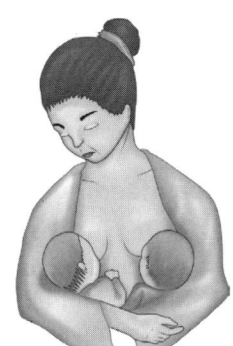

Questions you could ask if you suspect that the patient has a feeding problem[1,5,10,15,17,18]

Does your child gag when eating or drinking?
Does your child cough or choke when eating or drinking?
During feeding, has your child choked and become blue?
Does your child vomit often in relation to feeding?
How much does he or she vomit?
In toddlers ask if the toddler is excessively fussy or choosy with food (many are picky eaters), hence eats a very limited variety of food
The history of swallowing difficulties is important
Probe into slow weight gain
Ask if child refuses to swallow or tends to keep his or her food in the mouth
Ask about refusal to eat and difficulty progressing to adult type food (table food)

80   The Link: Pediatric History-Taking and Physical Examination

There is a recognized influence of early illness on the child's feeding. Early events can cause dysfunction to the mechanisms involved in the act of sucking and the act of swallowing. Incoordination of the act of sucking and the act of swallowing can result in feeding difficulties. Hence, these must be covered in history taking of a child with feeding problems.

Early illnesses or events that can result in feeding problems[1,18]

(Ask about problems that require seeking medical advice or admission into nursery or the neonatal intensive care unit)

Congenital anomalies that interfere with sucking and swallowing (e.g. cleft palate, micrognathia), gastroesophageal reflux (GERD)
Apnea or cessation of respiration for 20 seconds often associated with bradycardia and cyanosis
Necrotizing enterocolitis (NEC)
Premature birth
Bronchopulmonary dysplasia (BPD)
Prolonged tube feeding
Intraventricular hemorrhage

Breastfeeding History *(Refer to Chapter on Breastfeeding)*[1,15]

Breastfeeding has a major positive impact on the health of a child. Enquire briefly on mother's beliefs in breastfeeding and as to how she thinks breastfeeding is advantageous for the child.

Ask about the duration of breastfeeding and if it was exclusive breastfeeding, what was the duration of it. Enquire if the mother was fully informed about exclusive breastfeeding or also gave water and fruit juices during breastfeeding.

If actively breastfeeding, enquire on mother's exposure to infections like flu or flu like illness.

If duration of breastfeeding is inadequate or if not breastfed, enquire if colostrum was given early. If yes, enquire how much was given. Ask if the mother is working. Ask if she expresses her breast milk and how she stores the expressed breast milk.

If the child is not breastfeeding, enquire as to why the child is not being breastfed. Such reasons may include inverted nipples, her beliefs, her preferences, and family influences. This information can later be used for counseling.

It is an important part of history taking to ask about the introduction to solids or to complementary feeding; when and what type, was it rice-based or wheat-based. Ask when the child was given normal adult food.

LINKS IN THE FEEDING HISTORY[15]

Deficiency of micronutrients are common in children due to poverty, improper feeding habits and parental ignorance of infant's diet.

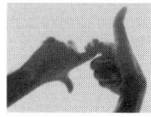

Cow's milk diet may be linked to iron deficiency anemia.[15]

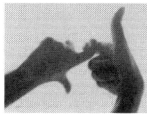

Goat's milk diet is linked to folate deficiency.[15]

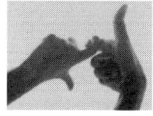

Pica is associated with iron deficiency.[15]

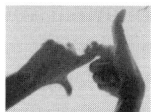

Cholestasis and malabsorption are linked to vitamin A,D,E and K deficiency.[15]

Iron deficiency can lead to symptoms and signs of anemia, lethargy and impaired learning and concentrating abilities. Ask about ocular symptoms as night blindness is the earliest symptom of vitamin A deficiency. This is followed by xerosis of the cornea and conjunctiva. Enquire about frequent infections as children with vitamin A deficiency are at increased risk of infections like measles.

If the history is suggestive of chronic liver disease, celiac disease, cystic fibrosis or abetalipoproteinemia, then ask about symptoms suggestive of sensory neuropathy as sensory and motor neuropathies are associated with vitamin E deficiency.

Enquire about excessive clothing or adequate exposure to sunlight or improper diet resulting in vitamin D deficiency; remember that skin pigmentation decreases the generation of vitamin D. Symptoms suggestive of chronic liver diseases, chronic kidney diseases, and malabsorption must be enquired into.

Enquire about maternal diet if fully breastfeeding. Ask about vegan diets, maternal folate intake; hemorrhagic disease of the newborn is more common among breastfed infants but is rare after prophylactic intramuscular vitamin K is given routinely soon after birth.

If bottle feeding, ask about type of milk, method of preparation; and heating of milk by boiling which destroys vitamins. Ask about prolonged phototherapy for hyperbilirubinemia.

Ask about the ingestion of milk other than cow's milk as goat milk is deficient in folate. Maternal alcoholism can result in micronutrient deficiencies. The family history of consanguinity may be discovered in some inborn errors of metabolism involving micronutrient deficiency.

When zinc deficiency is suspected as part of multinutrient deficiency or on its own, ask about anorexia, growth faltering, and repeated infections.

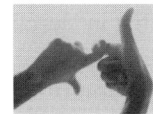

Moderate zinc deficiency is associated with delayed secondary sexual characteristics and signs on the skin. Mood swings, alopecia, diarrhea, night blindness, and photophobia are also relevant questions to ask.[15]

Vitamin Deficiencies and Historical Points to Consider[1,15,22]

Ascorbic acid	Scurvy	Unsupplemented cow's milk with inadequate fruits or vegetables	Irritability, purpura, bleeding gums, aching bones, periosteal hemorrhage
Thiamine (vitamin B_1)	Beriberi	Alcoholic mothers, infants with protein calorie malnutrition, infants receiving boiled milk, infants on unsupplemented hyperalimentation	Polyneuropathy, calf tenderness, heart failure, edema, ophthalmoplegia
Riboflavin (vitamin B_2)	Aribo-flavinosis	Poor socioeconomic conditions, diabetic children, children with chronic cardiac disease, infants under prolonged phototherapy	Anorexia, anemia, mucositis, cheilosis, nasolabial seborrhea
Niacin (vitamin B_3)	Pellagra	Diets low in tryptophan	Photosensitivity, dermatitis, diarrhea, dementia

Contd...

Contd...

Pyridoxine (vitamin B_6)	Heat treatment of infant milk formula Deficiency can also occur secondary to some drugs	Seizures, microcytic anemia, neuropathy, nasolabial seborrhea, hyperacusis
Vitamin B_{12}	In vegans, due to short gut syndrome, fish tapeworm, transcobalamine or intrinsic factor deficiency	Megaloblastic anemia, peripheral neuropathy, posterior and lateral spinal column disease, vitiligo
Biotin	Ingestion of raw eggs, biotinidase deficiency, bowel resection	Alopecia, dermatitis, hypotonia
Folate	Deficient in goat's milk, inactivated by heat, drug antagonists	Megaloblastic anemia, neural tube defects

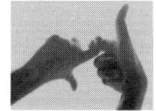

Link clinical picture to fat-soluble vitamin deficiencies[1,15,22]

• Xerophthalmia, nightblindness (earliest manifestation), xerosis of conjunctiva, cornea. • Untreated xerophthalmia leads to ulceration, keratomalacia and corneal scar. • Immunodeficiency, increased risk of infection like measles with increased mortality	Vitamin A
• Rickets is seen in children and osteomalacia is seen in adults • Craniotabes, enlarged, delayed closure of the anterior fontanelle and beading of the ribs as seen in rachitic rosary • Greenstick fractures, bowlegs, knocknees, scoliosis, exaggerated lordosis	Vitamin D
• Progressive sensory and motor neuropathy in children with fat malabsorption	Vitamin E
• Hemorrhagic disease of the newborn common in the breastfed. • Manifested by ecchymosis, gastrointestinal hemorrhage, umbilical stump bleeding • Bleeding from circumcision, uncommonly intracranial hemorrhage	Vitamin K

In 'picky' eaters, remember that the mother can use various strategies to cope with the poor feeding of her child such as distracting the child during meals or force feeding. Some mothers may reward the child by giving him or her the food that he or she prefers.

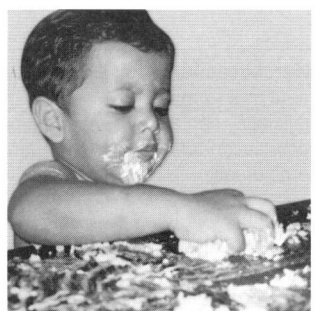

A young child in an Asian culture delights in the "mess" as he eats his meal on a banana leaf on an auspicious day. (Photograph with courtesy of VRK; reprint with permission)

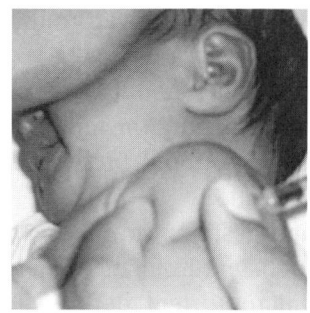

Vaccination (Photograph courtesy: Associate Professor Dr Loh Keng Yin, reprint with permission)

In a child with feeding problems, do not omit asking if the parents use punishment of any kind during periods of food refusal or if they positively reinforce the child if the child eats the required food.

Ask if food supplements or other high calorie formulae are offered as a consequence of suboptimal growth.

The Immunization History
(Refer Chapter on Immunization)[1,15,34]

The impact of childhood vaccination is appreciated in the following paragraph:

"The gasping breath and distinctive sounds of whooping cough; the iron lungs and braces designed for children paralyzed by polio; and the devastating birth defects caused by rubella:..infectious diseases, such as measles, diphtheria, smallpox, and pertussis topped the list of childhood killers. Fortunately, many of these devastating diseases have been contained, especially in industrialized nations, because of the development and widespread distribution of safe, effective, and affordable vaccines."

Alexandra Minna Stern and Howard Markel. The History of Vaccines and Immunization: Familiar Patterns. New Challenges Health Affairs. 2005;24(3):611-21.[25]

- Immunization history is the cornerstone in the pediatric preventive history and a good indicator of the future health with reduction in morbidity and mortality as a result of many vaccine preventable diseases.
- The single most important assessment of the vaccination status is to have written documentation of the vaccination; hence, it would be wise to begin the vaccination history by kindly requesting parents or caregivers for the vaccination card, which can then be studied.
- Learn the compulsory government immunization schedule.
- Know about important optional vaccines.
- Have a working knowledge on other important vaccinations available in special circumstances.

Start the immunization history by politely requesting to see the document of immunization, if any. Ask when the last immunization was taken. If immunization is not up-to-date ask for reason(s) including any reaction to immunization like high fever or inconsolable crying. Decide if reactions were attributable to immunization, especially if symptoms were within 3 days of vaccination. Ask when the next immunization is due. The Extended Program for Immunization (EPI) could be referred to as a good example for standard immunization schedules.[34] The vaccination card will give you the necessary information; politely request this if available.

It is important to remember that vaccination schedules can change from time to time, so you must always keep up-to-date with the latest immunization schedule recommended by the Health Ministry of your country.

Enquire about immunizations and if immunization other than those in the compulsory government immunization schedule, such as the extended program for immunization (EPI) schedule, Ministry of Health, Malaysia, were taken. In some countries, these may include the rotavirus, pneumococcal, influenza, or meningococcal vaccination.

Family History[1,15]

- This part is very relevant in the pediatric history as many childhood infections are transmissible and contagious. The source of an acute infection can often be traced back to a family member.

Other Components of the Pediatric History

- While family illnesses contribute to diseases, the impact of a child's illness especially if chronic can affect the family.
- Parental history of consanguinity is important in the investigation of inborn errors of metabolism. A family tree may reveal inherited and genetic diseases with clarity.
- The structure and functions of the family positively or negatively influence the health and development of children.
- Families are important for physical, emotional, educational and social support for their children.
- Failure to meet with the child's physical needs for protection or nutrition results in various forms of family dysfunction.
- The inheritance patterns of some diseases, if known, makes the family history a tool that can be used in arriving at inherited, familial or even mutifactorial diseases.
- The pedigree is the gold standard for the collection of the relevant family history, and is drawn clearly to illustrate patterns of inheritance.

HISTORICAL IMPORTANCE OF INHERITANCE[1,8,15-17,24]

The Pedigree is usually drawn as part of the family history during history-taking.

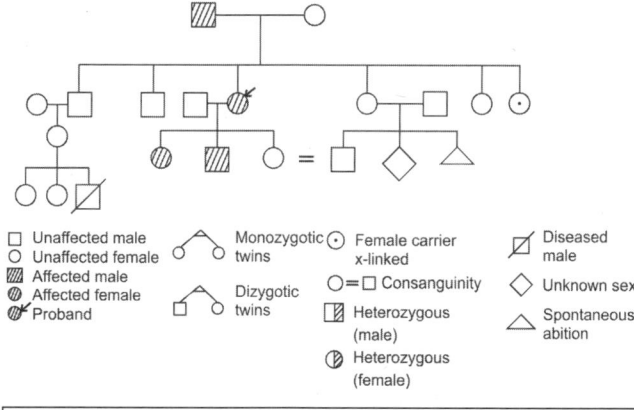

- ☐ Unaffected male
- ○ Unaffected female
- ▨ Affected male
- ⬤ Affected female
- ⬤⬋ Proband
- ⟨⟩ Monozygotic twins
- ⟨⟩ Dizygotic twins
- ⊙ Female carrier x-linked
- ○=☐ Consanguinity
- ▨ Heterozygous (male)
- ⊙ Heterozygous (female)
- ⧄ Diseased male
- ◇ Unknown sex
- △ Spontaneous abition

Importance of the family history[1,8,15-17,24]
- To identify single gene disorders
- To identify pattern of inheritance
- To elucidate the possible trigger of some diseases and as a tool to study the index patient if family history of neurocutaneous stigmata, bleeding, etc. are obtained
- As a patient education tool, e.g. counseling if family members of more than 2 generations have died from premature myocardial infarction
- To clarify with the patient or family regarding misconceptions on beliefs concerning the disease, such as if the particular disease affects only one gender.

Pattern of Inheritance[1,15]

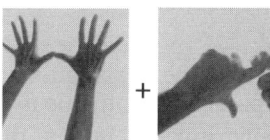

Use some **Cardinal Ten (Historical)** + link with the pedigree in the family history to know pattern of inheritance.

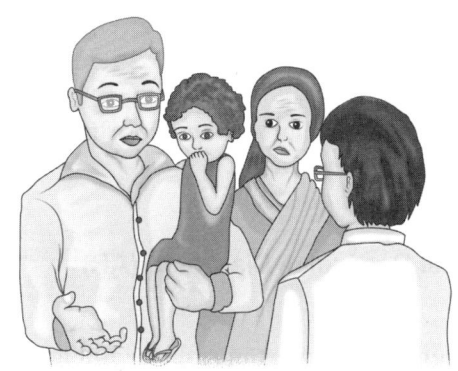

- First degree relatives are parents, children, and siblings
- Second degree relatives are aunties, uncles, nieces, nephews, and grandparents
- First cousins are third degree relatives.

LINK TO DISEASES[1,15]

Single Gene or Mendelian[1,8,15-17,24]

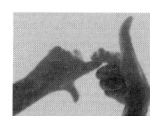

Autosomal Dominant Disorders (AD)

This inheritance is typified by a single copy of the mutated gene sufficient to cause disease. The parent with a mutation in one gene has a 50% chance of passing the mutated gene to each child. The heterozygous state is when one functioning and one nonfunctional gene is present and the homozygous state is when two copies of the gene are present.

When obligate carriers of a mutation known to cause an AD do not manifest clinical signs of the disorder, it is referred to as **incomplete penetrance** as opposed to complete penetrance in an AD where clinical signs are manifest.

When signs and symptoms differ in expression from one individual to another, differences of such expression in AD is termed variable expressivity.

Unrelated clinical findings in a condition caused by a mutation in a gene is called **pleiotropy**.

Rules
- Every child of an affected person has a 50% chance of being affected.
- The gender ratio is equal.
- The gene can be passed on from one male to another.
- Uncommon traits involve genes that code for structural proteins.
- In every generation, the traits are expressed.

Below are some common autosomal dominant disorders:
- Neurofibromatosis type 1.
- Huntington's disease.
- Marfan's syndrome.
- Achondroplasia (short-limbed dwarfism).
- Polycystic kidney disease.
- Von Willebrand disease.

Autosomal Recessive Disorders (AR)[1,8,15-17,24]

Rules

- The traits are manifest in siblings and are not seen in the parents.
- Every sibling at the time of conception has a 25% chance of being affected.
- A phenotypically normal sibling of an affected person has a two-third chance of being a carrier.
- Both genders are affected equally.
- Uncommon traits are associated with parental consanguinity.
- Traits involve genes that program for enzymes.

Below are some common AR disorders:
- Cystic fibrosis
- Tay-Sachs disease
- Hemochromatosis
- Phenylketonuria (PKU)
- Von Willebrand disease (certain types).

X-linked Dominant Disorders[1,8,15-17,24]

Rules

- Both sexes are equally affected
- The tendency is to less severely affect females than males due to X inactivation or lyonization where one of the X chromosomes present in females is inactivated.
- Some types of such disorders are lethal in males.

Examples are as follows:
- Incontinentia pigmenti
- Some forms of retinitis pigmentosa
- Fragile-X
- Chondrodysplasia punctata
- Most cases of Alport's syndrome
- Hypophosphatemic rickets (Vitamin D resistant rickets)
- Rett syndrome
- Charcot-Marie Tooth-Disease.

X-linked Recessive Disorders[1,8,15-17,24]

Rules
- Males manifest traits commoner than females.
- A carrier female who may manifest mild disease expression passes trait to half of her sons
- Trait is transmitted from males who are affected to all daughters and never to sons
- As the trait can be passed through many carrier females, it can skip generations
- The son of a carrier mother has a 50% chance of affection.

Examples are as follows:
- Duchenne muscular dystrophy
- Hemophilia A
- X-linked severe combined immune disorder (SCID)
- Lesch-Nyhan syndrome
- Some forms of congenital deafness
- Color blindness.

Multifactorial Inheritance or Polygenic Inheritance[1,8,15-17,24]

Features
- Cluster in families without a simple Mendelian pattern of inheritance
- Disorders occur more often in first and second degree relatives than would be expected by chance.
- Genetics and environment could both play a role.
- Concordance may be expressed in monozygotic twins.

Examples are as follows:
- Height
- Insulin dependent diabetes mellitus (IDDM)
- Neural tube defects
- Some malignancies
- Atopic reactions
- Spina bifida
- Anencephaly
- Pyloric stenosis
- Cleft lip
- Cleft palate
- Developmental dysplasia of the hip (DDH)
- Club foot
- Bronchial Asthma

- Autoimmune diseases, such as multiple sclerosis
- Some cancers
- Heart disease
- Hypertension
- Ulcerative colitis and Crohn's disease
- Mental retardation
- Anxiety and depression
- Obesity
- Refractive error.

Codominance[1,8,15-17,24]

ABO
Alpha I antitrypsin deficiency
Example: Blood type. If a parent has an A blood type and the other has B type then there is a possibility that their offspring will have AB blood type which is a combined influence of both.

Incomplete Dominance[1,8,15-17,24]

Example: Hair type. If someone with curly hair and someone having straight hair have children, their children will have wavy hair, the effect of a combination of the two types.

Mitochondrial Inheritance[1,8,15-17,24]

Features

- This is indeed a rare pattern of inheritance
- Affects organs with high-energy utilization such as the heart, skeletal muscle, liver, and kidneys.

Mitochondrial encephalomyopathy with lactic acidosis and stroke (MELAS) like episodes and Leber hereditary optic neuropathy are examples.

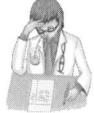

"I should try to link my knowledge of the rules and features of inheritance and inherited conditions when enquiring about the family history; if I cannot remember these conditions, I could refer standard textbooks and then utilize links to deduce patterns of inheritance. This may then help me make a logical diagnosis".

Enquire about any family history of similar illnesses, including coughs, flu, rash, febrile fits or epilepsy.

The family history has to be given due importance in respiratory diseases and should include questions about bronchial asthma, atopy, immune deficiencies, and cystic fibrosis.

Enquire about heart disease, diabetes, and hypertension. The family history of peptic ulcer disease, inflammatory bowel disease, biliary diseases, and migraine are relevant. Ask about a family history of drug reactions as ethnicity and genetics of drug reactions are important.

Parental consanguinity is important in Mendelian autosomal recessive diseases.

The family history of ambiguous genitalia is important in congenital adrenal hyperplasia (CAH), 46XY gonadal dysgenesis and 5 alpha reductase deficiency as these are inherited by autosomal recessive or familial patterns. Symptoms may be due to inadequate mineralocorticoids or excessive androgens.

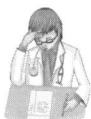

"For counseling, which is a part of effective management, the knowledge of the pattern of inheritance is important. In pediatrics, I appreciate that preventive counseling is an important tool. The family history contributes to an accurate diagnosis".

Enquire about sudden death among the siblings, the age of death and whether the cause was known. Sudden death among the siblings could suggest metabolic diseases or salt losing congenital adrenal hyperplasia. Vomiting and dehydration can occur.

The development of primary or secondary sex characteristics may be altered in some affected infants, children, or adults.

OTHER HISTORICAL POINTS[1,8,15-17,24]

In developmental delay, if there are members who are mentally retarded or require special schooling, this suggests possibility of environmental and hereditary risks factors. Questioning environmental causes of developmental disabilities,[26] including the prenatal history, postnatal history and exposure to toxins[27] are important.

In chromosomal disorders, enquire about maternal age. Advanced maternal age is a recognized factor in trisomy 21. Trisomy 21 is primarily caused by chromosomal nondisjunction occurring during the maternal meiotic division.

Sudden or unexpected early death of a family member is indicative of an inborn error of metabolism or a storage disease.

Enquire about family history of epilepsy. Sometimes, a family history suggestive of prominent multiple skin lesions (neurocutaneous stigmata) as in neurofibromatosis may be obtained.

In a case suspected of a hematological problem, enquire about bleeding problems and hemarthrosis in maternal uncles in hemophilia. Draw the family tree—this is vital in inherited or familial diseases.

Family History: Bleeding Disorders[1,15,28]

Inheritance	Types	Family members affected
Autosomal recessive disorders	Rare coagulation deficiency	Both sexes, consanguinity increases chance
Autosomal dominant traits	Von Willebrand disease	Both sexes
X-linked recessive inheritance	Osler-Weber–Rendu Hemophilia A and B	Male siblings Maternal uncles

Family History in Chronic Diseases[1,8,15-17,24,28]

(Always enquire about the impact of the disease on the family)

- Functions and activities of daily living
- Interfamily relationships
- Family stresses
- Socioeconomic impact
- Impact of disease on family dynamics

Note: Questionnaires to the child, adolescent and parent if family violence is suspected are available in standard pediatric textbooks.

Social History[12]

- It is important to determine the influence of sociocultural factors on etiology of diseases and their possible outcomes
- Social risk factors are important to identify in a given community as their health impact on children are significant
- Specific problems, such as failure to thrive, child abuse and emotional or physical neglect, involve psychosocial issues that need in depth understanding and detailed histories
- Environmental influences can also be included here

Ask if both parents work. If both are working parents, enquire as to the nature of their work and how far away from home they work. If they are unemployed, ask for how long they have been unemployed and if they are receiving any social benefits.

LINK BETWEEN THE SOCIAL HISTORY AND HEALTH[1,15]

Social factors are found to influence child health.[12]

These ten factors have to be further enquired into appropriately in each case. Make use of **The Cardinal Ten (Historical)** to help you think of questions to ask in your history.

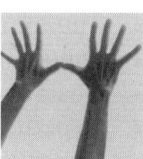

- Poverty
- Low parental education
- Single-parent household
- Race or ethnicity
- Maternal education
- Child health insurance coverage
- Maternal mental health
- Family structure
- Family conflict
- Neighborhood safety.

Ask about the type of house they live in and its proximity to construction sites or factories. Is the area damp or dirty? Ask about the environment. Enquire about extended family support, i.e. grandparents, aunties, etc.

The environmental history must include exposure to smoke, pets and pollutants. Enquire if the child is in contact with pets, including cats, dogs, birds or other animals. If the child has been in contact with these animals, find out about the duration of such contact and how often the contact has been.

Some studies have found that environmental exposure to certain substances in early childhood can contribute to diseases in later childhood. Identified environmental exposure to the following may contribute to the development of bronchial asthma.[13,23,29]

- Wood or oil smoke
- Dust mites
- Soot
- Exhaust smoke
- Cockroaches
- Herbicides
- Pesticides
- Farm crops
- Farm dust
- Indoor mold
- Animal dander
- Daycare centers usually due to exposure to other children with viral infections.

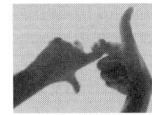

Link the major trigger factors of diseases in your environment to known preventable factors of diseases, for effective counseling, treatment, and prevention

Remember that dust mites are found in bedding, pillows, upholstered furniture, in areas of high humidity, house dust mites, cockroaches, and indoor mold.

Pets must be cleaned and vaccinated regularly.

Stuffed toys can be a source of dust mite-induced allergy.

Read around some of the factors that are allergenic in your environment. Such knowledge will sharpen your ability to take an effective history. Knowing the factors involved in exposure can help you counsel your patients practically and meaningfully.

During the embryonic period, there are many agents that can affect organogenesis.[29] Some of the known teratogens are antineoplastic drugs, diethylstilbesterol, lead and ionizing radiation. A significant percentage of aborted fetuses are either morphologically abnormal, karyotypically abnormal or both.

As the central nervous system, endocrine and other systems are still developing after the first trimester, exposure during this time can cause abnormalities in these systems. Organic mercury, lead and tobacco smoke can have adverse effects on the later part of pregnancy. Carcinogens can be transmitted transplacentally, and therefore, can affect the development of the fetus.

The toxins within tobacco smoke potentially adversely affect reproduction. Such toxins include nicotine, carbon monoxide, aromatic solvents and polynuclear aromatic hydrocarbons.[13,29] Smoking in the mother is linked to developmental anomalies in the fetus and reproductive difficulties in the mother.

Some of the common obstetric problems associated with exposure to tobacco smoke are premature delivery, intrauterine death of the fetus and infertility.

Neither is the fetus spared of deleterious effects. Among the fetal complications associated with exposure to tobacco smoke are small for gestational age and later, observed behavioral problems in infants.

The recognized constellation of anomalies in the fetal alcohol syndrome is linked to excessive intake of alcohol during pregnancy, especially during the critical early period of organogenesis. There is a link to sudden infant death syndrome and non-optimal growth, which may go on to possibly manifest its effects during adolescence.[13,29]

Exposure to toxins after birth can potentially cause a spectrum of developmental anomalies. Direct environmental exposure or indirect parental occupational exposure may be deemed to exert negative impact. High concentrations of low molecular weight (LMW) nonpolar substances, such as dichlorodiphenyl, polychlorinated biphenyls (PCBs) and trichloroethane (DDT)[13,29] could be passed into the lactating mammary gland and into breastmilk as a result of their concentration in maternal adipose tissue.[13,29]

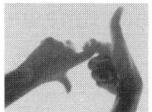

Link enquiries on toxic exposure in the high-risk environment to fetal anomalies or other abnormalities.

Group of toxicant, toxicant and type of hazard associated with adverse effects in the fetus, infant and women in the reproductive age[13]

Group of toxicant	Toxicant	Type of hazard	Adverse effects
Medication	Chemo-therapeutic drugs	Chemical	Teratogenic harm Abortion
	Anesthetic gases	Chemical	Reduced fertility Abortion
Gases	Tobacco smoke	Chemical	Abortion
	Carbon monoxide	Chemical	Abortion
Heavy metal	Mercury	Chemical	Neuro anomalies Abortion Developmental delay Menstrual disorders
	Lead	Chemical	Neuro anomalies Infertility
Metal	Arsenic	Chemical	Abortion Fetal mutation
Chemicals	Dioxins	Chemical	Defects at birth
	Polychlorinated biphenyls (PCBs)	Chemical	Low birth weight Intrauterine growth restriction
	Chlorinated by-products	Chemical	Abortion
	Solvents	Chemical	Abortion
	Alcoholic beverages (consumed prior and during pregnancy)	Chemical	Fetal alcohol syndrome Growth deficit Behavioral problem Mental function deficits
Magnetic fields	Electromagnetic fields	Physical	Cancers in childhood
Radiation	Ionizing radiation	Physical	Teratogenicity

Also enquire if the pets are well taken care of. You may enquire about vaccination of some domestic pets if relevant. In diseases that are specifically related to or caused by environmental factors, environmental history and exposure has to be taken in depth.

Who takes care of the child? If the child is placed in a nursery, ask how many other children are in nursery and their age groups. Ask if the child is happy with friends?

Does the child cry each time he or she is dropped off at nursery? Does the child show eagerness to go to the nursery?

Ask of any recent illnesses in the nursery. If a babysitter is taking care of the child, ask of how many other children are being taken care there and their age groups. Is the babysitter a responsible person or not?

Parental psychiatric disorders are sometimes relevant to the case. Unhappy parental relationships may need to be explored. Some social problems are more complex and referral to a social worker will be required. Sometimes, more than one medical discipline may need to be involved.

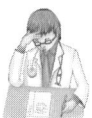

The behavioral history is incorporated in the history of the presenting illness as the child's behavior during the acute illness is important in pediatrics. Yet, in children with specific and more long-term behavioral problems, the behavioral history has to be taken in detail with many questions on the perinatal period, as well as the developmental and social history. Complex social problems can be deduced by a tactful, polite history, going into necessary details. This is important when deciding on appropriate referral.

Behavioral History[1,2,19]

- This aspect sheds light on how physical diseases affect the child's behavior and the behavior during the presenting illness such as inactivity, irritabilty or lethargy gives clues to the diagnosis of the child's acute illness.
- However, specific behavioral problems, if present, have to be dealt with in more detail, under this section.
- Some aspects of this part of the history may be closely linked to the perinatal, social and developmental history.
- Child factors, parental factors, environmental factors and parent-child interactions are all important to enquire in the history of behavioral problems.
- Behavioral, emotional, and functional problems or "disorders" can arise in these basic areas.[2,19] These areas need a detailed behavioral, social and environmental history.
- Referral to an expert is always recommended on these matters if the problem is complex.

The beginnings of behavioral disorders as mentioned by WB Carey, a clinical professor of pediatrics at the University of Pennsylvania's School of Medicine and senior physician in the Division of General Pediatrics at The Children's Hospital of Philadelphia, could be viewed as follows.[2]

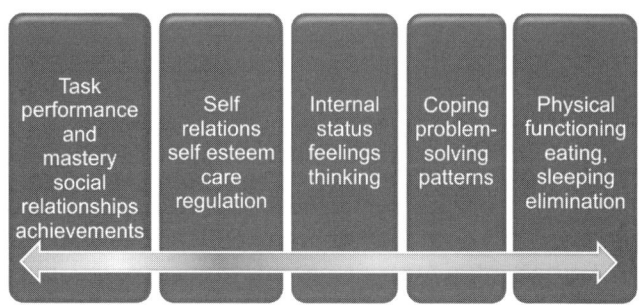

SPECIFIC BEHAVIORAL PROBLEMS AND TEMPER TANTRUMS[1,15,30-33]

Crying

Ask about the frequency and intensity of crying. Colic is often diagnosed using the rule of three, i.e. crying for more than 3 hours a day, for more than 3 days per week and for more than 3 weeks but this definition has its own limitation and hence can only be used as a very rough guide.

Type of Crying

Ask if the crying is paroxysmal, accompanied by facial grimacing, drawing up of legs or passing flatus. These signs are suggestive of colic in infant.

Unusual Behavior

Does the child manifest any unusual behavior such as thumb sucking, frequent bursts of temper tantrums, even excessive masturbation? If a child has temper tantrums, ask about the child's daily routine which may reveal associated problems like hunger, fatigue, inadequate physical activity or in need of attention. Also ask about exposure to abuse or violence at home.

Sleep Disturbances

Enquire about any sleep disturbances the child might have especially at night.

Learning Problems

Has the child been faring well in school or has there been a drop in the child's learning performance?

Abnormal Craving

Geophagia refers to the ingestion of dirt or clay, lithophagia is stone or gravel eating, trichophagia is hair eating, amylophagia is starch eating, pagophagia is ice eating and cautopyreiophagia is the ingestion of burned match.[30]

Does the child exhibit any abnormal cravings, such as pica, which is ingestion of substances other than food? In pica in children close questioning of eating habits, especially related to mouthing activities are useful where explicit questions with examples may be necessary. Ingestion of paint chips or plaster must be asked.

Abnormal Bowel Habits

Enquire about the presence of any abnormal bowel habits like stool holding. Children younger than 3 years can present with painful defecation, impaction and stool withholding. Constipation with soiling presents with uncontrolled defecation in the pampers or undergarment.

Ask about diarrhea due to soiling of liquid stool. Enquire about the passage of large-caliber bowel movements that sometimes block up the toilet.

Abnormal Micturition Habits

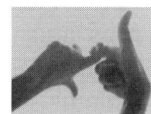

Link habits of micturition to achievement of normal milestones.

Primary and Secondary Nocturnal Enuresis[20]

Enuresis or bedwetting may be primary or secondary. In primary bedwetting the child has not had sphincter control at night or has not been dry during the night for a reasonable period of time. Secondary bedwetting is bedwetting that commences after the child has been dry at night for at least 6 months. The most common reason for primary eneuresis is a delay in development and parents can usually be reassured. In secondary enuresis, having been continent for a period of time, he or she becomes incontinent again. In such situations, certain conditions must be excluded such as a urinary tract infection or undiagnosed diabetes mellitus.

In enuresis, the family history and social history are important. The pattern of voiding is elucidated by asking questions about timing and associated factors linked to wetting the bed. How often does wetting occur? When does it occur—day, night or both? Are there any associated conditions with wetting episodes like bad dreams, drinking caffeinated beverages or tiring days? Does the child wake up after wetting the bed? During the day, does the child use the toilet to pass urine? Was a change in wetting pattern preceded by a stressful event? Has there been unnecessary punishments or humiliations in the past by friends, relatives or parents? Enquire further on other triggers such a social, environmental or even emotional causes for the change. Ask about recent bereavement, bullying and parental separation.

In secondary enuresis, ask if there are symptoms during the day such as abnormal frequency of urination or infrequent urination.

Ask about urgency, daytime wetting, straining with poor stream, or pain on urination. Is there constipation?

It may sometimes be useful information to ask for documentation of the amount of fluid taken, the trends of bedwetting and toileting.

Temper Tantrums[1,15]

These are extreme behaviors within the normal developmental spectrum and stage. A tantrum is how a young child may express his or her frustration when faced with the challenges of the moment. It occurs between 1 year and 4 years of age.

Examples are breath holding spells, head banging, hitting, screaming and sometimes even biting.

Head Banging[31]

Head banging and body rocking are rhythmic movements that usually involve the whole body. These movements are repetitive, stereotypical behaviors commonly seen in children around the time of sleep and may recur if they wake up throughout the night.

- Ask if there is associated injury or if the parents fear potential harm.
- Ask if there are concerns about the development of the child.
- Do you think the parents are concerned that it is a seizure?

Thumb Sucking[32]

Enquire about breastfeeding and duration. The natural rooting and sucking reflexes can cause some infants to put their thumbs or fingers into their mouths.

As thumb sucking soothes infants, some might eventually develop a habit of thumb sucking when they feel insecure, bored, tired or anxious.

Many children who suck their thumbs or fingers do so while holding a favorite object, such as a security blanket or pillow.

Stuttering or Stammering[1,15]

It is a repetition of syllables, a prolongation of sounds or a pausing of words. It is usually part of childhood development when children learn to speak or may also be due to a flight of ideas. Sometimes stammering is a pathological speech behavior.

Sleep Pattern

Enquire about the sleep pattern including snoring, parasomnias or sleep disturbances involving abnormal events or experiences, and timing of night-time urination. Enquire about furry toys, stuffed toys and teddy bears, usage of a particular blanket or pillow that could seldom be washed as the child could not do without it.

Pacifier usage

Enquire about the use of a pacifier. If the child has used one, ask since when and for how long.

Breath Holding Spells[33]

These are seen between 6 months and 3 years of age. The child may turn blue or cyanosed, pale or pallid and, can lose consciousness and have a fit. The child stops breathing and loses consciousness for a short period immediately after a frightening or emotionally upsetting event or a painful experience.

Breath-holding spells are differentiated from brief episodes of voluntary breath-holding by some children who voluntarily hold their breath, do not lose consciousness and go back to breathing normally after they get what they want.

Inattention, Hyperactivity and Related History

Ask about inattention, hyperactivity, impulsivity-these need to be further detailed using standard attention deficit hyperactivity disorder (ADHD) rating scales.

Munchausen's Syndrome and Munchausen's Syndrome by Proxy[1,5,6,8,15-17,24]

In Munchausen's syndrome, the child induces physical symptoms to be in the hospital or in Munchausen's syndrome by proxy, the parents induce physical symptoms as an excuse to take children to hospital.

LINKS TO BEHAVIORAL DISORDERS[1-3]

Some Recognized Risk Factors in Childhood Behavioral Disorders[1-3,10]

Gestation and birth	Difficulties during pregnancies, low birth weight and prematurity
Family life	Dysfunctional families; domestic violence at home, poverty, faulty parenting skills or substance abuse are a problem
Temperament	Children who are difficult to manage and who are temperamental and aggressive from an early age
Learning difficulties	Problems with reading and writing are often associated with behavior problems
Intellectual disabilities	Children with intellectual disabilities tend to have behavioral disorders
Brain development	Areas of the brain that control attention appear to be less active in ADHD

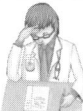

"This is nice to know"

Behavioral History in the Dysmorphic Child and in Conduct Disorders[1,3,7,19]

Some specific abnormalities in the patterns of sleep, such as nocturnal awakening and disturbed sleep seen in some syndromes like Smith-Magenis syndrome, personality traits, such as gregarious 'cocktail party' personality are linked to William's syndrome.

The recognized problems concerning difficulties with social interaction and other behavioral disorders can occur in Asperger's syndrome.

Certain conduct disorders like attention deficit hyperactivity disorder (ADHD), other hyperactive disorders and autism also have elements of behavioral abnormalities.[19]

A young boy has pharyngitis, painful neck swelling, and develops a generalized rash after being given oral ampicillin
Photography courtesy: Associate Prof Dr Loh Keng Yin, reprint with permission

Drug History[1,4,15]

- Many acute drug reactions are caused by predictable, nonimmunologic effects
- 'Drug allergy' as defined by the World Allergy Organization (WAO) is an immunologically mediated drug hypersensitivity reaction.[4]
- The mechanism of drug allergy may be either IgE or non-IgE mediated, where non-IgE mediated reactions are mainly T cell mediated.[11]
- The drug history may sometimes give a clue to diagnosis if adverse drug reactions have occurred in the patient. For example, ampicillin and amoxicillin are known to induce a maculopapular rash in infectious mononucleosis (See figure on previous page)
- The drug history is also important as it will guide management choices on alternative drugs to use in cases of allergy.

FACTORS IN DRUG ALLERGY

The following results are based on a study conducted by Bernard YH Thong and Teck Choon Tan on pediatric patients who experienced an acute reaction at a community-based tertiary care teaching hospital.[27]

More than half were deemed to be allergic/idiosyncratic in nature
About a quarter of all acute drug reactions (ADRs) were attributed to drug hypersensitivity reactions
Stevens Johnson Syndrome (SJS) occurred mainly from phenytoin and carbamezepine
Most frequently antibiotics were the cause of ADRs
Narcotic analgesics contributed to ARDs
Anticonvulsants also contributed to ARDs

Enquire about any use of drugs at present and in the past. If the child has a chronic illness, detail the type and duration of therapy. Also determine route of therapy i.e. oral, inhalational, parenteral, or intranasal. Remember that drug reactions to penicillin and cephalosporin are the most common allergic drug reactions in pediatrics. Be aware that approximately 6% to 10% of children are "penicillin allergic."

Enquire on all risk factors for drug allergy, including previous exposure, parenteral or topical administration and intermittent repeated exposure. Ask if the allergy occurred immediately or within 60 minutes of drug ingestion (anaphylactic reaction), if it occurred within 1 hour to 3 days of exposure to allergen (accelerated reaction) or if it occurred after 3 days of exposure to allergen (late reaction).

Factors influencing drug allergy[1,15]

Host factors in general
- Very young, very old
- Concomittant disease reactivation of herpes virus (Ebstein-Barr virus, human herpes virus (HHV) 6 and 7, cytomegalovirus)
- Ethnicity and genetics

Increased risks for children
- Capacity to metabolize drugs is usually not fully developed
- Premature birth; immature liver and kidneys
- Widespread use of drugs in general practice may sensitize children

Increased risks during pregnancy and breast-feeding
- Transplacental and breastmilk passage of maternal drugs

Drug factors
- Certain classes of drugs associated with a higher frequency of drug allergies
- Immunogenicity of drug to act as a hapten, a prohapten or to bind covalently to immune receptors
- Previous exposure
- Parenteral administration
- Topical administration and intermittent repeated exposure

IMPORTANCE OF DRUG INTERACTIONS IN THE DRUG HISTORY

Adverse effects of some drugs in the newborn and young child[1,15]

- Warfarin use for anticoagulation can lead to birth defects, and increased risk of bleeding problems in newborns and mothers
- Lithium, for bipolar disorder, can lead to defects of the heart, lethargy, reduced muscle tone, and underactivity of the thyroid gland
- Use of sulfonamides (antibiotic) can lead to jaundice and brain damage in the newborn
- Newborns cannot metabolize or eliminate chloramphenicol, an antibiotic
- Growth of cartilage is interfered with by quinolones in growing children
- Children younger than 18 months are at risk of developing Reye's syndrome if given acetylsalicylic acid (aspirin)

Ask for the presence of any skin lesions and the time frame of contact with drug.

Be aware that adverse reactions to drugs frequently manifest on the skin. Accelerated adverse drug reactions are usually dermatological or serum sickness type. Desquamating dermatitis, toxic epidermal necrolysis, serum sickness, and Stevens-Johnson syndrome are late adverse reactions to drugs. Enquire if a Medic Alert bracelet has been given to patient or family members.

Ask for history of maternal drug ingestion, such as danazol, steroids, and some traditional medicines and herbs that may contain steroids. This history may also be important in some rare clinical problems, such as the child with genital ambiguity.

Also remember that drugs can interact with one another.

If the child is on more than one medication, enquire about the nature of all medicines used. Drug interactions include incompatibility of drugs, interference of absorption, interference with drug distribution, augmenting metabolism, competition of excretion and transport competition.

These interactions may result in lower drug concentrations, decreased effectiveness or toxicity. Erythromycin increases blood levels when used with carbamazepine, digoxin and theophylline. Acetaminophen reduces serum chloramphenicol levels in patients treated for meningitis.

Hypoglycemia is an adverse effect of many medications, including salicylates, oral hypoglycemic agents, insulin, alcohol, propranolol, and valproic acid.

The drug history also can indicate the cause of the allergy. Some examples are as follows:[1,15]
• Oxidants cause hemolysis in glucose-6-phosphate dehydrogenase (G6PD) deficiency
• Immune mediated hemolysis is linked to penicillins
• Phenytoin increases the requirement for folate
• Bone marrow suppression occurs in chemotherapeutic drugs
• Prolonged paralysis or hyperthermia can be caused by succinylcholine in patients with abnormal pseudocholinesterase isoenzyme
• Extrapyramidal symptoms are associated with antiemetics such as phenothiazine
• There is a small risk of aplastic anemia caused by drugs, such as chloramphenicol, phenylbutazone and quinacrine. These drugs have very specific indications.
• Drugs known to cause megaloblastosis include anticonvulsants, antimetabolites and antituberculous drugs

Some teratogenic drugs include[1,29]
• Alcohol
• Aminopterin
• Coumarin
• Isotretinoin
• Lithium
• Misoprostol
• Penicillamine
• Phenytoin
• Radioactive iodine
• Radiation

Contd...

Contd...

• Retinoic acid
• Diethylstilbestrol
• Tetracycline
• Testosterone-like drugs
• Thalidomide
• Vitamin D
• Valproate

Allergic History[1,11]

- History must include nature of allergen.
- Try to determine type of allergic response.
- Food allergies are due to immunological reactions to glycoproteins and there is a link to genetic predisposition.

Enquire on all risk factors for allergic responses to known or suspected allergens, including previous exposure, parenteral or topical administration, intermittent repeated exposure and a positive family history. Be aware that multiple genes predispose to atopy.

Enquire if one or both parents have allergies both parents have allergies, which can predispose to similar allergies in the child. When there is a history suggestive of an atopic background, be aware that similar allergic diseases may be present within the family.

Enquire about family history if food allergies are suspected. Enquiries regarding food allergens must be asked in detail. **The Cardinal Ten (Historical)** is a tool to utilize. Ask questions in the context of the age of the child because the causes are different as food exposure is different. Be sensible and think through the dietary history when making enquiries.

The triggers of such allergy include:
- Cow's milk
- Peanuts
- Soybean
- Eggs
- Wheat
- Shell fish
- Fish.

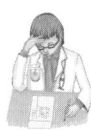

"I believe that I will be able to take an effective history fast enough in a medical emergency. That would require practice, but I have now learnt that an observational history (i.e. observing the young patient and using my other senses such as hearing) while I approach the case for history taking is the best way."

Insect allergies are commonplace in many children. These are usually mild and of little consequence. However, stings by the wasp, or red ant can be more severe.

Localized pain, swelling and redness at the site of sting could last a variable time. Find out how long it lasted, how severe it was and so on.

In atopic eczema, family history of allergies if obtained is a useful adjunct in diagnosis. Other symptoms of allergic diseases like sneezing or wheezing must be enquired.

When many such insects sting, serum sickness reactions including nausea, vomiting, nephrosis, neuritis and vasculitis can result. These are medical emergencies and a collateral history taken from the mother or caregiver must be focused and fast.

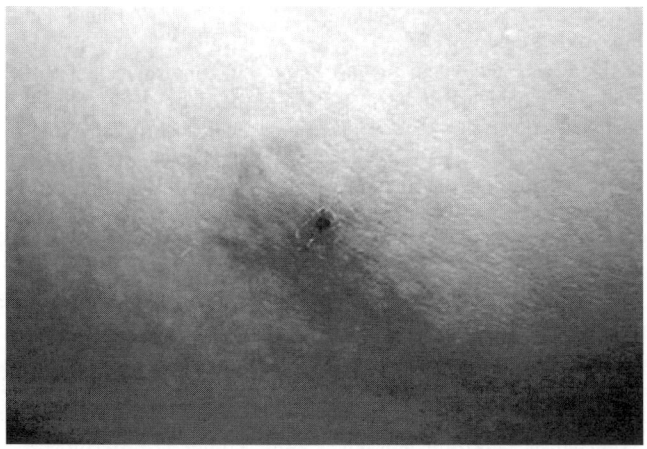

Atopic eczema. Photography Courtesy: Associate Prof Dr Loh Keng Yim, reprint with permission

Travel History[14]

This history is especially important when dealing with communicable diseases or epidemics of such diseases.

Enquire about history of travel including destination and date of travel. Also ask about the travel of family members and relatives who live with the baby. In epidemics, ask for history of specific diseases, whether quarantine was practiced, immunization and other relevant issues. One must know the diseases that are highly endemic in certain regions. This must be asked where relevant.

Respiratory diseases that are linked to air travel include the following:[14]
• Possibility of common colds
• Tuberculosis
• SARS or Severe acute respiratory syndrome (corona virus)
• Influenza
• Meningococcal disease
• Measles
Food-borne linked to air travel and other forms of travel include the following:
• Salmonellosis
• Staphylococcus
• Food poisoning
• Shigellosis
• Cholera, during an epidemic of cholera
• Viral enteritis
Vector-borne diseases linked to travel include the following:
• Malaria
• Dengue
• Yellow fever (No outbreaks since disinfection of aircraft)
Bioterrorism agents include:
• Smallpox (before eradication)

REFERENCES

1. Richard E. Behrman (comps). Robert M Kliegman, Waldo E Nelson, Victor C Vaughan III. (eds). Nelson's Textbook of Pediatrics (14th ed). Philadelphia: WB Saunders; 1992.
2. Carey WB. Normal Individual Differences in Temperament and Behavioral Adjustment, in Developmental-Behavioral Paediatrics (4th ed). Philadelphia, Pennysla: Saunders/Elsevier; 2009.
3. Centre for early childhood mental health consultation. Available at:http://www.ecmhc.org.
4. Drug Allergies—World Allergy Organization. Available at http://www.worldallergy.org/professional/allergic_diseases_center/drugallergy/
5. Sidwell R, Thomson M. Easy Paediatrics. Royal Society of Medicine Press, 2011.
6. Elizabeth KE. Clinical Pediatrics for Undergraduates. India: Jaypee Brothers Medical Publishers (P) Ltd. 2009.
7. Genetic Home Reference. Available at http://ghr.nlm.nih.gov. Accessed in April 2013.
8. Goel KM, Gupta DK. Hutchinson's Paediatrics (1st ed). India: Jaypee Brothers Medical Publishers (P) Ltd; 2009.
9. Hoff E, Naigles L. How children use input in acquiring a lexicon. Child Dev. 2002;73(2):418–33.
10. Illingworth, Ronald S. The Development of the Infant and Young Child Normal and Abnormal (9th ed). London: ELBS; 1989.
11. Johansson SG, Bieber T, Dahl R, Friedmann PS, Lanier BQ, Lockey RF, et al. Revised nomenclature for allergy for global use: Report of the Nomenclature Review Committee of the World Allergy Organization, October 2003. J Allergy Clin Immunol 2004;113:832–36.
12. Kandyce L, Shirley RA, James JC, Halfon Neal Influence of multiple social risks on children's health. Pediatrics. 2008;121(2):337-44.
13. LaDou J. Approach to the diagnosis of occupational illnesses. In: LaDou J (comps) Occupational and environmental medicine. United States of America: Lange McGraw Hill; 1997.
14. Mangili A, Gendreau MA. Transmission of infectious diseases during commercial air travel. Lancet. 2005;365:989-96.
15. Marcdante K, Kliegman RM, Jenson HB, Behrman RE (eds). Nelson's Essentials of Pediatrics (6th ed). Saunders Elsevier; 2010.
16. Mason S, Swash M (eds). Hutchinson's Clinical Methods (17th edn). A Bailllere Tindall book published by Cassell Ltd; 1980.
17. Milner AD, Hull D. Hospital Pediatrics. 3rd edn. ELBS with Churchill Livingstone. 1998.
18. Paediatric feeding and swallowing. Feeding History Questionnaire. The Children's Hospital of Philadelphia. Available at http://www.chop.edu. Accessed in April 2013.
19. Parens E, Johnston J. "Troubled Children: Diagnosing, Treating, and Attending to Context," Special Report, Hastings Center Report. 2011;40(2):S1-S320.
20. Nocturnal enuresis in children. Available at http://www.patient.co.uk/doctor/nocturnal-enuresis-in-children. Access in December 2014.
21. Risley TR, Hart B. Meaningful differences in the everyday experience of young American children. Baltimore: Brookes; 1995. pp. 304.
22. Robinson MJ & Lam LE. Paediatric Problems in tropical countries. Pelanduk Publications (M) Sdn Bhd;1994
23. Salam MT, Li YF, Langholz B, and Gillilan FD. Early-life Environmental Risk Factors for Asthma: Findings from the Children's Health Study. Environ Health Perspect. 2004;112(6):760–65.
24. Stephenson T, Wallace H (eds). Clinical Paediatrics for postgraduate examinations. UK: Churchill Livingstone; 1991.
25. Stern AM and Markel H. The History of Vaccines and Immunization: Familiar Patterns, New Challenges. Health Affairs. 2005;21 (3):611-21.
26. Walker SP, Wachs TD, Gardner JM. Child development: risk factors for adverse outcomes in developing countries. Lancet. 2007;369 (9556):145-57.
27. Thong BYH, Tan TC. Epidemiology and risk factors for drug allergy. Br J Clin Pharmacol. 2011;71(5):684-700.
28. Trotter TL, Martin HM. Family History in Pediatric Primary Care. Pediatrics 2007;120 (suppl. 2) S60 -S65.

29. Chung W. Teratogens and their effects. Available at http://www.columbia.edu/itc/hs/medical/humandev/2004/Chpt23-Teratogens.pdf. Accessed in December 2014.
30. Johnson BE. (1990) Pica. In Walker HK, Hall WD, Hurst JW. (Eds). Clinical Methods: The History, Physical, and Laboratory Examinations. 3rd edition. (Page 709-710) Boston. Butterworths
31. Head Banging and Body Rocking. Available at http://my.clevelandclinic.org/. Accessed in January 2015.
32. Mayo clinic staff. Thumb sucking: Help your child break the habit. Available at http://www.mayoclinic.org. Accessed in February 2015.
33. Breath-Holding Spells. Available at http://www.merckmanuals.com. Accessed in January 2015.
34. The Extended Program for Immunization (EPI) Schedule, Ministry of Health, Malaysia. Accessed in Dec 2014.

The essence of the relevant chapters in the following books have also been numbered as references in this chapter. We recommend for further reading, the rich text in these books for greater integration and deeper understanding.

1. Carey WB. Normal Individual Differences in Temperament and Behavioral Adjustment, in Developmental-Behavioral Paediatrics, 4th edn. Philadelphia, Pennysla: Saunders/Elsevier. 2009.
2. Goel KM, Gupta DK. Hutchinson's Paediatrics, 1st edn. India: Jaypee Brothers Medical Publishers (P) Ltd. 2009.
3. Illingworth, Ronald S. The Development of the Infant and Young Child Normal and Abnormal, 9th edn. London: ELBS. 1989.
4. LaDou J. Approach to the diagnosis of occupational illnesses. In: LaDou J (Eds). Occupational and environmental medicine. United States of America: Lange McGraw Hill. 1997.
5. Marcdante K, Kliegman RM, Jenson HB, Behrman RE (Eds). Nelson's Essentials of Pediatrics, 6th edn. Saunders Elsevier. 2010.
6. Mason S, Swash M (Eds). Hutchinson's Clinical Methods, 17th edn. A Bailllere Tindall book published by Cassell Ltd. 1980.
7. Milner AD, Hull D. Hospital Pediatrics, 3rd edn. ELBS with Churchill Livingstone. 1998.
8. Behrman RE (comps). Kliegman RM, Nelson WE, Vaughan VC III. (Eds). Nelson's Textbook of Pediatrics, 14th edn. Philadelphia: WB Saunders. 1992.
9. Robinson MJ, Lam LE. Paediatric Problems in tropical countries. Pelanduk Publications (M) Sdn Bhd.1994.
10. Sidwell R, Thomson M. Easy Pediatrics. Royal Society of Medicine Press, 2011.
11. Stephenson T, Wallace H (Eds). Clinical Paediatrics for postgraduate examinations. UK: Churchill Livingstone; 1991.

Chapter 6

Clinical Links Relevant to Breastfeeding

REASONS AS TO WHY BREAST MILK PROTECTS FROM DISEASES[1-23]

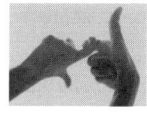

The following are important links to exclusive breastfeeding[1-22]

• The undergraduate pediatric medical student must know about the immunoprotective effects found within breast milk
• The student must be aware that breast milk contains important cells and other constituents for the protection and immunological growth of the infant
• The student must appreciate the growing body of scientific information on the role of breast milk in mucosal protection, which is an early arena of protection in the body's defence system
• Continued and sustained breastfeeding during rotavirus diarrheas and influenza virus infections should be emphasized where the benefits conferred must be understood as these are two examples of diseases of the gastrointestinal and respiratory tracts where mucosal protection is important
• The student must know that this is an expanding and fascinating area of research and must keep himself or herself updated on this vital information regarding the benefits of breast milk conferred to the breastfed child
• With the understanding of the nutritive and immunoprotective potential of breast milk, the student should enrich the details of the feeding history with many important questions on breastfeeding and be able to formulate the differential diagnosis linked to the history of breastfeeding (or the absence of it) and its duration in the individual patient

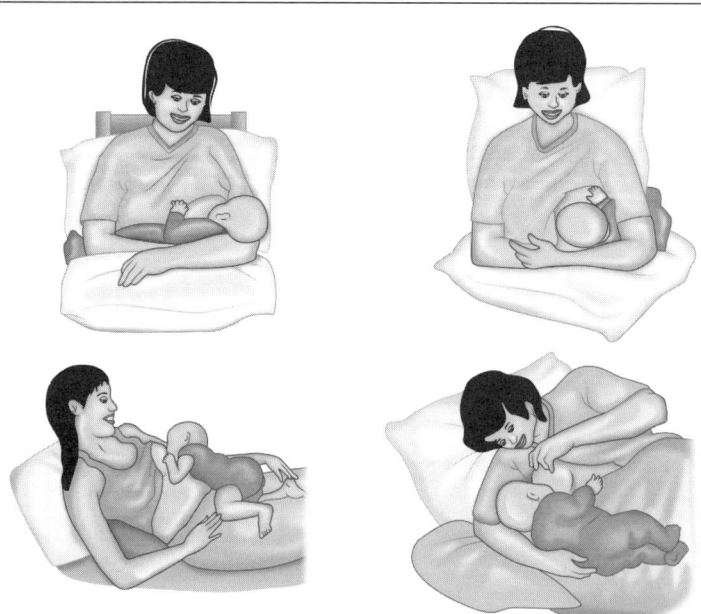

As far as possible do not disrupt exclusive breastfeeding for six months; hence advice wisely and do not unnecessarily discontinue breastfeeding.

Characteristics of Breast Milk

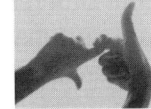

The links to knowing about the characteristics of breast milk include the importance of colostrum in preventing early neonatal infections.[2,14-16]

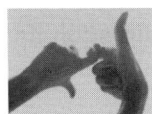

The infant is nursed as per his or her wish on one breast and then fed on the other breast to ensure that both foremilk and the high-calorie hindmilk is obtained.[3,8,17] This is so that the infant achieves satiety and grows optimally. Can you think of other links that could be advantageous to the suckling infant pertaining to the knowledge of the characteristics and "types" of breast milk?

Breastfeeding benefits to the baby and mother[1-22]	• To the baby, it prevents deaths, improves growth and nutritional status, lowers risk of short-term and long-term diseases, reduces obesity risk and enhances cognitive and motor development.[1-3,8,17] • To the mother, it acts as a contraceptive in the early months, lowers risk of breast and ovarian cancers, enhances maternal postpartum recovery and weight loss and tends to positively foster the mother's psychological wellbeing after delivery.[1-3,8,17]
Colostrum[3]	• A pivotal early component of breastmilk in the first few postpartum days • Rich in immunoglobulin especially sIgA (secretory immunoglobulin A) and many anti-infective constituents [4-6] • Caloric density is about 67 calories/100 mL
Transitional milk[3]	• Produced several days postpartum • Greater in volume than colostrum. Increased amounts of water and soluble vitamins. Caloric content higher than in colostrum • Immunoglobulin content is less than colostrum
Mature milk[3]	• Biologically varies between the individual breastfeeding mother herself at different times and between a single breastfeeding mother and another at different phases of lactation[7-12] • Changes in accordance with the baby's nutritional needs • Contains mainly water but its fat content is not constant • Caloric value is about 75 calories/100 mL
Foremilk[3]	• Produced during the initial phase of feeding • More dilute than hindmilk and contains less fat
Hind milk[3]	• Produced in the later part of feeding • More concentrated and contains more fat hence contributes to satiety in the suckling infant • Energy content is high • Because of the above reasons, the mother must empty the breast completely during feeding

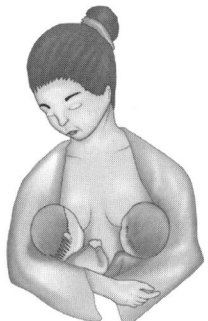

A mother who takes a well-balanced diet can feed her twins effectively.

Good Feeding Positions[4-13]

Good attachment of the baby to the mother's breast is indicated by recognizable features in an infant who suckles. The following suggests good attachment.[4-13]

• Baby's chin is comfortably in contact with mother's breast
• Baby's tongue is beneath the lactiferous sinuses and nipple is against the palate
• Widely opened mouth with lower lip turned outwards
• The areolar is seen mainly above the tongue much more than below it
• Sucking is regular, slow and deep
• Baby's cheeks are full
• Comfortable without pain

Breast Milk Protection against Diseases[8,14-18]

- It is established that exclusive breastfeeding is at least partially protective against some diseases of the newborn and influences the health of the child in later life.
- The incidence of diarrhea, upper and lower respiratory tract infections including otitis media and allergies are less common in the breastfed infant than in the infant fed on artificial formula.
- The advantages of breastfeeding, including the socioeconomic and nutritional advantages that it confers to the suckling infant are well-known. Breast milk in immunological protection is now well recognized.
- Breast milk is globally recognized to be the sole exclusive nutrient for the first six months of the infant's life and as an additional nutrient for a further eighteen months.[4]
- In breast milk, its constituents that are important for immunological protection and to support infant nutrition, provide both short term and lasting benefits. Subjects deprived of breastfeeding in infancy suffer from a higher incidence of some

illnesses which can occur immediately or after some time.[4]
- Breastfeeding programmes potentially positively influence breastfeeding, timely initiation of breastfeeding and continued breastfeeding for up to two years.[7]

Protective Components in Breast Milk

- The newborn infant depends on maternal immunoglobulin via transplacental transfer as means of protection from diseases. The immunity conferred by mothers on their newborn is by placental transfer of immunoglobulin G (IgG) and subsequently by colostral immunoglobulin A (IgA) during breastfeeding.
- The infants' own immune system lacks many vital constituents that are necessary for adequate immunological protection against the diverse types of organisms the infant is challenged with.[14-16]
- Mucosal surfaces are the entry point of many infections of the respiratory tract and the gastrointestinal tract. Here, breastfeeding is pivotal by providing innate substances, cells, and mucosal protection.

Bioactive Factors[8,14-18]

- Components in breast milk that are biologically active, generally do not have any intrinsic immunological memory but contribute towards the protective values of breast milk, such as its nutritive, growth, cognitive, developmental and immune benefits.

Bioactive factors[8,14-18]
• Lysozymes
• Lactoferrin
• Lactoperoxidase
• Free fatty acids
• Folic acid binding protein
• Complement cascade
• Cobalamin binding protein (Vitamin B12)
• Oligosaccharides
• Bifidus factor
• Mucins

Cellular Defenses in Breast Milk

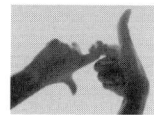

Breast milk contains macrophages, neutrophils and lymphocytes. Ask yourself how these cells function in blood and link your knowledge to how they may function in breast milk.

The quantity of these cells will depend on the timing and duration of lactation. Different types of leukocytes are present in colostrum and mature breast milk with macrophages forming more than half of total breast milk cells, neutrophils, a third and lymphocytes, 5–10%. Viable breast milk leukocytes from the feces of suckling infants remain antigenically intact and importantly reflect resistance to digestion and mucosal protection in breast milk.[14]

Appreciate that a drop of breast milk carefully examined under the microscope has:

• Macrophages
• Neutrophils
• Lymphocytes

Breast Milk can Modulate Immune Cells and Reduce Allergies[8,14-18]

- The macrophages in breast milk regulate lymphocytes through their activation markers.[14]

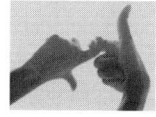

Breast milk contains B lymphocytes for humoral protection and T lymphocytes for cell-mediated protection.[14-16]

Breast Milk Protects against Atopy and Allergy[8,14-18,21]

- The incidence of eczema in children is reduced if they are breastfed, and a clear relationship exists between artificial cow's milk based formula feeding and cow's milk allergy in infancy, a possible reduced number of T cells with a spectrum of problems with immune regulatory function, and increased IgE levels in such infants.[14-16]
- Breast milk has proteins that are species specific. Exclusive breastfeeding delays the introduction of foreign proteins, hence, delays untoward allergic responses.

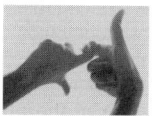

Link the history of atopy to the history of feeding, the family history, the drug history and the social and environmental history.

Neutrophils in Breast Milk are Immunocompetent [14,17,18]

- Neutrophils in breast milk have special features that augment immunological activity and express various markers such as an impressive number of CD11b and lower levels of L selectin.

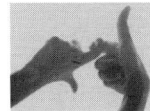

Immunological memory is important in preventing a reinfection. It is a method of lasting protection offered by immunization. Link this knowledge to the history of breastfeeding.

The Much Needed Immunological Memory in Breast Milk[14-16,19,20]

- Breast milk lymphocytes have greater numbers of CD8+ expressed receptors. CD4+ cells with specific surface markers are found in human milk indicating the presence of active immunological memory.

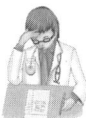

It is amazing that breast milk has so much immunological potential.

Breast milk cells[14-16,19,20]	Functions[14-16,19,20]
• Macrophages	• Immunocompetent with phagocytic and immunoregulatory functions
• Neutrophils	• Immunocompetent with prior activation before secretion into breast milk
• Lymphocytes	• Immunocompetent with production of immunoglobulins and cytokines • Immunological memory

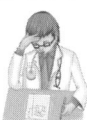

So it is the secretory piece that prevents the vital secretory immunoglobulin A (sIgA) from gastric and enzymatic degradation in the infant's gastrointestinal tract. It is interesting how nature nurtures the essentials for survival!

Protection Conferred via Antibodies[14-16,19,20,21]

- Secretory immunoglobulin A (IgA) is the vital immunoglobulin in mucosal protection.
- The secretory piece (SC) confers increased resistance to enzymatic degradation.
- There are two forms of IgA:
  - IgA1 mainly in the serum and the secretions produced above the diaphragm
  - IgA2 that forms most of the IgA within the lumen of the gastrointestinal tract.[14,21]
- Abundant IgA are produced at the mucosal surfaces of the respiratory and gastrointestinal tract and other epithelial layers.
- Breastfeeding enhances mucosal immunity by quantitatively and qualitatively augmenting IgA at mucosal surfaces.
- The prime, early defense aims to prevent the microbes from binding to the mucosae. Binding to the mucosae is an important step for penetration of microbes into the body.
- In order to prevent this at mucosal surfaces in the body, in addition to the innate mechanism of mucus production, immunoglobulin A is manufactured by lymphoid aggregates, both organized (adenoids, tonsils, Peyer's patches) and less organized (urogenital tract, lung, and lamina propria) which together form the mucosal-associated lymphoid tissue (MALT).[14,21]
- The binding of the pathogens to the mucosae, as an important early step of microbial pathogenesis, is greatly reduced when it is covered by sIgA.

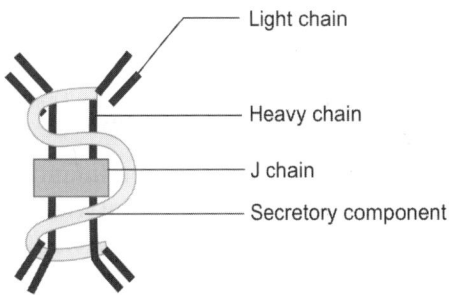

The most important immunoglobulin in breast milk is sIgA (molecular structure)[14,21]

The lactating mammary gland which provides important childhood protection is a part of mucosal immunity and the mucosa associated lymphoid system or MALT [14-16]

- The mother's gut when sensitized by a foreign antigen will produce specific sIgA.
- Activated lymphocytes within the gut-associated lymphoid tissue (GALT) produce sensitized T cells in the MALT. As the lactating mammary gland is part of the MALT, the link between the maternal gut and the lactating mammary gland or the enteromammary axis will ensure that the breastfeeding infant is provided specific protection via specific sIgA.

100 *The Link*: Pediatric History-Taking and Physical Examination

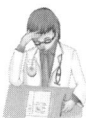

Mucosal-associated lymphoid tissue (MALT) seems "separate" from the systemic lymphoid system, yet, so interlinked in physiological processes.

MALT includes: [14,21]

Lymphoid tissue[14,21]	Representations[14,21]
• NALT	• Nasopharyngeal-associated lymphoid tissue • Palatine tonsils and adenoids
• BALT	• Bronchial and tracheal-associated lymphoid tissue
• LALT	• Larynx-associated lymphoid tissue
• GALT	• Gut-associated lymphoid tissue
• SALT	• Skin-associated lymphoid tissue
• CALT	• Conjunctiva-associated lymphoid tissue
• VALT	• Vulvo-vaginal-associated lymphoid tissue
• Lactating mammary gland and products of lactation	• Enteromammary axis and others

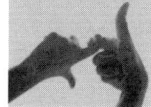

Mucosal protection is an extremely relevant route of infant protection through breastfeeding.

This further emphasizes that the infant's mucosae are protected in the breastfed infant via the enteromammary axis which links the mother's gut to the lactating mammary gland. Apart from that, adaptive immunological memory is also found in breast milk.

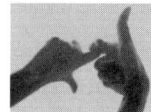

Link breastfeeding to the history of protection from respiratory infections.

Breast Milk and Transplacental Protection[14-16,19,20,21]

- Maternal antibodies delivered to the fetus transplacentally, are also due to the mother's immunological exposure and are useful to the immature immune system of the infant.
- The placental receptor specificity preferably transfers IgG which offers short-term protection to the neonate.
- One of the functions of IgG antibodies passively transferred from mother to fetus includes active protective priming of the immune system of the neonate.
- The neonatal immune system is directed by immune exposure via maternal flora that is encountered during a vaginal delivery.
- Although the fetal immune system is immature, there are some fetal immune responses that help the fetus in immunological protection. Such an example is its ability to mount immune responses via anti-immunoglobulins. Protection is also transferred via anti-idiotypic antibodies by the mother to the fetus and the infant to stimulate the naïve immune system. Anti-idiotypic antibodies transferred through the placenta or via breast milk have antiviral potential.[16]

Breast Milk Protection against the Influenza Virus[14-16,19,20,21]

- IgA is important to protect against respiratory tract illnesses such as defense against the influenza virus in the upper respiratory tract. Nasopharyngeal-associated lymphoid tissue (NALT) produces anti-influenza virus responses.[16]
- The cells of the NALT produce specific antibodies and are triggered when there is maternal exposure to the influenza virus. This in turn generates influenza-specific antibodies which pass through the mother's breast milk.[16]
- When a mother has been exposed to the influenza virus, her influenza-specific antibodies are transferred to the infant through breast milk and can be crucial in protecting the infant. The local immunity is not affected by these antibodies.[16]

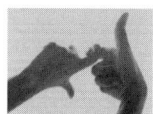

Breastfeeding has proven benefits for protection against gastrointestinal infections. Innate protection by breast milk factors and adaptive protection via maternal exposure are transferred to the suckling infant. Interestingly, the microflora of the breastfed infant's gut is different from that of the formula fed infant and these beneficial microflora are protective.

Breast Milk and Rotavirus Diarrheas[2,14-16,19-22]

- Viral neutralization by antibodies in breast milk and transplacental antibodies can confer protection against the commonest causes of childhood diarrheas.

- Several studies have indicated that the duration of breastfeeding was important in protection against rotavirus (Yap et al., 1984)[22] with noted ethnic differences.
- Serotype specific antirotaviral activity expressed in the milk of some mothers were mainly antibody-mediated (Bell et al., 1988).[2]
- Antigen-antibody mediated neutralization renders these viruses incapable of producing significant clinical disease.
- Rotavirus strains that infect neonates may be different from the strains in the community. During breastfeeding, the lactating mother who encounters pathogens such as unusual strains of the rotaviruses actively produces sIgA in the mammary gland via the enteromammary axis already described. This is how breast milk can dynamically protect the infant when the protection is most needed.

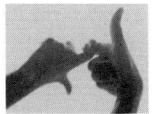

Link the overall breastfeeding history, past history of illnesses and maternal postpartum history to breastfeeding. Remember that there is reason to believe that the "quality" of maternal milk and its protective potential is optimal when the breastfeeding mother is relaxed and happy.

Cytokines in Breast Milk Confer Protection to Infants[14-16,19-22]

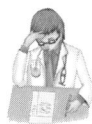

So in breast milk there is innate protection, specific protection and a link between both for enhanced protective potential. There is certainly a strong case to support and counsel exclusive and continued breast-feeding in every child.

Actions of Cytokines[2,8-11,14-17,20]

Common benefits of cytokines[2,8-11,14-17,20]	Benefits and maternal features[2,8-11,14-17,20]	Benefits in the child[2,8-11,14-17,20]
For many useful clinical responses, it is worthwhile to know that breast milk cytokines are links between innate and adaptive immunity	Respond appropriately to the breastfeeding mother's exposure to antigens. Levels in the individual mother can vary with stress, mood, anxiety and depression	There is a basal cytokine level in colostrum and unprimed milk
Multipotent polypeptides that function in an autocrine or paracrine manner via specific receptors	The breast associated lymphoid tissues of the MALT can produce important antibodies that enter breast milk	Useful soluble receptors in breast milk that augment its biological activity
Complex immunomodulatory potential can protect against some viruses	Maternal exposure can direct and influence crucial immune mediators	Exerts effects on the nasopharyngeal associated lymphoid tissue (NALT) and the gut-associated lymphoid tissue (GALT) of the newborn
For protection, it is useful to realize that cytokines influence epithelial barrier integrity (esp. IL-10 and IFN-γ) while TGF alpha and epidermal growth factor are important for the development of epithelium		It is clinically useful to understand that cytokines including interleukins, interferon gamma are found adequately in breast milk. A spectrum of growth factors at least partially make up for the immune deficiency in neonates, especially in preterm infants
Epithelial barrier integrity is influenced by specific cytokines such as IL-10 and IFN-α		Intestinal epithelial barrier integrity can be enhanced by the action of specific cytokines, such as IL-10 and IFN-γ

102 *The Link*: Pediatric History-Taking and Physical Examination

Breastfeeding Confers Long-term Protection Against Some Diseases[2,8-11,14-17,20-22]

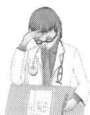

Although some long-term benefits of breastfeeding are not fully proven, there is so much to think about and link in this vast ocean of knowledge in the protection of breast milk.

- Although the exact mechanisms of disease are controversial in diseases such as insulin dependent diabetes mellitus (IDDM), Crohn's disease, other autoimmune diseases, and certain malignancies breastfeeding may have long-term protective effects.[4]
- Immunological memory in breast milk may contribute to its capacity for long-term protection.
- Some constituents of breast milk also contribute to tumor surveillance, e.g. Human Alpha-lactalbumin Made LEthal to Tumor cells (HAMLET).
- Studies indicate that the immune responses in infants towards certain vaccinations like the *Haemophilus influenzae* type b-tetanus toxoid conjugate vaccine[18] (HIB) and BCG vaccine responses are found to be enhanced.[12]

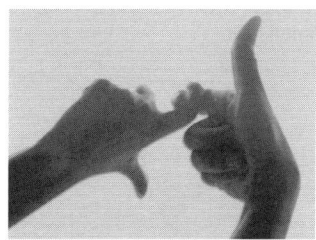 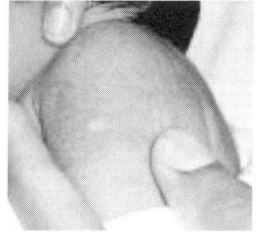

Breastfeeding enhances the effect of some vaccinations. Photograph courtesy: Dr Loh Keng Yin, Associate Professor, reprint with permission.

BREASTFEEDING HISTORY

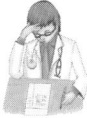

The breastfeeding history is an important component in the pediatric nutritional history which will influence the differential diagnosis to be considered.

This is part of the dietary and feeding history but is clarified further in this chapter as breastfeeding confers many immediate and some long-term health benefits to the child.

> **Learning Points**
> - A part of the dietary and feeding history. The influence of maternal diet on breast milk is not fully elucidated in the literature; hence, a good history may help in some clarification of uncertain areas. This topic in the pediatric history requires specific and in depth knowledge of the constituents in breast milk.
> - Allude to the following questions when necessary.

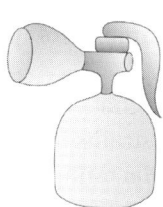

Breast pumps to express breast milk

Expressed breast milk (EBM) can be given if the mother is unable to directly breastfeed her child. If the child is premature or too ill to suck, EBM should be given through the nasogastric tube.	EBM can be stored in the fridge for up to 5 days (at 4°C or at lower temperatures). In the freezer, it lasts for up to 6 months.

Historical questions in breastfeeding and mixed feeding

Important reflections in the history include some of the following:
• How long was much breastfeeding given?
• Was it given exclusively?
• Was it given with artificial formula?
• Was the baby given stored breast milk when the mother went to work?
• Did the child suffer any problems like vomiting, diarrhea, skin rashes, colic, cough with phlegm, wheezing or any other abnormal symptom(s) after the introduction of artificial formula?
• Why did the mother have to introduce artificial formula?
• Did the mother get family support for her breastfeeding practices?
• What was the mother's diet like during breastfeeding?
• What was her state of health during breastfeeding?
• Was she on any form of medication?
• If so, explore type(s) of medicines and why?
• Was she on traditional medication?
• What sort of traditional medicines or herbs was she on, why and for how long?
• Did the child have prolonged jaundice or any other problem(s)?
• If child was never breastfed or if breastfeeding was stopped earlier than six months, explore reason(s) why. Enquire on the mother's knowledge, understanding and beliefs about breastfeeding.

There are not many contraindications to breastfeeding. Some considerations and contraindications (many are relative contraindications) for the mother and child include the following:

Maternal considerations and contraindications[1,4,10,17,19]	Child considerations and contraindications[1,4,10,17,19]
• Active tuberculosis (TB) in mother. Treat mother with active TB with anti-TB medication for 2 weeks and give TB prophylaxis to the infant. During these 2 weeks, breastfeeding should not be given.	• Galactosemia (Contraindicated)
• Maternal HIV (Contraindicated in many parts of the world)	• Phenylketonuria (May consider partial breastfeeding)
• HTLV-1 • HTLV-2 (contraindicated) • Active maternal herpes lesions in the breast. Interrupt breastfeeding until lesions are healed or crusted. Practice good hand hygiene	
• Varicella Zoster • Continue breastfeeding; for perinatal infection, give Varicella Zoster Immunoglobulin (VZIg); for postpartum, give Varicella Zoster Immunoglobulin (VZIg)	
• Mastitis • Discard pus from the infected breast and continue breastfeeding.	
• Selected medications transmitted through the breast milk which could be harmful to the baby[19] **High-dose metronidazole:** Stop breastfeeding for 12 h to 24 h to allow excretion of dose **Chloramphenicol:** Can potentially cause unpredictable or idiosyncratic bone marrow suppression **Trimethoprim/ sulfamethoxazole, sulfisoxazole, dapsone:** These medications must be used with extreme care and vigilance if the breastfeeding infant has jaundice or G6PD deficiency, and also if ill, stressed or premature **Primaquine, quinine:** Contraindicated during breastfeeding if mother or baby has Glucose 6-phosphate dehydrogenase (G6PD) deficiency	

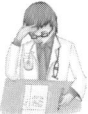

"I must know about breast milk acting as a vehicle for the transmission of a few diseases. In these cases, breastfeeding is contraindicated. But, I must look at many other factors like the stage of such maternal diseases, the treatment of the mother, socioeconomic factors and many more in disallowing breastfeeding. In such situations, do the risks of breastfeeding outweigh its many benefits? ... this is the question I must ask myself."

Viruses found in breast milk[17,23]

• Human immunodeficiency virus (HIV)
• Moloney murine leukemia virus (MMLV)
• Sarcoma virus
• Mammary tumor virus
• Cytomegalovirus
• Rubella
• Herpes simplex
• Hepatitis B in the event of active maternal hepatitis B infection
• Epstein-Barr virus
• Human herpesvirus 6 (HHV 6)
• Hepatitis C

Some drugs to avoid during breastfeeding include:
(also refer databases with maternal drug information which are updated from time-to-time)[1,10,19]

What maternal diseases will require the usage of such medication? Use the **The Cardinal Ten** to ask about such conditions where indicated
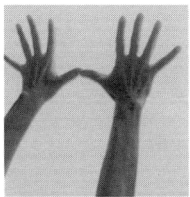
Nonsteroidal anti-inflammatory drugs (NSAIDs)
• Aspirin
Tetracyclines
• Minocycline
• Tetracycline
• Fluoroquinolones
Anticonvulsants
• Lamotrigine
• Phenobarbitone
Cardiovascular
• Amiodarone

Contd...

Contd...

• Atenolol
Antifungals
• Fluconazole
Radioactive isotope—discontinue breastfeeding until the milk is clear of radioactivity
Chemotherapy agents—specific agents, discontinue breastfeeding until the milk is clear of these agents
Social drugs
• Nicotine
• Cannabis
• Ethanol
• Excessive caffeine
Metronidazole – discontinue breastfeeding until at least 12-24 hours after cessation of medication
In G6PD deficiency, breastfeeding mothers should avoid the following:
• Sulfasalazine
• Nitrofurantoin
• Sulfamethaxazole and trimethoprim (Bactrim)
• Antimalarials—Primaquine and Quinine
• Herbs the constituents of which are unknown (e.g. may contain salicylate)

Drug Therapy of the Lactating Mother[1,10,19]

As a general practitioner, it is important to know some basic principles of prescribing drugs to a mother who is breastfeeding. Many drugs are found in breast milk but not all are documented to be harmful.

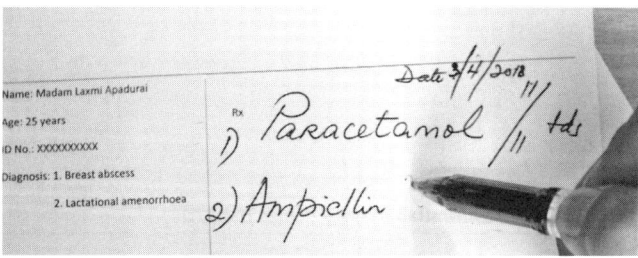

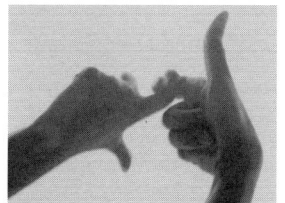

When prescribing drugs to the lactating mother think about the following by linking to your knowledge of basic pharmacology.

Appreciate how the interactions of a drug in the body in terms of its absorption, distribution, metabolism, and excretion in clinical pharmacokinetics can be applied to the principles of safe and effective therapeutic management of drugs in a lactating mother and her infant.

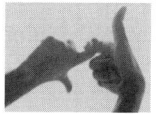

In clinical practice think of links comprising simple clinical questions you must consider.

Considerations on drug usage[1,10,19]
• How important is the drug?
• Can the mother do without the drug?
• Is there specific data available on drug use in a lactating mother?
• Is the drug chosen the safest option available?
• What are the pharmacokinetics of the drug?
• Is the dosage correct, and is it the minimum effective dose?
• Is there a possibility that a drug that has to be used for the mother may present a risk to the infant?
• Are there specific factors in the infant that require extra caution when using the drug? An example is prematurity. If so consider measurement of blood concentrations in the nursing infant.

• While you must exercise caution in prescribing a drug to a nursing mother, thoughtful selection of medications can usually allow nursing to continue without fear or interruption
• While it is well known that teratogenic effects of a minority of drugs taken during pregnancy exist, be aware that on the other hand, the majority of maternal medications are safe during breastfeeding
• The mother ultimately decides on whether to continue nursing and to comply with prescribed medications; therefore, she should be educated regarding the potential risks of nursing while taking a specific medication
• She should also be advised on the potential impact that interruption of lactation can have on herself and her baby.

REFERENCES

1. Alison E Dillon, Carol L Wagner, Donald Wiest, Roger B Newman. Drug therapy in the nursing mother. Obstetrics and Gynecology Clinics of North America. Vol. 24(3):675-96.
2. Bell LM, Clark HF, Offit PA, Slight PH, Arbeter AM, Plotkin SA. Rotavirus Serotype—Specific Neutralizing Activity in Human Milk Am J Dis Child. 1988;142:275-78.
3. Definitions of common breastfeeding terms. Available at www.007b.com/breastfeeding_terms.php.
4. Edmond, K, et al. Delayed Breastfeeding Initiation Increases Risk of Neonatal Mortality. Pediatrics. 2006 Mar;117(3):e380-6.

5. Elizabeth KE. Clinical Pediatrics for Undergraduates. New Delhi: Jaypee Brothers Medical Publishers (P) Ltd.; 2009.
6. Goel KM, Gupta DK. Hutchinson's Pediatrics, 1st edn, India: Jaypee Brothers Medical Publishers (P) Ltd; 2009.
7. Fatimah S, Siti Saadiah HN, Tahir A, Hussain Imam MI, Ahmad Faudzi Y. Breastfeeding in Malaysia: Results of the Third National Health and Morbidity Survey (NHMS III) 2006. Mal J. Nutr 2010;16(2):195-206.
8. Marcdante K, Kliegman RM, Jenson HB, Behrman RE (eds). Nelson's Essentials of Pediatrics (6th ed). Saunders Elsevier; 2010.
9. Mason S, Swash M (eds). Hutchinson's Clinical Methods (17th edn). A Baillere Tindall book published by Cassell Ltd; 1980.
10. Maternal Infectious Diseases, Antimicrobial Therapy or Immunizations: Very Few Contraindications to Breastfeeding. Canadian Paediatric Society. Can J Infect Dis Med Microbiol. 2006 Sep-Oct;17(5):270-2.
11. Milner AD, Hull D. Hospital Pediatrics. 3rd edn. ELBS with Churchill Livingstone. 1998.
12. Pabst HF, Godel J, Grace M, et al. Effect of breastfeeding on immune response to BCG vaccination. Lancet; 1989;1(8633):295-7.
13. Phua Kong Boo, Janil Puthucheary, Tan Cheng Lim, Tan Ten Hong. The Baby Bear Book. A Practical Guide on Pediatrics. 2008.
14. Prameela KK, Mohamed AEK. Breast milk immunoprotection and the Common Mucosal Immune System. Review. Mal J Nutr. 2010;16(1):1-11.
15. Prameela KK, Vijaya LR. The importance of breastfeeding in rotaviral Diarrheas. Mal J Nutr 2012;18(1):103-11.
16. Prameela KK. Breastfeeding -Anti-viral Potential and Relevance to the Influenza Virus. Pandemic Med J. Malaysia 2011;660.
17. Behrman RE (comps), Kliegman RM, Nelson WE, Vaughan VC III. Nelson's Textbook of Pediatrics, 14th Edn. Philadelphia: WB Saunders;1992.
18. Silfverdal SA, Ekholm L and Bodin L. Breastfeeding enhances the antibody response to Hib and Pneumococcal serotype 6B and 14 after vaccination with conjugate vaccines. Vaccine. 2007;25(8):1497-502.
19. The Transfer of Drugs and Other Chemicals into Human Milk. Pediatrics 2001;108 (3):776-89.
20. Stephenson T, Wallace H (eds). Clinical Paediatrics for Postgraduate Examinations. UK: Churchill Livingstone; 1991.
21. Woof JM, Kerr MA. The function of immunoglobulin A in immunity. J Pathol. 2007;208(2):270-82. Review.
22. Yap KL, Sabil D, Muthu PA. Human Rotavirus Infection in Malaysia. A Hospital-based Study of Rotavirus in Children with Acute Gastroenteritis J Tropic Pedia. 1984;30:131-5.
23. Michie CA. Breast feeding and the risks of viral transmission. Arch Dis Child. 2001;84:381-2.

The essence of the relevant chapters in the following books and articles in the stated journals have also been numbered as references in this chapter. We recommend for further reading, the rich text in these books and journals for greater integration and deeper understanding.

1. Goel KM, Gupta DK. Hutchinson's Pediatrics, 1st edn, Jaypee Brothers Medical Publishers (P) Ltd, India 2009.
2. Marcdante K, Kliegman RM, Jenson HB, Behrman RE (Eds). Nelson's Essentials of Pediatrics, 6th edn. Saunders Elsevier. 2010.
3. Mason S, Swash M (Eds). Hutchinson's Clinical Methods, 17th Edn. A Baillere Tindall book published by Cassell Ltd; 1980.
4. Milner AD, Hull D. Hospital Pediatrics. 3rd Edn. ELBS with Churchill Livingstone. 1998.
5. Phua Kong Boo, Janil Puthucheary, Tan Cheng Lim, Tan Ten Hong. The Baby Bear Book. A Practical Guide on Pediatrics. 2008.
6. Behrman RE (comps), Kliegman RM, Nelson WE, Vaughan VC III. Nelson's Textbook of Pediatrics, 14th edn. Philadelphia: WB Saunders.1992.
7. Stephenson T, Wallace H (Eds). Clinical Paediatrics for Postgraduate Examinations. UK: Churchill Livingstone.1991.
8. Prameela KK, Mohamed AEK. Breast milk immunoprotection and the Common Mucosal Immune System. Review. Mal J Nutr. 2010;16(1):1-11.
9. Prameela KK, Vijaya LR. The importance of breastfeeding in rotaviral Diarrheas. Mal J Nutr 2012;18(1):103-11.
10. Prameela KK. Breastfeeding—Anti-viral Potential and Relevance to the Influenza Virus Pandemic Med J. Malaysia. 2011;660.

Chapter 7

Immunization

INTRODUCTION[1-25]

Sanitation and immunization are the two most effective methods of reducing morbidity and mortality due to infections. Immunization is one of the single most useful preventive method in today's healthcare industry. They either totally prevent some important diseases which is primary prevention, or substantially reduce severity.[1-9]

In 1796, it was demonstrated by Jenner that when he inoculated the vesicular fluid from cowpox lesions into the skin of susceptible individuals, they were conferred smallpox protection, and that noted association of the two diseases marked the beginning of the era of immunization. The first ever vaccine was developed in 1796 for smallpox.[10]

Today, modern vaccines are relatively safe and effective.

In many countries, vaccinations recommended during childhood are available in government health clinics, private clinics and hospitals and are associated to school entry where reporting of vaccination status is required. If there is a missed dose, parents are encouraged to attend the nearest government clinic to receive the catch up doses. Children who lag behind in immunization should receive catch up immunizations as fast as possible.

Over the years, immunization programs have successfully prevented the spread of vaccine preventable diseases. This is evidenced by the few vaccine preventable diseases or the total absence of some of them. Vaccination also indirectly protects the community from many infectious diseases (Chang HG et al, 2008).[6] As vaccine preventable diseases become less common, the adverse effects of vaccines may take relatively greater importance.

Therefore, since disease and their complications may produce increased morbidity and even mortality compared to the adverse effects of vaccination, we have to educate the public at large, especially parents or caregivers on the benefits of vaccination. Effective communication will encourage and educate parents to get their children immunized.

It is our responsibility to find out the immunization status of our patient and offer any vaccination that have been missed or that are due. The missed vaccinations doses must be given at the earliest opportunity.

It is advisable to address the parents' concerns while emphasizing the benefits as well as the risks involved with not vaccinating their children and reassuring parents about the safety of vaccines.

IMMUNIZING AGENTS[10]

These agents include preparations containing antibodies, vaccines and toxoids from human or animal donors.

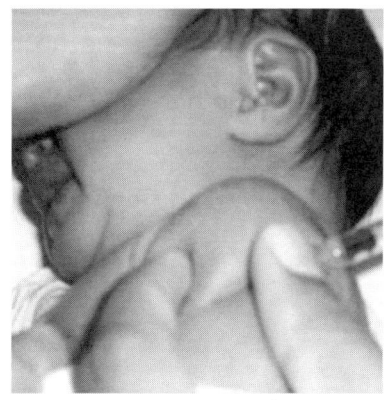

Photograph courtesy: Dr Loh Keng Yin, Associate Professor, reprint with permission

The important definitions are as follows:

Definitions of vaccine, toxoid, immunoglobulin and specific immunoglobulin[7,10-18]	
Vaccine	• A suspension of killed or live attenuated microorganisms or fractions of the microorganisms, naturally produced or artificially engineered, given to a subject to induce immunity
Toxoid	• A bacterial toxin modified and rendered nontoxic but has the potential to encourage the formation of antitoxin
Immunoglobulin	• A sterile solution containing antibodies. • Given intramuscularly. • Primarily indicated for protection of immunodeficient patients and for passive immunization, especially after exposure. For example, measles and hepatitis A • Intravenous immunoglobulin (IVIg) is indicated for replacement therapy in immunoglobulin G (IgG) deficiency, treatment of Kawasaki disease (in order to prevent cardiac involvement), and idiopathic thrombocytopenic purpura (ITP)
Specific immunoglobulin	• Special preparations obtained from donor pools. It has high antibody content, e.g. hepatitis B immune globulin (HBIG)

ACTIVE AND PASSIVE IMMUNIZATION

Immunization artificially produces or stimulates immunity or produces protection from disease either actively or passively.

Active immunization is said to occur when toxoids or vaccines given, produce antibodies or cell-mediated immunity or both, which protect against the infectious agent.

Passive immunization occurs by providing temporary protection through the administration of exogenous antibody, such as transplacental transfer of antibodies to the fetus, which may protect the individual against the disease in the initial 6 months of life or via the injection of immunoglobulins for specific preventive purposes. However, the protection is short-lived.

VACCINES AND VACCINATION

A vaccine is an immune biological product and its antigenicity is such that it confers desired protection against a specific disease without it in itself causing the disease. Vaccination is a procedure of administering an antigen to stimulate the immune response through the route of active immunization and is aimed at producing specific protection against a given disease.

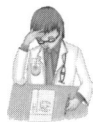

Innate protection is important as it is the first line of defense. It also provides vital defenses until the body mounts more specific defenses. The specific defenses are long lasting and more targeted.

How do innate (inherent) and adaptive (acquired) immunity differ?[7,10,19]	
Adaptive immunity[7,10,19]	*Innate Immunity[7,10,19]*
• Known as antigen-specific immunity	• Is non-specific immunity
• Protection provided by vaccination	• Protection at the first line of defense or portal of entry of the pathogen.
• More complex than the innate response	• Consists of non-specific cells and host defense mechanisms
• Includes a "memory" that makes future responses against a specific antigen more efficient	• Generic recognition of pathogens
• First it recognizes an antigen, then creates an armamentarium of immune cells specifically designed to attack that antigen hence its specificity	• Lasting protective immunity not conferred

108 The Link: Pediatric History-Taking and Physical Examination

Basic mechanisms of innate and adaptive immunity[2,3,5,7,10]

The criteria when choosing the antigenic material from the particular pathogen for vaccine preparation are as follows:
- Safe to administer
- Induces the desired type of immunity
- Affordable by the target population.

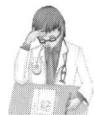

Children who are not immunized are at risk for many vaccine preventable diseases. The benefits of vaccination clearly outweigh the risks.

Reasons for not Immunizing Children

- Healthcare providers miss the opportunity to vaccinate due to lack of knowledge, lack of motivation or other reasons.
- Forgetful caregivers (e.g. parents or grandparents).
- Parents with conflicting beliefs against vaccination due to misguided information. Others oppose vaccination with complete knowledge. They are known as conscientious objectors.

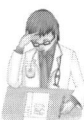

Effective counseling on all available vaccines at every given opportunity is one way to overcome misconceptions; proper education to all healthcare workers is another.[19,20]

Frequently Encountered Wrong Beliefs Regarding Vaccinations in Some Parts of the World

- Parents believe that vaccination may bring danger to their child
- Natural immunity via disease is best
- Safe and effective complementary and alternative pathways of treatment

Ensuring safe and efficient vaccines[2,5,11,12]	
Areas influencing safety and efficacy of vaccines	*Solutions*
Cold chain	Vaccines must be kept in functioning refrigerators designed for vaccine storage in line with the manufacturers' instructions. Do not freeze vaccines. Refrain from using a vaccine if in doubt of its cold chain storage
Prevent immunization errors	Constant effective monitoring of the cold chain reduces efficacy
Observation after vaccination	Individuals receiving vaccination are advised to stay in the health facility for a minimum of 15 minutes. Children can play in the play area while they are observed. Anaphylaxis, though rare, potentially occurs with any vaccine. Ensure intramuscular adrenaline is available for resuscitation

Vaccination Techniques[19]

Before Immunization

- Minimize physical and emotional distress when giving vaccines as injections.

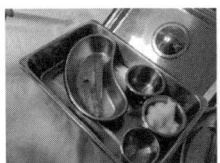 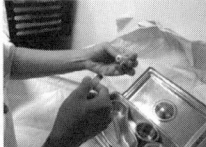 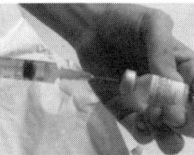

Preparation for vaccination.

During Immunization[19]

Use pain-relieving techniques appropriate for age, such as the following:

- Stress reducing techniques: Passive (watching a robotic toy in motion) or active (building a castle using Lego)
- Give fun toys or colorful stickers to keep the child happy
- Pharmacological agents may be used to reduce or stop pain due to immunization (e.g. oral sucrose for infants, topical anesthetic agents, etc.)
- For every injection, it is mandatory to use a fresh new needle and syringe
  - Injections given subcutaneously or intradermally as well as those used in premature children less than 2 months should be of small gauge.
- When giving intramuscular injections deep into the muscle, ensure that the needle is angled at 90°. For infants (≤12 months of age), give into the anterolateral thigh pointing towards the knee. For toddlers and children aged ≥12 months of age, give an intramuscular injection into the deltoid pointing it to the shoulder
- If many vaccines have to be given: 2 vaccinations may be given in one limb at a distance of at least 25 mm. Another method is to give one vaccine in each limb.

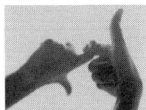

Link the nature of the vaccine to the dosage schedule when counseling parents.

Live vaccines versus killed vaccines[7,10,19]

Live vaccines[10]	Killed vaccines[10]
Confer life-long protection	Do not induce permanent immunity with one dose
Examples[6] BCG Measles Mumps Rubella Oral polio Rotavirus Nasal influenza	**Examples[6]** Diphtheria Tetanus Rabies Typhoid
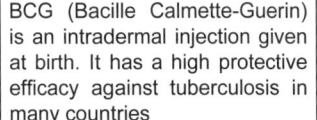 *To know the diseases that vaccines prevent, the incubation period of the disease and the nature of vaccines used for specific diseases is useful. The vaccine schedule, contraindications and temporal side effects depend on these facts.*	Repeated vaccination and subsequent boosters necessary to develop and maintain high levels of antibody
BCG (Bacille Calmette-Guerin) is an intradermal injection given at birth. It has a high protective efficacy against tuberculosis in many countries	Exceptions are as follows: - Hepatitis B vaccine (has long-term immunologic memory, for at least 10 years post vaccination)

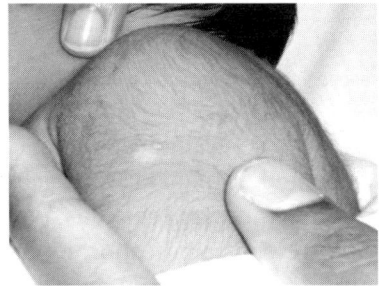

Photograph courtesy: Dr Loh Keng Yin, Associate Professor, reprint with permission.

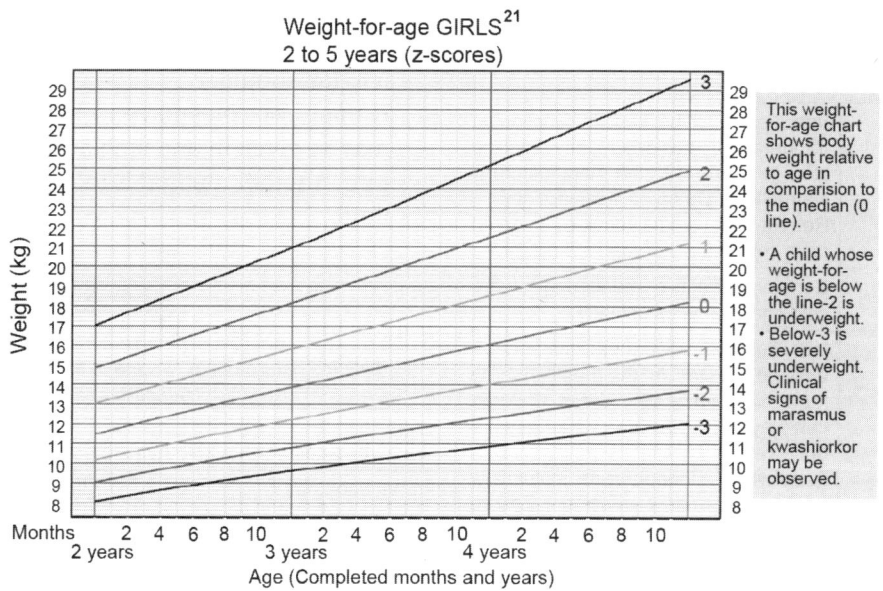

Growth must be measured and plotted at each vaccination visit.[21]

When vaccinating children, explain to the mother the following[7,10,19]

- The disease(s) to be prevented
- The nature of vaccine
- The number of doses needed to complete the schedule
- The anticipated common adverse side effects and how to handle them
- Due date for next immunization
- Advice the mother and baby to wait for about 15 minutes or so before leaving the clinic to be able to look out for adverse reactions.

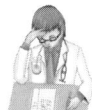

Contraindications to vaccination are very few.

- Individuals with contraindication for vaccination must be exempted from taking the vaccine to avoid unwanted serious adverse reactions.[1]
- When a relative contraindication or precaution is present, further assessment on a case to case basis and a risk-benefit analysis may be necessary.

Avoid false contraindications to vaccination[1,7,10,19]
Vaccination must be given despite the following circumstances:
• Have minor infections without fever or systemic upset
• A low grade fever (<38.5°C) with or without an upper respiratory illness
• Post-vaccination adverse effects in members of the family
• Seizures in the family
• Past history of pertussis-like illness, measles and rubella or mumps infection
• Prematurity (vaccination should not be postponed)
• Have an established or nonprogressive neurological condition such as cerebral palsy or Down syndrome
• Contact with communicable or infectious diseases
• Recovering from an infection
• Suffering from a spectrum of allergies, e.g. bronchial asthma or atopic eczema
• Being treated with antibiotics
• On steriod inhalers or topical steroid therapy
• A healthy person who is thin
• An immediate past history of surgery or scheduled for surgery
• Exclusively breastfeeding
• The mother is pregnant

Immunization

Vaccinations: Absolute Contraindications[1,5,7,10,19]	
Vaccine	*Contraindication*
• Any Vaccine	• Fever >38.5°C, defer vaccination
	• Anaphylactic reaction to a previous dose of the same vaccine or a vaccine component becomes a contraindication for that particular vaccine
• DTaP 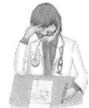 "Cerebral palsy is not a contraindication to DTaP but epilepsy is. Why is that so? I must try to link my knowledge of pathophysiology to this so that I do not forget this fact. A dynamic evolutionary process in nerve pathology of the brain in epilepsy must have something to do with it."	• Encephalopathy within 7 days of previous DTP vaccination • Neurological reactions within 3 days of DTP that contraindicate further doses • Shock like syndrome—a contraindication to DPT • An acute febrile illness • An evolving or suspected neurologic event • Severe reaction to prior dose of DPT • Remember that a static neurological disease like cerebral palsy is not a contraindication An extracranial cause of a seizure such as a febrile seizure is also not a contraindication
Live vaccines (e.g. MMR, varicella)	• Immune-suppression due to high-dose corticosteroids (2 mg/kg for more than 2 weeks). • Allow a gap of 3 months after immune-suppressive therapy before administering MMR and varicella. • Individuals who have received blood products • If live vaccines need to be given on the same day, give at different sites. You may also delay administering one live vaccine by 4 weeks. (This does not apply to any killed vaccines). Reducing the number of injections to be given will help with the compliance of the patient. A good example is the mumps, measles, rubella and varicella (MMRV) vaccination given between 12 months and 12 years of age • Pregnancy
• Influenza, yellow fever, and one of the rabies vaccines • Mild egg allergy is not a contraindication to routine MMR vaccine	• Anaphylaxis to egg
Other vaccines	• Severe adverse reactions (extremely rare)

A relative contraindication makes the vaccination possibly inadvisable under certain circumstances in the patient.

Vaccinations: Relative contraindications[1,5,7,10,19]	
Vaccine	*Relative contraindication*
All vaccines	Avoid vaccination 2 weeks before an elective surgery

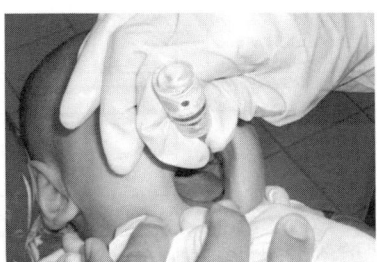

Photograph courtesy: Dr Loh Keng Yin, Associate Professor, reprint with permission.

Oral Vaccines

General contraindications of live vaccines are applicable if they contain live organisms. Breastfeeding and vaccination enhance immunological protection. SIgA in breast milk is important for protection. Secretory IgA (sIgA) is important in mucosal immunological protection (Refer to Chapter 6). Some studies indicate that sIgA in breast milk is important for protection. In addition, be aware that breastfeeding immediately before, after or during the administration of oral vaccines can interfere with the immunogenicity of the vaccine and render the oral vaccine inactive.[18] This is due to the interaction of secretory immunoglobulin A (sIgA) breast milk which potentially neutralizes the antigen in the oral vaccine via an antigen antibody reaction.[18] Timing oral vaccines with breastfeeding (i.e. breastfeeding one hour after administration of the oral vaccine) may somewhat overcome this problem.[18] But this is not conclusive and many studies show no benefit of this.[22,23]

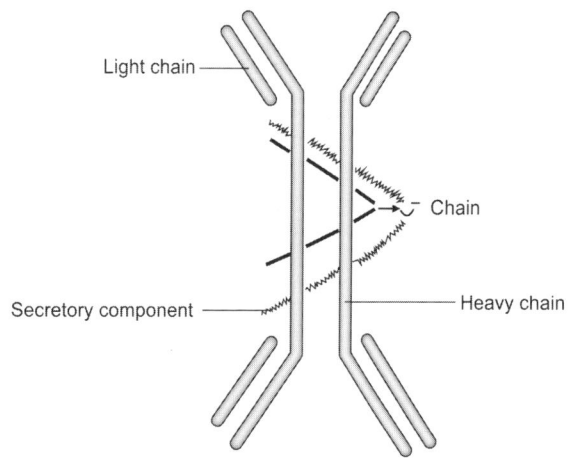

Secretory immunoglobulin A in breast milk is important for mucosal immunity in many diseases. Could its presence enhance some vaccine reactions?

Types of Vaccines[1,5,7,10,19]

Live, attenuated
Virulent pathogens are made to be attenuated and avirulent while still being antigenic. They are unable to induce a full-blown disease but retain their immunogenicity.

Inactivated (killed)
Inactivated vaccines are manufactured by killing the pathogenic microbe using heat chemicals or radiation.

Subunit
Subunit vaccines include only antigens that stimulate the immune system. One such example made of a recombinant subunit vaccine is hepatitis B virus.

Toxoid
These vaccines are used when a bacterial toxin is the main cause of illness.

Conjugate
A special type of subunit vaccine, which contains the outer coating of polysaccharides.

DNA
These vaccines contain the DNA of the organism. DNA vaccines use genes that code for antigens. It stimulates a very strong antibody and cellular response.

Recombinant vector
Here, an attenuated virus or bacterium is used to introduce microbial DNA into cells via these experimental vaccines. The virus or bacterium used as the carrier is the "Vector".

Live Attenuated (Avirulent) Vaccine[1,5,7,10,19]

Virulent pathogenic organisms are treated to become attenuated and avirulent but are able to stimulate an antigenic response. They have lost their potential to cause full-blown disease but are still immunogenic.

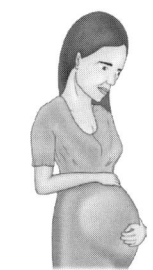

Pregnancy is a contraindication to live vaccines.

Contraindications to Live Attenuated Vaccines[1,5,7,10,19]

A definite contraindication to live attenuated vaccines is suppressed immunity. Examples are:
- Leukemia
- Lymphoma
- Immunosuppression due to congenital immunodeficiency, receiving corticosteroids (>2 mg/kg/day for more than 2 weeks) and anti-metabolic agents
- Human immunodeficiency virus (HIV) with low CD4 counts
- Radiation
- Pregnancy.

Live attenuated (avirulent) vaccine	
Organism	Disease
Virus	• Polio for oral polio vaccine
	• Measles
	• Yellow fever
	• Rubella
	• Mumps
	• Varicella zoster
	• Influenza for nasal influenza vaccine
Bacteria	• Tuberculosis

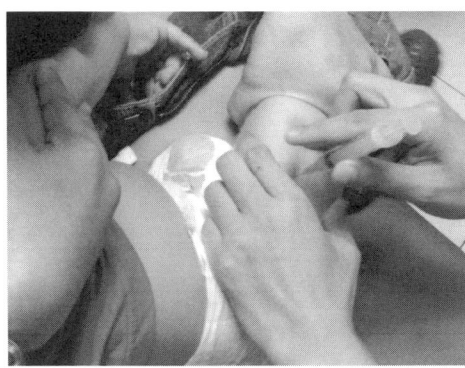

Giving the Hepatitis B vaccination.

Killed vaccines are being used despite their inferior efficacy compared to live attenuated vaccines. There has been success with the rabies, salk polio vaccine, typhoid, cholera and influenza but debatable value in the vaccines in diseases such as plague and typhus.

Below are some examples of killed vaccines:

Organism[1,5,7,10,19]	Disease[1,5,7,10,19]
Virus	• Intramuscular polio (safe in immuno-compromised individuals)
	• Rabies (can be given post-exposure, with passive antiserum), intramuscular influenza (strain specific)
	• Hepatitis A (also attenuated vaccine)
Bacteria	• Pertussis
	• Typhoid (confers approximately 70% protection)
	• Cholera, plague (short-term protection)
	• Q fever

Tetanus and diphtheria are the most efficacious of all bacterial vaccines.

Toxoids[1,5,7,10,19]

Organism[1,5,7,10,19]	Vaccine[1,5,7,10,19]
Clostridium tetani *Corynebacterium diphtheria*	Inactivated toxin (booster every 10 years, usually given with tetanus)
Vibrio cholerae	Toxin, B subunit
Clostridium perfringens	Inactivated toxin

Counseling on Reactions to Immunizations[1,5,7,10,19]

Primary Objectives

- To allay parental anxiety.

The reactions:
- Are genuine concerns to many parents
- Most reactions occur within 48 hours of the immunization
- Reactions are usually mild and short lived and include the following:
  - Feeling unwell
  - Irritability
  - A low grade fever.
  - Soreness around the injection site (e.g. reaction to the MMR vaccine might occur 6–12 days after the injection due to the measles component of MMR and may include feeling unwell, being irritable, having a low grade fever, a faint rash, a runny nose or a cough. Swelling of the lymph nodes of the neck may occur about 3 weeks after the injection. This is due to the mumps component of the vaccine).

Practical Tips to Reduce Reaction due to Vaccination[1,5,7,10,19]

- Put a damp, cool cloth on the injection site if it is red or swollen
- Paracetamol or ibuprofen helps the fever or the pain
- Ensure adequate fluid intake (step up breastfeeding)
- Lots of tender loving care.

Routes and Sites of Administration[19]

- Oral—OPV (sabin), live typhoid vaccine, rotavirus vaccine (live attenuated vaccine)
- Intradermal—BCG (deltoid area—4 fingerbreadth below acromion-proximal to deltoid muscle insertion)
- Deep subcutaneous, intramuscular injections—all vaccines except those mentioned above.

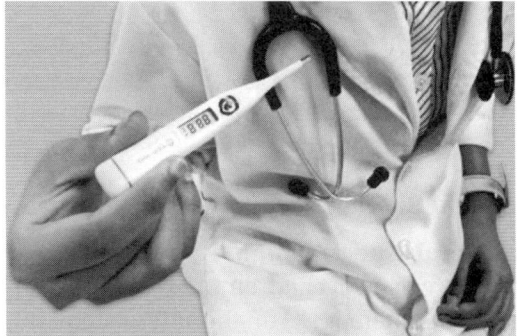

Parents must be reassured if their child develops a low-grade fever post-vaccination.

114 *The Link*: Pediatric History-Taking and Physical Examination

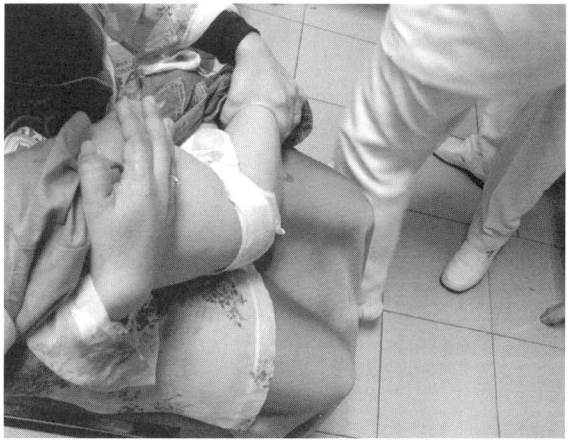

Subcutaneous injections can be given at this site.[19]

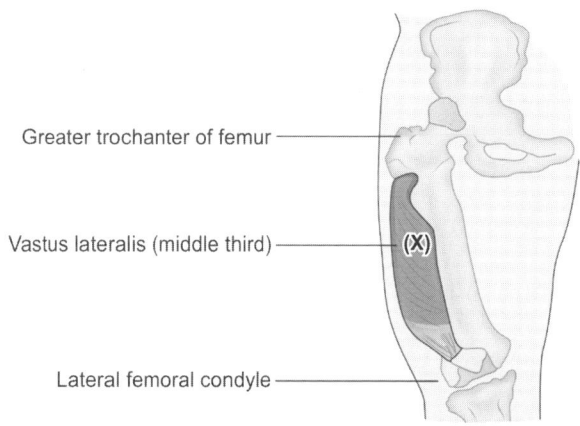

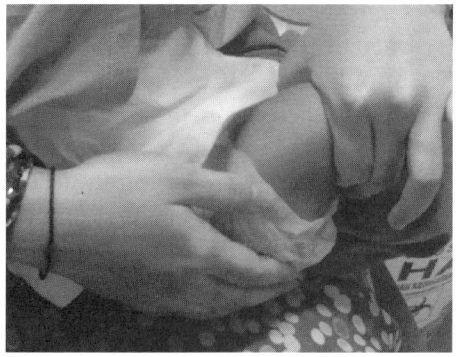
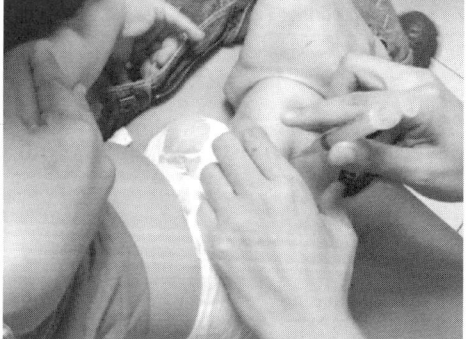

Intramuscular route of vaccination at the middle third of the vastus lateralis.

Anatomical Sites of Vaccination[19]

Anterolateral aspect of thigh—
- The favored site in children
- The vastus lateralis (X) on the anterolateral thigh

Upper arm—
- Preferred site for older children and adults
- The site of injection is in the upper 1/3rd of the arm, midway between the acromion and deltoid tuberosity
- Subcutaneous injections can be given here.

Ventrogluteal injection

- At any age, a preferred site when multiple injections are required.

While specific positions are useful, parents may also naturally keep the child as comfortable as possible.

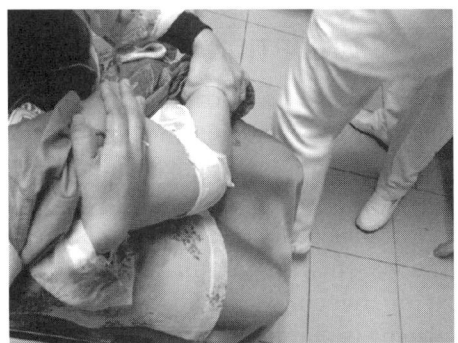

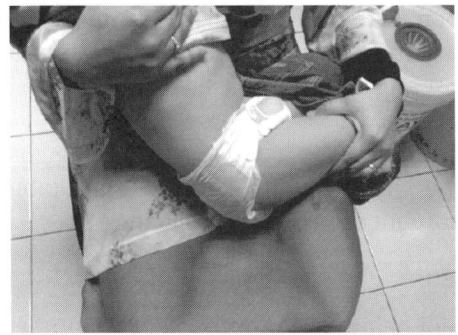

Here the mother naturally hugs the child for comfort and kindly helps to clear the field exposing the vastus lateralis.

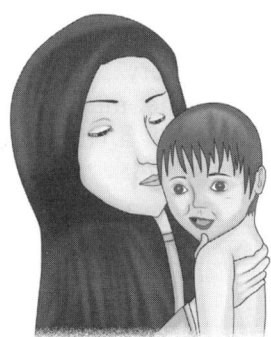

The mother's embrace comforts the child.

- Additionally, the Australian Immunisation Handbook[19] has recommended some practical and child-friendly positions during vaccinations according to different age groups, such as the cuddle position for infants, the cuddle position in an older child, the straddle position in a child and the solo sitting position for deltoid injections (The Australian Immunisation Handbook; 10th edition).

These positions are, perhaps, best to keep the child as comfortable as possible and to make the experience of vaccination least traumatic.

Special Circumstances

A child with bleeding disorders

Use the subcutaneous route for children who have bleeding disorders (e.g. hemophilia or thrombocytopenia).

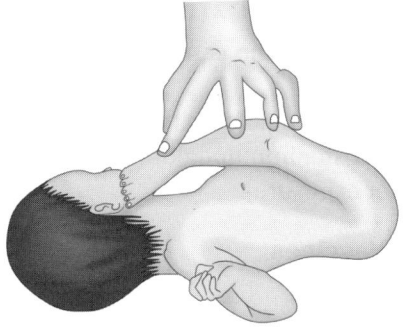

A preterm infant. Picture demonstrating hip flexibility. Generally, in preterm infants, all vaccines can be given as per schedule.

Immunization in Preterm Infants[1,5,7,10,19]

As a general rule, all vaccines can be given according to schedule following the chronological age irrespective of birth weight or period of gestation. Preterm babies who are very-low birth weight (VLBW) (refer to Chapter 12) can be given immunizations after stabilization. Hepatitis B vaccine (HBV) is given when the baby is 2 kg.

Vaccinating Children Receiving Corticosteroids[1,5,7,10,19]

Do not administer a live vaccine to children who are on a course of high doses of oral corticosteroids (2 mg/kg/day or more for more than 14 days) until cessation of the steroids for at least four weeks. Topical or inhaled steroids have no such precautions or contraindications.

Vaccination in Children with Human Immunodeficiency Virus (HIV) Infection

Generally, vaccinations are safe. However, the T4/T8 lymphocyte ratio at time of vaccination will determine whether to give the immunization or not. When the lymphocyte ratios are altered memory responses can be inadequate. Hence, immunization upon improvement of their immune status following antiretroviral therapy must be considered.

Vaccinating Children with Splenic Dysfunction, Asplenia or Awaiting Splenectomy[1,5,7,10,19]

They are at risk of infection from specific organisms particularly capsulated organisms. Hence, they must be vaccinated against important organisms including the following:
- *Meningococcus*
- *Haemophilus influenzae* type B (Hib)
- *Pneumococcus*
- *Influenza*.

For those children who cannot receive live vaccines consider using:
- Measles immunoglobulin (post measles exposure)
- Varicella-zoster immunoglobulin (post varicella and herpes zoster exposure).

Individual Vaccines

OPV

Booster of IPV can be given to a person who has taken OPV before. Hence, OPV is interchangeable with IPV. Repeat the OPV dose if the vaccine is vomited out soon after administration.

MMR

This vaccination can be given to those who have had measles, mumps or rubella infection in the past.

Global Immunization Programs

The cornerstone of primary prevention and a tool to achieve global health is immunization.

In any community, doctors and other healthcare providers including allied healthcare professionals should make certain that the latest immunization schedule is followed by referring to updated national or international websites on vaccination (Immunization Schedule: For Infants as Recommended by the WHO Expanded Program on Immunization (EPI).[20]

COUNSELING ON OPTIONAL VACCINES[7,10,20]

- Parents must also be informed of other important vaccines that are available in the country but are not in the compulsory government vaccination schedule.
- The importance of such vaccines must be discussed with the parents or guardian of the child in the context of the child's health and its significance must also be explained.
- The significance of such diseases must be discussed in the context of sociodemographic factors.
- Counseling must include all common side effects of the vaccine.
- You may need to counsel the rough cost of the vaccine when it is not yet made available by the government as in optional vaccines.

Examples[1,5,7,10,19]

- A child below six months sent to nursery could beneficially take the rotavirus vaccine.
- A young child could be offered the pneumococcal vaccine especially if living in a family with a large number of people, with siblings of school going age or if being sent to nursery.
- The influenza vaccine must be discussed with parents of a child with a chronic lung disease or congenital heart disease.

Other important vaccines[1,5,7,10,19]	Description[1,5,7,10,19]
Varicella vaccine	• A live attenuated vaccine • Given subcutaneously • Given as a single dose to infants, toddlers and children aged 12 months to 12 years. • Given in 2 doses, 28 days apart for children aged 12 years and above. • Immune-compromised children such as leukemia in remission for a year having an acceptable level of circulating lymphocytes, should be given this vaccination.
Hepatitis A	• Given intramuscularly • 2 doses 6 to 12 months apart • An inactivated vaccine • Approved for children more than one year old
Cholera	• Oral inactivated vaccine • Children aged 2 – 6 years • Booster dose after 2 years

Contd...

Contd...

Pneumococcal polysaccharide vaccine	• Given as a single dose • Given either intramuscularly or subcutaneously • Booster given 3 – 5 years for high risk persons • Stimulated appropriate immune response in children equal to or more than 2 years • Beneficial for children with asplenia, nephrotic syndrome as these children are susceptible to infections by capsular organisms. In chronic lung diseases, immunosuppression, including asymptomatic HIV • For infants < 2 years old, give conjugate vaccine
Pneumococcal conjugated vaccine *Conjugation of a polysaccharide to a protein carrier triggers a T cell dependent response in infants. Such effective vaccines are available for H. influenzae type B, S. pneumoniae, N. meningitidis.... hence, conjugated vaccines are effective in young children.*	• Given intramuscularly • Consist of 3 doses, given 4–8 weeks apart • As early as 6 weeks
Meningococcal A, C, Y, and W –135 vaccine Rabies vaccine	• Single dose intramuscularly • Immunity up to 3 years • Given by intramuscularly • Pre-exposure immunization: 3 doses at on the day of exposure, after a week and after a month • Boosters given every 2–3 years • Post-exposure treatment
Japanese encephalitis vaccine	• An inactivated vaccine • A booster is given at 4 years

Typhoid vaccine	• 2 vaccines available:
	  – Vi polysaccharide vaccine—single dose intramuscularly booster every 3 years
	  – Oral typhoid vaccine (Ty21a vaccine)
	• 3 doses 2 days apart
	• Booster every 3 years
	• A live attenuated vaccine

Human papilloma virus (HPV)	• 2 vaccines are available. The bivalent and quadrivalent • 3 doses (0, 1-2 months and 6 months) • Indicated for females aged 9 years to 45 years Prevents against HPV infection and disease. • Is not protective for existing or past HPV infection
Influenza vaccine	• It is given intramuscularly as a single dose • Minimum age is 6 months • Require yearly vaccination due to antigenic variation • Beneficial for children with chronic respiratory or cardiovascular system disorders, e.g. cyanotic heart disease, chronic pulmonary disease[23]
Rotavirus[25] *The rotavirus is ubiquitous, has a minute infectious dose, and is environmentally stable. These factors facilitate transmission of the rotavirus.* *Diarrhea due to rotaviruses is common in infants and can cause severe dehydration. The rotavirus vaccine must be given early to all children at risk especially those in nurseries. The combination of exclusive breastfeeding and vaccination has an important health impact on the individual and the community.*[6,16,25]	• Given orally • 2 vaccines are available • Live-attenuated vaccine • Earliest age is 6 weeks • Ideally completed by 6 – 8 months • Report early link of vaccine associated with intussusception but benefits outweigh the risks neutralization of oral vaccine by IgA in breast milk

Anaphylactic Reaction[1,5,7,10,19]

Anaphylaxis: A rare but fatal side effect of vaccination
• Anaphylaxis after a vaccine can be fatal if untreated urgently • It is important to recognize the early possible symptoms and signs of anaphylaxis • Convulsions and fainting can look similar but must be clinically differentiated
Features that characterize an anaphylactic reaction are:
Onset: • Rapid
Main features: • Laryngeal edema leading to acute dyspnea and cardiovascular collapse and/or circulatory collapse
Early signs are: • Involvement of the skin-generalized erythema, urticaria with or without angioedema • May involve the gastrointestinal tract with symptoms, such as diarrhea and vomiting
Severe cases have: • Hypotension, cardiovascular compromise and acute respiratory distress • If anaphylaxis is suspected, include the airway, breathing, circulation (ABC) of resuscitation and management, including the immediate administration of adrenaline without hesitation or fear of over treatment

VACCINATION AND BREASTFEEDING[1,5,7,10,19]

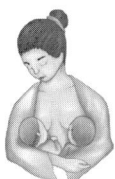

• Vaccination and breastfeeding both benefit children greatly
• Vaccination is a means of primary prevention of many diseases
• Breastfeeding offers a continuum in protection of the infant by strengthening and enhancing the immune system both short-term and long-term
• Some studies indicate that children exclusively breastfed for longer periods might be better protected against Hib and to specific serotypes of the pneumococcus (Silfverdal SA et al. 2007).[17]
• Some studies indicate that breastfeeding significantly enhances cell-mediated immune response to BCG vaccine given at birth, without much effect if given after four weeks (Pabst HF et. al. 1989)[15]

KEY POINTS

- Some background knowledge of immunization and vaccinations are important before history taking of the pediatric patient.
- Primary prevention of diseases and a tool to achieve global health is immunization.
- The history of immunization against a particular disease can never completely exclude the possibility of the child currently having, or previously having had, the disease.
- The information obtained from the immunization history is a tool for parental education and to narrow down the differential diagnosis.
- The reasons for missed or declined or withheld vaccinations are mostly due to misconceptions regarding vaccination.
- It must be reemphasized that the single most important evaluation of the vaccination status is up-to-date documentation; hence, it would be wise to begin the vaccination history by kindly requesting parents or caregivers for the vaccination card which can then be studied.

REFERENCES

1. Contraindications and Routine Precautions. CDC Immunization Program Section IIB. Available at http://www.bccdc.ca/NR/rdonlyres/22AB8B06-E83B-4159-BA23-0A51717E386B/0/SectionIIB_Contraindications_and_Precautions_April.pdf. Accessed on 26.1.2015.
2. Marcdante K, Kliegman RM, Jenson HB, Behrman RE (Eds). Nelson's Essentials of Pediatrics. 6th edn. Saunders Elsevier, 2010.
3. Milner AD, Hull D. Hospital Pediatrics. 3rd edn. ELBS with Churchill Livingstone. 1998.
4. Stephenson T, Wallace H (eds). Clinical Paediatrics for Postgraduate Examinations. UK: Churchill Livingstone; 1991.
5. Behrman RE (comps), Kliegman RM, Nelson WE, Vaughan III VC. (Eds). Nelson's textbook of pediatrics (14th ed). Philadelphia: WB Saunders; 1992.
6. Chang HG, Smith P, Markey K, et al. Reduction in New York hospitalization for diarrhea and rotavirus. October 23, 2008, Atlanta, Georgia. Available at http://www.who.int/immunization.
7. Clinical Practice Guidelines. Childhood Immunization. 2004. Ministry of Health, Malaysia.
8. Elizabeth KE. Clinical Pediatrics for Undergraduates. India: Jaypee Brothers Medical Publishers (P) Ltd; 2009.
9. Goel KM, Gupta DK. Hutchinson's Pediatrics, 1st edn. India: Jaypee Brothers Medical Publishers (P) Ltd; 2009.
10. Malaysian Immunization Manual, 2nd ed. College of Paediatrics, Academy of Medicine of Malaysia. 2008.
11. Mandell, Douglas, Bennett (Eds). Principles and Practice of Infectious Diseases (7th ed). Philadelphia: Churchill Livingstone/Elsevier; 2010.
12. Mason S, Swash M (Eds). Hutchinson's Clinical Methods (17th edn). A Bailllere Tindall book published by Cassell Ltd; 1980.
13. Groome MJ, Moon SS, Velasquez D, et al. Effect of breastfeeding on immunogenicity of oral live-attenuated human rotavirus vaccine: a randomized trial in HIV-uninfected infants in Soweto, South Africa. Bulletin of the World Health Organization 2014;92:238-245.
14. Milner AD, Hull D. Hospital Paediatrics (2nd ed.). ELBS with Churchill Livingstone. 1992.
15. Pabst HF, Godel J, Grace M, Cho H, Spady DW. Effect of breast-feeding on immune response to BCG vaccination. Lancet;1989;1(8633):295-7.

16. Prameela KK, Vijaya LR. The importance of breastfeeding in rotaviral diarrheas. Mal J Nutr 2012;18(1):103-11.
17. Silfverdal SA, Ekholm L, Bodin L. Breastfeeding enhances the antibody response to Hib and Pneumococcal serotype 6B and 14 after vaccination with conjugate vaccines. Vaccine. 2007;25(8):1497–502.
18. Moon SS, Wang Y, Shane AL, et al. Inhibitory Effect of Breast Milk on Infectivity of Live Oral Rotavirus Vaccines. Pediatr Infect Dis J. Oct 2010;29(10):919-23.
19. The Australian Immunization Handbook, 10th edition, 2013. ISBN: 978-1-74241-861-2.
20. The Extended Program for Immunization (EPI) Schedule, Ministry of Health, Malaysia. Accessed in Dec 2014.
21. Training Course on Child Growth Assessment. WHO Child Growth Standards. Available at http://www.who.int/childgrowth/training/girls_growth_record.pdf and http://www.who.int/childgrowth/training/boys_growth_record.pdf. Accessed on 14.8.2013, with kind permission.
22. Vaccines. United States, Me: National Institute of Allergy and Infectious Diseases, 2012. National Institute of Health. 2012.
23. Vesikari T, Karvonen A, Puustinen L, et al. Efficacy of RIX 4414 live attenuated human rotavirus vaccine in Finnish infants. Pediatr Infect Dis J. 2004;23:937-43.
24. Weiss LN. The diagnosis of wheezing in children. Am Fam Physician. 2008;77(8):1109-14.
25. Detailed review paper on Rotavirus vaccines. April 2009. Available at http://www.who.intl/immunization.

The essence of the relevant chapters in the following books have also been numbered as references in this chapter. We recommend for further reading, the rich text in these books for greater integration and deeper understanding.

1. Elizabeth KE. Clinical Pediatrics for Undergraduates. Jaypee Brothers Medical Publishers (P) Ltd, India 2009.
2. Goel KM, Gupta DK. Hutchinson's Pediatrics, 1st edn. Jaypee Brothers Medical Publishers (P) Ltd, India 2009.
3. Malaysian Immunization Manual, 2nd edn. College of Paediatrics, Academy of Medicine of Malaysia. 2008.
4. Mandell, Douglas, Bennett (Eds). Principles and Practice of Infectious Diseases (7th ed). Philadelphia: Churchill Livingstone/Elsevier; 2010.
5. Marcdante K, Kliegman RM, Jenson HB, Behrman RE (Eds). Nelson's Essentials of Pediatrics, 6th edn. Saunders Elsevier, 2010.
6. Mason S, Swash M (Eds). Hutchinson's Clinical Methods, 17th edn. A Bailllere Tindall book published by Cassell Ltd; 1980.
7. Milner AD, Hull D. Hospital Paediatrics, 2nd edn. ELBS with Churchill Livingstone. 1992.
8. Milner AD, Hull D. Hospital Pediatrics, 3rd edn. ELBS with Churchill Livingstone. 1998.
9. Behrman RE (comps), Kliegman RM, Nelson WE, Vaughan VC III. (Eds). Nelson's Textbook of Pediatrics, 14th edn. Philadelphia: WB Saunders. 1992.
10. Stephenson T, Wallace H (Eds). Clinical Paediatrics for Postgraduate Examinations. UK: Churchill Livingstone. 1991.
11. The Australian Immunization Handbook, 10th edn 2013. ISBN: 978-1-74241-861-2.

Chapter 8

Analysis and Deduction in the Layout of a Complete Pediatric History

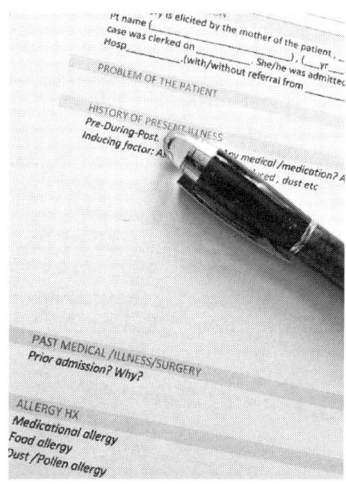

We have discussed history-taking in detail so far. Having extensive medical knowledge alone is of limited use if you are unable to extract accurate information about the ailment from the patient, from his or her family or from both.[1-3]

In any branch of medicine, including the field of pediatrics, a rational plan of management will depend on the correct diagnosis or sensible, differential diagnosis and this can be obtained when a comprehensive and complete history is available.

In all patients except in acute emergencies, comprehensive and complete history-taking should precede physical examination. In emergencies too, a focused history to direct the physical examination is needed without delay.

A medical history is the first step in making a diagnosis which will direct the doctor to do the appropriate physical examination and determine investigations that are appropriate. The correct diagnosis is mainly suggested by the history and confirmed by the physical examination.

Investigations are additional tools to reach a definitive diagnosis.

The presentation of the history has to be systematic, rational and understandable. There is a standard layout to follow. You must analyze the history in depth before you present the history in its standard layout. As mentioned in the previous chapters, the process of thinking and discerning the differential diagnosis must start early on during history-taking. You consciously go through a series of thought processes by attentive listening, then asking the many questions in the different ways that we have discussed. The **Cardinal Ten (Historical)** and the historical links are very useful tools to initiate proper thinking.

PROCESS OF ANALYSIS

There must always be a standard format for the presentation of the history. You may divide this standard layout into 10 components as follows:
1. Chief complaint and history of present illness and history of the presenting problem
2. Review of systems
3. Past medical/surgical history
4. Pregnancy and birth history and history of neonatal period
5. Developmental history
6. Feeding history
7. Immunization history
8. Drug and allergy history
9. Family history
10. Social, behavioral and travel history.

These components can be further expanded as follows to make it simpler for you to obtain an accurate history.

Content by headings of the pediatric history
• The presenting problem or the chief complaint
• History of the presenting problem
• The symptomatic enquiry of systems
• History of the past medical or surgical problems
• History of relevant prepregnancy events and pregnancy
• History of the delivery or birth history
• History of the neonatal period
• Development history
• Dietary or feeding history
• Immunization history
• Drug history
• Allergic history
• Family history
• Social history
• Behavioral history
• Travel history

Your own process of thinking, questioning and analysis starts early in history-taking. From the early stages, after listening to the chief complaint, you start to think logically from the information you obtain. You then listen again and question the parents, the patient or the caregiver in order to sharpen your logical assessment of the patient's problem or problems.

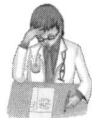

"In history-taking, there is listening, thinking, questioning, linking and thinking again. There is science and sense in this whole process of thinking....layer by layer I reaffirm and consolidate my thoughts on my patient's problems. Such systematic analysis can never be done by the most ingenious computer !!!! The training of the human mind is the only way to make a human diagnosis."

Remember to use **The Cardinal Ten (Historical)** in any part of the history as a tool for in depth enquiry.

1. **T**ime of onset — When
2. **N**ature of onset — What
3. **T**rigger of onset — How
4. **I**ntensity at onset — How much
5. **D**uration of symptoms — How long
6. **C**hange in intensity — How much less or how much more
7. *****A**ssociated factor(s) — ******W**hat else
8. **E**xacerbating factor(s) — Worsened by
9. **R**elieving factor(s) — Lessened by
10. **A**ction factor(s) or intervention(s) — What was done?

Presenting problem or the chief complaint
• **History of the presenting problem**
• At this point you formulate 5 reasonable early impressions or differential diagnoses based on the anatomical site of the disease, the pathophysiological process of the disease and the etiological agent causing the disease
• **Symptomatic enquiry of systems**
• At this point you sharpen your thinking by asking questions of all systems, to reinforce the system in question . By your questions you make one system more likely and try to exclude all other systems as the primary anatomical site of the disease
• **History of the past medical or surgical problems**
• Support or negate the 5 early differentials. Sometimes reveals the severity of the presenting problem, may help in categorization of a disease and enhances knowledge of pathogenesis and prognosis of the likely disease.
• **History of relevant prepregnancy events and pregnancy**
• Support or negate the 5 differentials. Bear in mind that early insults may affect organogenesis, weight gain and physical growth.
• Insults such as maternal infections, drug consumption and dietary intake during pregnancy can affect the health of the patient.
• **History of the delivery or birth history**
• Support or negate the 5 differentials and for deductions, forming clinical links, strengthening one impression and weakening another.
• Events such as prolonged labor or premature rupture of membranes are important to note as they predispose to asphyxia and infection respectively.
• Presence of meconium stained liquor indicates fetal distress.
• Instrumental deliveries increase the chances of birth injuries and asphyxia.
• **History of the neonatal period**
• Support or negate the 5 differentials, for information and deductions, sometimes useful in the pathophysiological diagnosis .
• Inquire about health in the first 28 days of life.
• **Development history**
• Support or negate the 5 differentials, for a complete clinical story of the patient's milestones and achievements. Ask about all 4 aspects of development.
• **Dietary or feeding history**
• Support or negate the 5 differentials and for a complete clinical story, clues on predisposition to diseases and for cues in the physical examination. It is advisable to take a full dietary history to rule out or to consider malnutrition and its type.
• **Immunization history**
• Support or negate the 5 differentials, for a complete clinical story and for counseling if needed.
• It is important to note that the immunization status is up-to-date. If immunization is not up-to-date, the patient may be predisposed to infections that they are normally protected from. Immunizations may be rarely omitted from the schedule for certain patients due to ailments that contraindicate specific vaccinations. Such information may help strengthen the differential diagnosis.

Contd...

122   *The Link*: Pediatric History-Taking and Physical Examination

Contd...

• **Drug history**
• Support or negate the 5 differentials and for important clinical information and management decisions.
• **Allergic history**
• Support or negate the 5 differentials and for important clinical information on choice of treatment, prevention, counseling and further management.
• **Family history**
• Support or negate the 5 differentials for clinical deductions and counseling, strengthening early impressions. • Bringing up a child is related to the parent's upbringing, age, educational level, occupation and household income. • History of consanguinity and infections especially among first degree relatives may have a role to play in the ailment the patient presents with.
• **Social history**
• Support or negate the 5 differentials and for information, counseling and referrals. Details on housing, environment, water supply and waste disposal may be a cause of the presenting complaint/s.
• **Behavioral history**
• Support or negate the 5 differentials strengthening the early impressions and making others less possible. The child's behavior gives clues to the underlying anatomical, pathophysiological and etiological diagnosis. In specific behavioral issues, in depth enquiry is imperative.
• **Travel history**
• Support or negate the 5 differentials, sometimes providing information on etiology and various medical and public health considerations in the patient's diagnosis of infectious diseases.

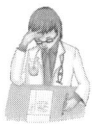

"A systematic history is a guiding tool to possibly excluding diagnoses. Every part of its format supports or weakens my impression and knowledge of pediatric illnesses, for example, in a child with a chronic cough, the absence of recurrent symptoms of nocturnal cough or wheeze would make bronchial asthma unlikely, the absence of oxygen requirement in the neonatal period could make chronic lung diseases such as BPD unlikely, completion of pertussis vaccination would make pertussis unlikely while no BCG taken will make me want to exclude tuberculosis. A family history of a close contact with chronic cough would make an infection likely, the absence of specific allergens or pets would make an allergy to triggers of some diseases less likely and a history of breastfeeding would exclude CMPA. If used with clinical sense and with proper linkage, the history is a vital tool for diagnosis."

When you complete your history you have probably reduced the number of differential diagnoses to one, two or three. This will then guide you in the physical examination, to further deduce the provisional diagnosis and then the definitive diagnosis. This may or may not require additional investigative tools.

Therefore, students must have an understanding of how to state a complete and comprehensive medical history
• Only the truth must be spoken
• Provide cues to search for relevant physical findings pertaining to the case. Provide information on the clinical problems of the patient
• Shed light on all differential diagnosis that should be considered. Provide a clue to the definitive diagnosis
• Furnish insight on possible management strategies. Give clues on the requirement or the involvement of other related medical or paramedical disciplines
• Give some idea on preventive strategies. Provide relevant information on the need for counseling

HISTORY-TAKING REQUIRES PRACTICE AND PRACTICE MAKES PERFECT

A good physician–patient relationship will give you a good history. Putting the patient at ease right from the start will help you build a rapport so that history-taking does not become a great bother.

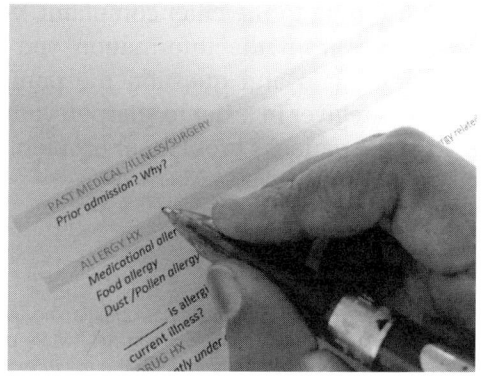

Patients' First Impression of You[4-12]

It must be always realized that the treatment of a patient begins when he walks into the consultation room or when you reach the bedside.

First impressions are vital and therefore I would like to stress this point. Their first impressions of your professional manner will have a lasting effect. Therefore, leave a good lasting effect that will not cause harm (primum non nocere) in any way.[4,13]

The Hippocratic injunction of primum non nocere or above all, to do no harm, constantly reminds us that every medical and pharmacological decision must be taken dutifully and has the inherent potential for harm.[4,13] A rough, unkind, careless method of approach to history-taking and physical examination of a patient can cause more harm than benefit even before treatment. Always aim to leave the patient feeling better

Analysis and Deduction in the Layout of a Complete Pediatric History 123

after your visit. The technique is difficult to teach but must be cultivated as practice on a daily basis for it to become natural to you. Each doctor has to develop his or her own method, guided by experience and the time you spend practicing in the wards. It is best learnt during your undergraduate days.

Ensuring a Good Doctor-patient Rapport in the Wards and in the Clinic

- As explained earlier, you must make an attempt to introduce yourself and explain your role to the patient and his or her family. This is especially relevant for undergraduate students posted at government health clinics and hospitals. You may say 'Good morning, Miss Liza. My name is Azhar, a 4th year medical student. I am a medical student from..... May I kindly take a bit of your time? I would like to ask you a few questions about your child, if you don't mind.'

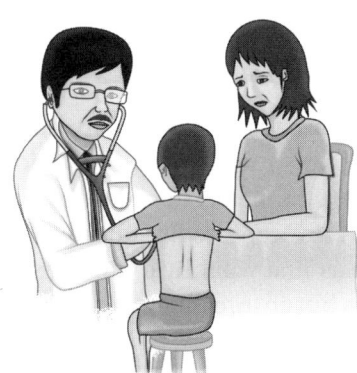

- If you are at the clinic, ask the patient to come in and sit down, showing him or her, the chair. Close the door for privacy or draw the curtains if you are in the ward.
- Sit down beside or reasonably near the patient so that you are at eye level with the patient and impress upon the patient that you are not in a hurry.
- Address the patient respectfully, calling him or her by name and title.
- Allow the patient to tell the whole story uninterrupted. Ask questions to fill in the gaps. When parents or guardians are the historians, their interpretation of the signs and symptoms may be exaggerated or otherwise. Therefore, if a child is able to express himself or herself, history is better taken from them. Bear in mind that the parents' or guardian's observation may vary from time-to-time. When you take history, use appropriate words.

- Listen attentively. Look at the historian with keenness on hearing the story and with eye contact.
- Record the entire interview and physical examination in full detail. If you are using a computer do not look entirely at the computer screen throughout the interview as the patient might feel offended and ignored. Looking continuously at the computer screen instead of the patient reflects poorly on your level of concern towards the patient.
- Observe the relationship between child and parent or guardian. This will give you a clue to the relationship they have fostered. The quality of the relationship does have an impact on the child's well-being.
- The final history recorded must be in chronological order.
- Follow a systemic approach to history-taking and recording your history to help you stay on track with the relevant history as some patients, due to anxiety or false belief, may tend to emphasize irrelevant points.

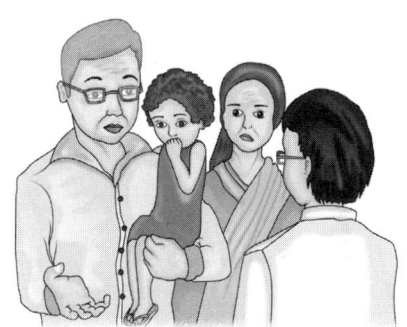

Note non-verbal cues as what is not said can be as vital as what is said

How to obtain a good history[11]
• Establish a good relationship
• Interview in a logical manner
• Listen carefully
• Interrupt appropriately
• Note non-verbal cues or body language
• Correct interpretation of information obtained

Initiating an Interview and a Follow-up

- For a new consultation, attempt a conversational approach. Ask the patient 'What has been troubling you lately? or 'When was the last time you were well?'
- For a follow-up consultation, make some reference to the last visit. For example: 'How is your health

or how are you?' or 'It has been ......days/weeks/ months since I last saw you, isn't it?' How has your health been since then?'
- You can also start with general questions or some basic open ended questions about life, but ensure that they are not intrusive. Be sensitive to the circumstances and the body language. Distracted parents do not give an accurate history. Therefore, it is important to ensure that you have the parents' undivided attention.
- You may also insert general questions in the 'social history' section.

LAYOUT OF A COMPLETE PEDIATRIC HISTORY

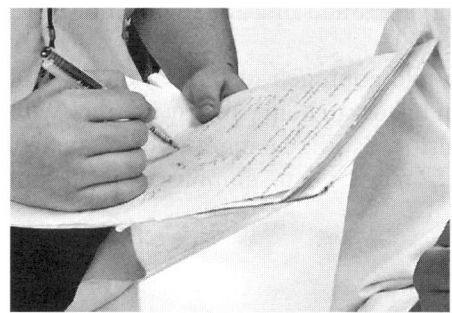

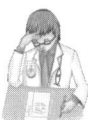

"Now it is time I use my analytical mind."

Layout of a complete pediatric history is as follows:[10,14-18]

| This case was clerked at |
| Date: |
| Time: |
| Note: State from whom the history is elicited and the relationship to the patient. (Opening: Verbal consent from the parent for history-taking and assurance of confidentiality must be gently made) |
| This case was admitted through ER/OPD/casualty department |
| If referred case, state by whom, which hospital and the reasons for referral as stated in the referral letter |
| **Patient's particulars**
Name:
Address:
Gender:
Date of birth:
Race (remember ethnicity is far more important in relation to diseases than nationality): |
| **Presenting problem/chief complaint:** Include who is narrating the history, e.g. in the mother's or caretaker's own words. State the duration of the chief complaint |

Contd...

Contd...

History of the presenting problem The symptomatic enquiry of systems (ROS) History of the past medical or surgical problems History of relevant prepregnancy events and pregnancy (especially in neonate, brief and relevant) History of the delivery or birth history (brief and relevant) History of the neonatal period The development history
The dietary or feeding history The immunization history Drug history Allergic history Family history Social history Behavioral history (usually part of the history of the presenting problem) Travel history.
Note: *Closing: Always politely enquire if the historian has any questions to ask. Politely and professionally thank the historian and the patient (patient who partook in the history-taking no matter how young)*

SOME POINTS TO REITERATE

- You must learn to listen with an open mind
- Do not jump to a diagnostic decision before the patient has completely described all the symptoms
- Try to avoid repeatedly questioning the same symptom as that would vary the description of the symptoms but ensure that you have taken it in depth in the first place
- Ask follow-up questions which are usually closed ended, when necessary. Such an example is 'Can you show me precisely where the pain is?' and 'What do you mean by dull pain?'
- Some older patients may be so overwhelmed by their own health that they may not want to talk too much about it
- You must recognize that some patients may have difficulties, such as deafness. You must be empathetic and understanding about it
- Do not hurt your patient in thought, word or deed directly or indirectly
- Treat the information given to you with strict confidentiality.

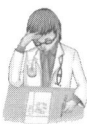

"I understand that patient confidentiality is my utmost priority."

Documentation of the History[10,14-18]

Written history is a confidential document

As mentioned earlier in Chapter 1 on symptoms, the history based on symptomatology given to you by the historian, and obtained by you utilizing your knowledge and historical links and organized in the standard format, is an important patient document that must be treated with strict confidentiality. It is important to keep patients' records private and confidential.

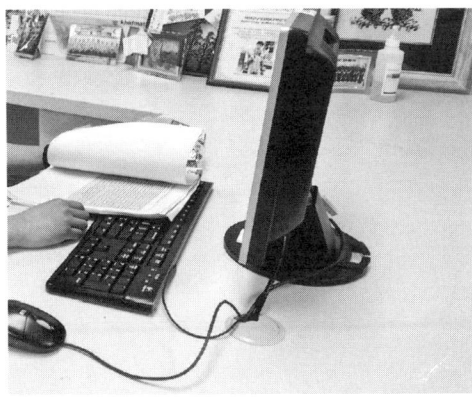

Patients' Records

- Clearly and legibly document using an ink pen the history under specific headings. If you are in a "paperless" system, you may make a soft copy of the history and keep the records in a confidential folder to be used only by the attending medical team
- State who the historian is, name and relationship to the patient
- Document the date and time of taking the history
- Document all aspects of the history under specific headings
- Include all temporal details of the history in your notes
- The relevant observations made during history-taking about mother-child and other family interactions may also be written down at the end of the history.

REFERENCES

1. Barrier P, et al. Two words to improve physician-patient communication: What else? Mayo Clin Proc. 2003;78:211-4.
2. Bellet PS, Maloney MJ. The importance of empathy as an interviewing skill in medicine. JAMA. 1991;266:1831-32.
3. Blau JN. Time to let the patient speak. BMJ. 1999;298:39.
4. Brewin T. Primum non nocere? Lancet. 1994;344:1487-88.
5. Coulehan JL, et al. 'Tell me about yourself': The patient-centered interview. Ann Intern Med. 2001;134:1079-84.
6. Elizabeth KE. Clinical Pediatrics for Undergraduates. India: Jaypee Brothers Medical Publishers (P) Ltd. 2009.
7. Fogarty L, et al. Can 40 seconds of compassion reduce patient anxiety? J Clin Oncol. 1999;17:371-9.
8. Goel KM, Gupta DK. Hutchinson's Pediatrics, 1st edn. India: Jaypee Brothers Medical Publishers (P) Ltd; 2009
9. Longson D. The clinical consultation. JR Coll Physicians Lond. 1983;17:192-5.
10. Marcdante K, Kliegman RM, Jenson HB, Behrman RE (Eds). Nelson's Essentials of Pediatrics. 6th edn. Saunders Elsevier, 2010.
11. Nardone DA, Johnson GK, Faryna A, et al. A model for the diagnostic medical interview: Nonverbal, verbal and cognitive assessments. J Gen Intern Med. 1992;7:437-42.
12. Platt FW, McMath JC. Clinical hypocompetence: The interview. Ann Intern Med. 1979;91:898-902.
13. Smith CM. Origin and uses of primum non nocere-above all, do no harm! J Clin Pharmacol. 2005;45(4):371-7.
14. Smith RC, Hoppe RB. The patient's story: Integrating the patient-and physician-centered approaches to interviewing. Ann Intern Med. 1991;115:470-7.
15. Mason S, Swash M (Eds). Hutchinson's Clinical Methods (17th edn). A Bailllere Tindall book published by Cassell Ltd; 1980.
16. Milner AD, Hull D. Hospital Pediatrics. 3rd edn. ELBS with Churchill Livingstone. 1998.
17. Richard E. Behrman (comps). Robert M Kliegman, Waldo E Nelson, Victor C Vaughan III. (eds). Nelson's textbook of pediatrics (14th ed). Philadelphia: WB Saunders; 1992.
18. Stephenson T, Wallace H (eds). Clinical Paediatrics for Postgraduate Examinations. UK: Churchill Livingstone; 1991.

The essence of the relevant chapters in the following books have also been numbered as references in this chapter. We recommend for further reading, the rich text in these books for greater integration and deeper understanding.

1. Goel KM, Gupta DK. Hutchinson's Pediatrics, 1st edn. Jaypee Brothers Medical Publishers (P) Ltd, India, 2009.
2. Marcdante K, Kliegman RM, Jenson HB, Behrman RE (Eds). Nelson's Essentials of Pediatrics, 6th edn. Saunders Elsevier. 2010.
3. Mason S, Swash M (Eds). Hutchinson's Clinical Methods, 17th edn. A Bailllere Tindall book published by Cassell Ltd; 1980.
4. Milner AD, Hull D. Hospital Pediatrics, 3rd edn. ELBS with Churchill Livingstone. 1998.
5. Behrman RE (comps), Kliegman RM, Nelson WE, Vaughan VC III (Eds). Nelson's Textbook of Pediatrics, 14th edn. Philadelphia: WB Saunders. 1992.
6. Stephenson T, Wallace H (Eds). Clinical Paediatrics for Postgraduate Examinations. UK: Churchill Livingstone, 1991.

SECTION 2

COMPREHENSIVE PEDIATRIC PHYSICAL EXAMINATION

- An Approach to the Pediatric Physical Examination
- Pediatric Physical Examination
- Layout of a Complete Pediatric Physical Examination

Chapter 9

An Approach to the Pediatric Physical Examination

BUILDING A RAPPORT[1-9]

At most times, young children will not cooperate during physical examination.

General observation is best noted while the child is at play alone or with siblings or friends.

Many factors influence the approach to the pediatric patient. Children are impulsive, unpredictable, interesting, and loving all at the same time. Your approach towards the child is vital to a good start in the physical examination.

Communicating effectively with the pediatric patient and their parents who have varying communication abilities and are busy with many duties is a daunting task by itself. A healthy patient-doctor relationship is itself therapeutic in many ways. It is enhanced by the conduct of a productive clinical encounter.

Therefore, you have to build a rapport with the child before you start any part of the examination. Rapport is quite easily established during the child's first visit. Achieving a rapport enhances the likelihood that the child will comply with the management plan.

It is the pediatric patient that will dictate:[1-4]

- The order you will follow in the physical examination. You may not be able to follow the traditional sequence of physical examination as done in the adult patient.
- The position you will choose during the physical examination.
- The way in which you conduct the examination.

The examination method of the pediatric patient is very age dependent.[1-9]

- In early infancy, it is best to examine the child on the examination couch with a parent nearby.
- A toddler is most comfortable when held against the mother's shoulder or seated on the mother's lap.
- Preschool children can be preliminarily assessed and examined while at play.
- Teenage girls should be examined in the presence of the mother.
- If you need the child to be undressed, ask the parent to do it, or to kindly help you with it.
- Throughout the examination, communicate appropriately according to the age and stage of development of the child.

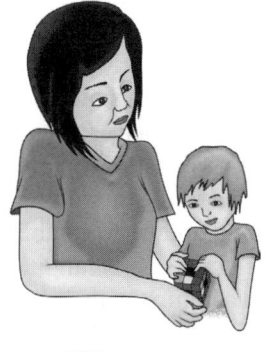

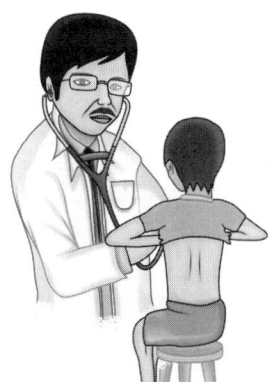

A friendly approach to examination is important

- Always ensure that your hands and instruments, such as the stethoscope are warm to the touch.
- Use small but safe child friendly little gadgets, building blocks or toys to warm the child's heart too.

Respect the:
- Privacy especially among the teenage patients.
- Cultural sensitivities of different ethnic groups.

Other age considerations when establishing and maintaining rapport, respect, and a professional relationship between yourself and the pediatric patient which can be used as a guide are stated below.

Infants and Babies[1,6]

How babies behave in a given encounter will depend on if they are hungry, sleepy and so on. It is also determined in part by the cumulative experience of each visit.

- Keep the infant or baby in the secure cuddle of the mother initially and as far as possible. As observation is the most important part of the physical examination, observe the infant closely. It is best to observe in this position the respiration and to count its rate.
- While approaching the child, keep movements slow and to the minimum.
- Pay attention to the caregiver's complaints in the history of the child carefully.
- Babies are very sensitive to body language as it is their primary form of communication.
- Do not invade the child's space.
- Smile at the parents; speak softly.
- When seated, try to ensure you are able to see eye to eye with the child while maintaining your distance.
- Smile at the child and try to establish eye contact.
- Try to read the child's body language.
- Try to perform as much of the physical examination while the child is in the parents' arms.
- Restraining a child to perform the physical examination should be the last resort.

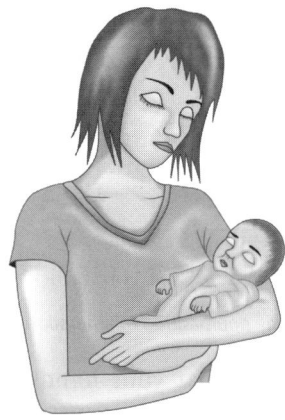

Keep the infant or baby in the secure cuddle of the mother during observation

Toddlers and Children[1,6]

- Do not take them away from the safe arms of their parents until it is necessary to do so.
- Do not take away any item the child may be playing with.
- Observe the child for the level of activity (e.g. active, lethargic) and the developmental milestones.
- Perform the less invasive examinations first while building the child's trust.
- You may allay the child's fears by pretending to examine their stuffed toy, or examine their parent to demonstrate what you are doing.
- Conduct the most unpleasant parts of the examination last.
- Offer the child a safe sweet or sticker as a 'peace offering' at the end of the visit.
- Wave goodbye or give a high five as the child is leaving the room.

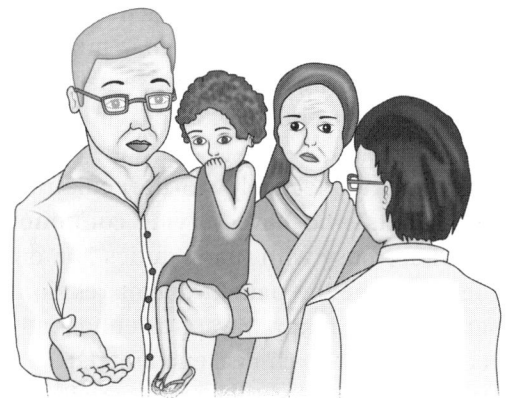

Do not take them away from the comfortable arms of their parents

Teenage or Adolescent Patient[1,6]

"Maturity is when your world opens up and you realize that you are not the centre of it."

—MJ Croan

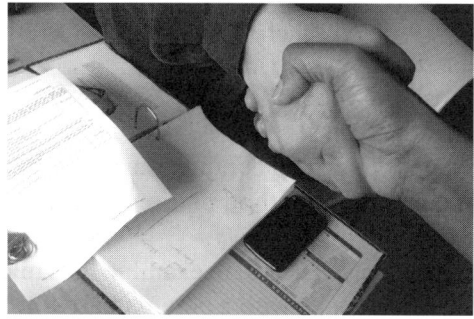

A friendly smile and a firm handshake will instill confidence in the adolescent patient

Adolescents[1,3,4,6]

- Allow the parents of the adolescent patient to verbalize their thoughts and concerns about their child.
- Politely request the parents to wait outside while you complete the physical examination.
- Greet the adolescent patient with a smile and a firm handshake while maintaining good eye contact.
- Involve the patient in conversation if he or she is shy and quiet.
- The HEEEADSSS technique (modified from HEADSS) is a helpful way to structure the interview in a thorough and time-conserving manner.[3,4]
- Thank the patient at the end of the examination.

The HEEEADSSS Technique[3,4]

The rapidly maturing phase of physical and mental development between childhood and adulthood is adolescence where there are changes ranging from physical to psychosocial and cognitive growth. This period must be covered with a different set of questions in the history which span from home issues, to education and to questions about emotion and feelings as well as various safety issues.

The HEADSS approach, first developed by Dr Harvey Berman in 1972, was refined by Dr Cohen.[3,4] This approach is now commonly used to take a developmentally-appropriate psychosocial history.[4]

Apart from the interviewee, nobody else should be present unless requested or given permission to be present by the interviewee.

The norms of an interview are followed, i.e. the introduction and the issue of confidentiality.

The HEEEADSSS interview questions[3,4]	
Link the phase of adolescence to their clinical history	
H	Questions about harmony and home environment, the family relationship, the health of family members, the parents occupation
E	Questions about early learning experience, such as formal and informal education, the school the interviewee attends and the relationship with teachers and peers and where relevant, queries on employment
E	Questions about extracurricular activities that are directly related to behaviour and that may affect pyschosocial development
E	Questions about eating habits, unusual habits or cravings
A	Questions about daily activities, social life and hobbies
D	Questions about drug abuse. If suspected, must be asked tactfully and in a nonjudgmental manner, without offending or alarming the patient
S	Questions about sexual relations, menses, breast/testicular self-examination
S	Questions about suicide or depression, self-esteem, abnormal fears or any unusual feelings of concern seemingly beyond normal limits
S	Questions about their safety during activities such as sports, being sexually abused or bullied or involved in physical violence

Examination of adolescents must be done respecting their privacy, and, as always, with a chaperone. Parents and friends will usually be asked to kindly wait outside.

Suggested methods in the approach of conducting the examination of the child

- In a child above one to two years of age, you may want to approach the physical examination by the organ system.
- In an infant or small child, conduct the head-to-toe approach of physical examination.
- For both age groups, however, you present the general observation as positives and absence of important negatives.
- Although the approach is conducted in the way the child dictates, present the findings of the systems by inspection, palpation, percussion and auscultation.
- To emphasize on the main problem, you may want to present the findings of the system(s) with abnormal findings first or the system(s) relevant to the history first before you present the other systems, to complete the presentation of your physical examination.

THE CARDINAL TEN (PHYSICAL)

The Cardinal Ten (Physical) is a tool that will help you define a positive finding in detail. It takes you to the depth of the problem.

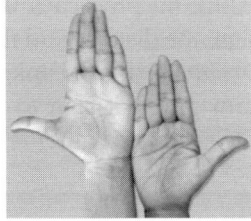

As the pediatric physical examination depends a lot on observation, it is useful to base the general observation of the patient using some guidelines as follows:

1. **A**lertness.
2. **A**ppearance.
3. **A**ppreciation (by sense of smell, sense of hearing and sense of touch).
4. **A**ctivity (of patient).
5. **A**djunct or surroundings.
6. **A**symmetry.
7. **C**olor.
8. **P**osture.
9. **S**welling.
10. **M**ovement (of specific parts of body).

If **The Cardinal Ten (Physical)** detect or discover signs that are positive, you must examine the relevant organ system(s) using appropriate physical links.

A visible or palpable mass or swelling must be defined based on the following objective parameters.
- Site
- Size
- Shape
- Edge
- Tenderness
- Surface
- Contour
- Consistency
- Mobility
- Ability to get above the swelling
- Pulsatility (pulsatile or not)
- Maneuvers to define exact location and nature e.g. intra or extra abdominal, transilluminability
- Comparison with other masses, if present, e.g. (on other limb)
- Percussion note over the swelling (done over nontender masses to differentiate cystic from solid)
- Auscultation.

PHYSICAL LINK

Like the historical link, the physical link is a tool to make you think of the sign, the disease and the complications in broad terms. Like the historical link, the physical link uses one important physical sign to direct a focused examination and to search for other relevant signs.

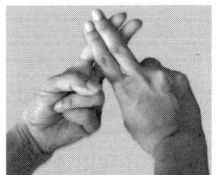

To Obtain the Correct Physical Link

- The initial physical observation must be thorough and accurate
- Knowledge of pathophysiology underlying related to physical signs must be known
- Basic knowledge of signs and major symptoms as expression of clinical diseases must be understood.

Example 1

Take for example yellow discoloration.

First look at the child as a whole. Is the child active or ill-looking? By observation, try to make out if it is an acute or chronic problem. If there is yellow discoloration of the sclera, it is jaundice. If the skin alone is involved and the sclera spared, it is carotenemia, not jaundice, as seen in some healthy children and is linked to the diet. If it is jaundice, observe and ascertain its severity. If the jaundice is mild or described as "a tinge of", see if it is associated with an enlarged spleen. Look for such causes considering pathophysiology. Deep icterus may be associated with hepatomegaly or a shrunken liver in cirrhosis. Ascertain this by examination of the liver. Link to signs associated with chronic liver diseases. If you have decided that it is a chronic process.

When **The Cardinal Ten (Physical)** is used, more information about the yellowness can be obtained. Additionally, important signs are not missed. The overall appearance and activity of the child is undoubtedly the most important observation.

Physical links can be found within the system in question (i.e. the abnormal system) and outside the system in question. Physical findings could be part of the disease or could be as a result of complications of the disease. The approach to the physical examination via the physical links will encourage you to search for relevant physical signs as well as encourage you later, to read further on pathophysiology and related clinical findings.

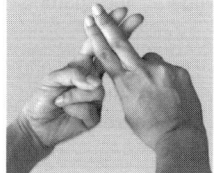

The wards are your greatest clinical teachers and physical links guide you to understand and diagnose the vast, extent of diseases afflicting the human body and the complications of diseases.

The physical links will lead you so that you conduct a complete physical examination without missing important clinical findings of a particular disease. A positive finding must make you search for all related findings in all systems.

- Remember what the mind does not know the eyes will not see and what the eyes do not look actively for can be missed.
- The associated abnormal physical links are found in the system that has the abnormality.
- The related abnormal physical link(s) can also be found outside the primary system of abnormality.
- Other associated clinical signs that are normal must be mentioned.
- However, it would be good practice to think of common things first. A child with chronic malnutrition is more likely to have the pallor of iron deficiency than manifest the Casal necklace of niacin deficiency!

Example 2

Taking a case of jaundice again, *a case of chronic jaundice* in a child must prompt you to look for the following: First study the jaundice itself in detail using **The Cardinal Ten (Physical)**.

The physical links within the abnormal system (i.e. within the hepatobiliary system)

It would be vital to palpate the liver and spleen to look for hepatomegaly or splenomegaly. Remember that fluctuating jaundice in a well child could also be due to a choledochal cyst where the jaundice is of the obstructive type. You must also actively look for all signs of chronic liver disease. Thus in jaundice, clubbing, koilonychias, onycholysis, infections of the skin and ecchymoses are important. Lymph node enlargement as well as dilated veins, palmar erythema, spider nevi, clubbing and scratch marks are all relevant positives or negatives that should be mentioned. These are links within the system that has the abnormality.

The physical links outside the hepatobiliary system (i.e. external to the system that has the abnormality)

Search for physical signs of nutritional deficiencies including growth failure or failure to thrive, pallor and enlargement of the metacarpophalangeal joints at the wrist, a smooth tongue, angular stomatitis and gum swelling. Dermatitis of the skin and perianal area, association of perianal excoriation linked to chronic diarrheas and signs seen in deficiencies of niacin or zinc, as multinutrient deficiencies tend to occur together and can affect a child who is chronically ill. The findings of deficiencies of vitamins A, D, E and K due to malabsorption of fat affecting the eyes, the bones and causing coagulopathy, are the physical links outside the primary system of abnormality.

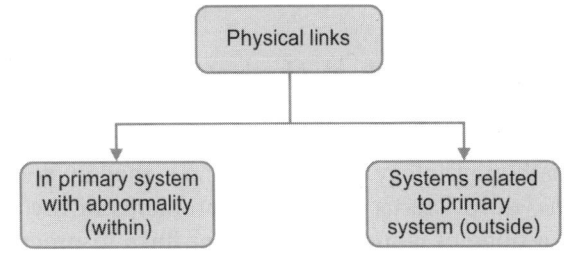

Physical links may be simply thought of as within or outside the abnormal system

Example 3

As a third example, consider a heart murmur **[The Cardinal Ten (Physical)]**—(Appreciation by hearing of murmur) must make you look for adequate growth, presence or absence of cyanosis or pallor. Examine all pulses, the precordial palpation, maneuvers of positioning the child, sitting or lifting up legs, (if venous hum) to check for the disappearance of the murmur with change in position, as well as auscultating the back, the axilla and below the clavicles, the lung bases and palpate the liver. These are physical links that you use to determine if the murmur is physiological or pathological.

Hence, if it is pathological, you will determine the cardiac lesion in broad clinical terms, the clinical significance and the type of murmur heard, the impact of the murmur on cardiac function, such as whether or not the child is in heart failure.

In this example, the physical link was used as a route to confirm the clinical diagnosis, and to include or exclude the important association of heart failure in the child.

Appreciate in the above examples how one positive sign must make you look for all findings that can help you reach a complete differential diagnosis based on anatomy, pathology, and etiology.

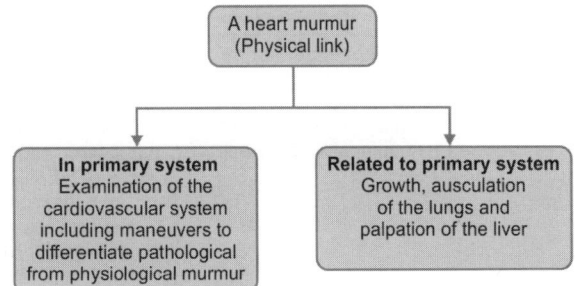

134 *The Link*: Pediatric History-Taking and Physical Examination

The search for associated signs allows meaningful links to pathophysiology that you have learnt in preclinical medicine as you use your basic knowledge to apply it in a relevant manner to the patient.

Example 4

You may also look at physical links this way. In jaundice, see if the jaundice is deep or light and look for other known associated signs that can lead you to pathophysiology. You must know that in general terms, deep icterus is linked to problems of the liver and a tinge of jaundice with pallor links to processes involving hemolysis including hemolytic anemias typically associated with enlargement of the spleen. Then ask yourself what the possible causes of jaundice are. You know that there are four core processes leading to jaundice. You also know that a tinge of jaundice with pallor differs in etiology to deep icterus with pruritis. How do you use this information properly in the examination? The physical link has helped you here.

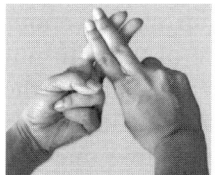

- Hepatocellular jaundice
- Hemolytic jaundice
- Obstructive jaundice
- Mixed jaundice with hepatocellular and obstructive element
- So how would you use the physical links to do an accurate focused examination?

PERTINENT NEGATIVES

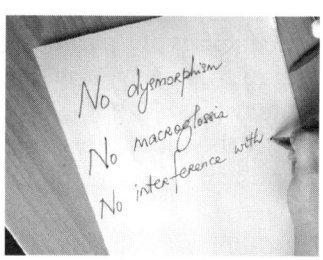

Negative signs are just as important as the positive signs in arriving at the diagnosis
Pertinent negatives have the following features: • Negative signs of another system that overlap with the system that is affected by the disease, e.g. tachypnea can be a sign of both respiratory and cardiovascular system. So, in tachypnea of likely respiratory origin, one also checks to exclude hepatomegaly and cardiomegaly seen accompanying tachypnea due to cardiac failure. In other words, no hepatomegaly and no cardiomegaly indicate that the tachypnea is not cardiovascular in origin
• To look for signs that are expected but not found. When physical signs are looked for in a case where there is overlapping presenting signs such as hematuria, no hypertension and no reduced urine output will exclude acute glomerulonephritis and make a diagnosis of urinary tract infection to be considered in the differential diagnosis. These negatives are important guides to an accurate clinical diagnosis
• The absence of important signs that point to a disease in one system. This gives greater weightage to the positive symptoms experienced in another system and greater accuracy in the diagnosis of that system. (e.g. a 3-year-old febrile child who is not drowsy or lethargic before or after the post ictal period of a fit. This makes a CNS infection as a cause of the fit less likely and a febrile fit a more likely diagnosis)
• Useful to eliminate more unlikely etiological diagnosis. When stridor is not associated with toxicity, not associated with high fever and not associated with drooling of saliva, it is less likely that the stridor is due to an acute bacterial etiology. This sharpens or focuses the more likely etiological diagnosis

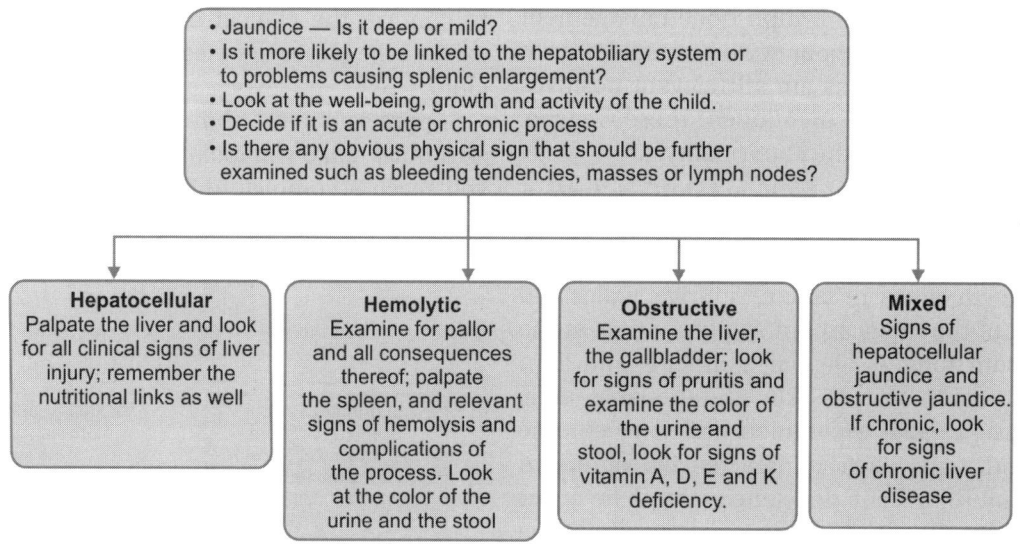

CCCC

Correlate, Compare, Capture and Confirm

The four C's that will help elucidate your physical findings clearly are to correlate, to compare, to capture and to confirm your findings.

Correlation

- Always think of the pathophysiological process of the presenting complaint and the presenting history, refer to that knowledge when looking for physical signs.
- The history must make you look for all related findings in all systems or from head to foot depending on the age of the child.
- Look for and mention all important negative findings guided by your history and physical examination.

Comparison

- Always compare the normal side to the abnormal side or normal skin to abnormal skin, comment on the abnormal right eye in comparison to the normal left eye, as you also examine both eyes, both ears and both nostrils.
- Palpation, percussion and auscultation of the lung must be compared on both sides.
- Limb appearance can only be confirmed by comparison of both limbs and establishing if either limb is normal first as a yardstick for comparison to the abnormal side, e.g. a swollen leg on the left should be compared to the normal limb on the right.
- Measurement of limb length from standard points, limb tone and reflexes must be done and compared on both sides.

Capture by Accurate Description

- Always describe visibly or palpably abnormal findings based on site, size, shape, distribution, surface, color, fluctuancy, transillumination or any other special characteristic based on the system involved. Ascertain the abnormality by apt description.

Confirmation

- An observation must be accompanied by measurement, palpation, percussion or auscultation for clinical confirmation. For example, a big head or macrocephaly must be measured and plotted in an age and gender appropriate head chart.

Remember the rules in arriving at a diagnosis

Correlate the history with the complete physical examination, compare both sides when necessary, on examination (both limbs, both sides of chest, both ears, etc.), then capture the clinical diagnosis and **confirm** your findings with the necessary measurements and clinical examination and finally, if necessary, do relevant investigations.

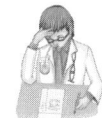

"I must use a thorough approach without taking short cuts to conduct a complete physical examination without missing the clinical signs".

In conducting the correct approach to the examination of the pediatric patient, ask yourself:
• What is the age of the patient?
• How ill is the patient?
• What is the expected level of cooperation?
• Has the history given me an idea on the complete and focused examination that I will conduct?
• Are there important historical links that direct me to think of specific physical examination links?
• How do I approach the child so as to cause no discomfort and maximal cooperation?
• In what way can I involve the parents in the physical examination, if the child is at an age where parental cooperation is useful?
• What innovative methods can I use? (within safe and reasonable limits).

This process of thinking makes for a sound approach to a good clinical examination.

REFERENCES

1. Behrman RE (comps), Kliegman RM, Nelson WE, Vaughan VC III (Eds). Nelson's Textbook of Pediatrics (14th Ed). Philadelphia: WB Saunders; 1992.
2. Elizabeth KE. Clinical Pediatrics for Undergraduates. New Delhi: Jaypee Brothers Medical Publishers (P) Ltd. 2009.
3. Goldering J, Cohen E. Heading into adolescent heads. Contemporary Pediatrics. 1988;75-80.
4. Goldering JM, Rosen DS. Getting into adolescent heads: An essential update. Contemporary Pediatrics. 200421:64
5. Goel KM, Gupta DK. Hutchinson's Pediatrics, 1st edn. Jaypee Brothers Medical Publishers (P) Ltd, India. 2009
6. Marcdante K, Kliegman RM, Jenson HB, Behrman RE (Eds). Nelson's Essentials of Pediatrics. 6th edn. Saunders Elsevier, 2010.

7. Mason S, Swash M (Eds). Hutchinson's Clinical Methods (17th edn). A Bailllere Tindall book published by Cassell Ltd; 1980.
8. Milner AD, Hull D. Hospital Pediatrics. 3rd edn. ELBS with Churchill Livingstone. 1998.
9. Stephenson T, Wallace H (eds). Clinical Paediatrics for Postgraduate Examinations. UK: Churchill Livingstone. 1991.

The essence of the relevant chapters in the following books have also been numbered as references in this chapter. We recommend for further reading, the rich text in these books for greater integration and deeper understanding.

1. Goel KM, Gupta DK. Hutchinson's Pediatrics, 1st edn. Jaypee Brothers Medical Publishers (P) Ltd, India. 2009
2. Marcdante K, Kliegman RM, Jenson HB, Behrman RE (Eds). Nelson's Essentials of Pediatrics, 6th edn. Saunders Elsevier, 2010.
3. Mason S, Swash M (Eds). Hutchinson's Clinical Methods, 17th edn. A Bailllere Tindall book published by Cassell Ltd; 1980.
4. Milner AD, Hull D. Hospital Pediatrics, 3rd edn. ELBS with Churchill Livingstone. 1998.
5. Behrman RE (comps), Kliegman RM, Nelson WE, Vaughan VC III (Eds). Nelson's Textbook of Pediatrics, 14th edn. Philadelphia: WB Saunders. 1992.
6. Stephenson T, Wallace H (Eds). Clinical Paediatrics for Postgraduate Examinations. UK: Churchill Livingstone. 1991.

Chapter 10

Pediatric Physical Examination

INTRODUCTION[1-41]

- Many factors will influence the approach to the pediatric patient which is most important in conducting a proper and complete physical examination.
- Children are impulsive, unpredictable, interesting and loving.
- A good approach toward the child is vital to a good start in the physical examination of the child.

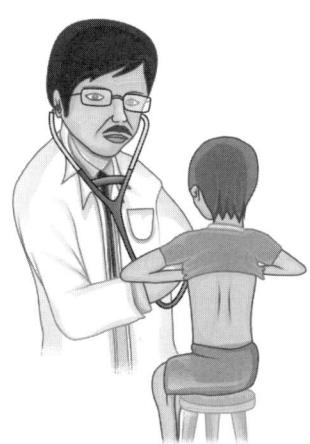

When approaching the pediatric patient, remember that each patient will dictate the following:

- The order you will follow in the physical examination.
- The position you will choose during the physical examination.
- The way you conduct the examination.

Consider these too….

The age-dependent examination may be as follows:[20,24,25,32,34,36,39]

- In the early infancy, it is best to examine on the examination couch with a parent nearby.
- A toddler is most comfortable on the mother's lap or over a parent's shoulder.
- Preschool children can be preliminarily assessed and examined even while at play.
- Teenage girls should be examined in the presence of the mother.
- When undressing the child, ask the parent to do it, unless the child is very cooperative.
- Throughout the examination, make sure that you communicate appropriately in accordance with the age and stage of development of the child.
- Always make sure that your hands are warm and that your stethoscope is warm too.
- Use child friendly little gadgets, bricks or toys attempting to warm the child's heart as well.

You need to be conscious of the following:
- Aware of the concerns of privacy of the teenager.
- Aware and give due respect to the cultural sensitivities of different ethnic groups.

Remember too that your hands must be clean and warm, your nails short, that you remove watches, bangles and bracelets that may hurt your patient. You must have a bright toy with you.

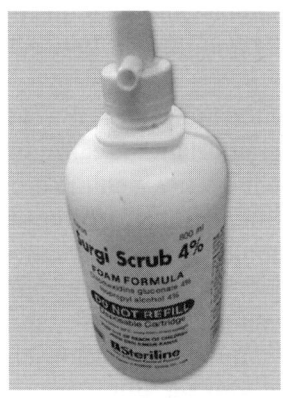

Use the appropriate scrub. Remove rings and bangles

138 *The Link*: Pediatric History-Taking and Physical Examination

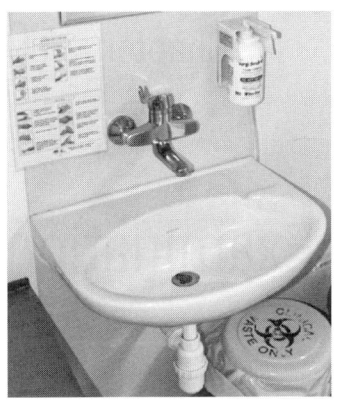
Wash hands with lots of water

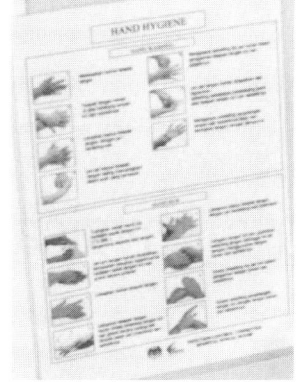
Hand washing is an effective way to reduce nosocomial infections

GOOD CLINICAL PRACTICE

MEASUREMENTS[20,24,25,32,34,36,39,41]

Obtaining maximum cooperation from the child is very important in maximizing the yield of your physical examination.

Make the child happy from the very beginning of your physical examination.

Measurement of weight and height are important and must be routinely done in the examination of children. The height, weight and head circumference are taken to see growth of the child in response to health, illness or treatment. Take the weight, height and head circumference at the most convenient time. In the pediatric examination, this is usually kept to the end.

The normal growth, development and behavior patterns of children are important to monitor. Progress of development, delays in development and abnormalities of development must be noted.

The child's growth and development are also influenced by parent–child relationships, relationships within the family and rapport between the family and community.

Growth is a good indicator of the overall wellbeing of a child and it is important to realize that psychological stresses can also influence a child's growth.

All measurements taken in the pediatric physical examination should be made under standard conditions.

Heights, weights and head circumferences are compared with standards of healthy children of similar gender and age and for this purpose the percentile charts are invaluable.

In general terms of growth, 'normal' growth indicates healthy growth patterns. Statistically, a normal set of values produce a normal distribution. This is the case with anthropometric milestones like age of independent standing. Serial measurements over a period of time, rather than growth at a single point in time, are essential in assessing changes in growth.

There is a range for height, weight and head circumference but the trend of growth is most important.

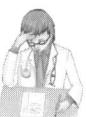

Just like in the history of illnesses where the overall trend of the illness is important, in measurements too, the observation of the trend of growth is vital. The interpretation of the trend of growth is much more meaningful than studying a single reading of growth. Plot these three measurements of growth at each visit.

The process of measurement has 2 steps—measure and record. Meticulous weighing and measuring have 3 critical components—technique, equipment, and trained measurers. You must use the appropriate techniques for each measurement. Today, metric units are used.

Measuring Weight[20,24,25,32,34,36,39,41]

Children, who can stand alone, should be weighed standing on the scale. Otherwise, the mother is weighed alone and then again with the child and her weight is subtracted to determine the child's weight. Another method used is tared weighing.

Tared weighing may be used to weigh a child who cannot yet stand alone or one that will not stand still alone on a weighing scale. In tared weighing, the caregiver (preferably the mother) stands first on the scale and the weight reading in the display panel is brought to zero. The child is then handed to the carer to carry while still on the weighing scale. The reading on the display panel is taken as the weight of the child who has been adequately exposed for weighing.

Advantages of tared weighing include the following:
- There is no need to subtract weight to determine the child's weight alone
- The child is more likely to remain calm in the mother's arms.

Children should be weighed unclothed. Explain to the parents or caregiver that the outer clothing will have to be removed in order to obtain an accurate weight.
- Infants and babies are weighed naked

- Older children are weighed with the bare minimum clothing.

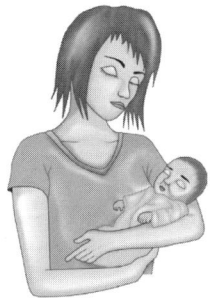

The mother's arms are the best place to keep the child calm-weigh mother and child together by tared weighing.

If it is socially unacceptable to undress the child, remove as much of the clothing as possible. Remove any hair clips or hair accessories that may interfere with the height or weight measurement. This is done to avoid any delay between measuring the weight and length of the child that might upset the child.

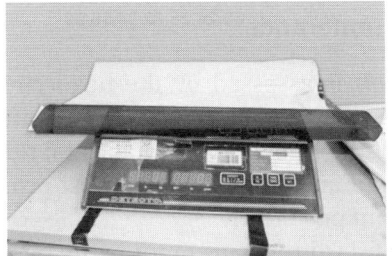

Infant weighing scale.

Normal trend in weight gain[24,25,32,34,36,41]	
Age	Average weight
At birth	3 kg (7 lbs)
At 5 months	6 kg (14 lbs)
At 2 years	13 kg (28 lbs)
At 7 years	22.5 kg (49 lbs)

Weight gain trends[24,25,32,34,36,39,41]	
Age	Trend in weight gain
At approx. 2 weeks	Regains birth weight; then gains about 0.6–0.9 kg (1.5–2 lbs)
At approx. 3 months	Gains 0.45 kg a month
At approx. 5 months	Doubles birth weight
At approx. age 1 year	Triples birth weight and then gains approx. 0.2 kg a month (0.5 lbs)
At approx. age 2 years	Quadruples birth weight and then gains about 1.8–2.2 kg a year (4–5 lbs)
At age 9–10 years	Increases weight as puberty approaches, often about 4–4.5 kg a year (10 lbs)

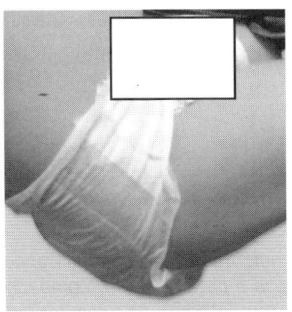

Remove wet diapers before weighing the child; it can contribute to a significant increase in weight.

Measuring Height[20,24,25,32,34,36,39,41]

Measure the length or height immediately after weighing, while the clothes are still off. In a naked child, a dry diaper can be on while measuring length. In an exposed infant, always ensure that the child is nice and warm when placed on an infantometer.

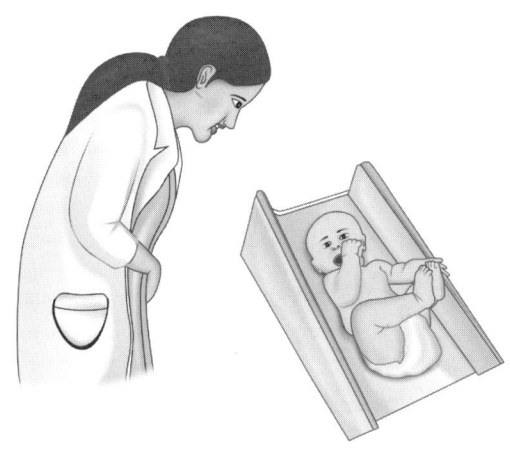

It is best to have the mother around to soothe and comfort the infant while measuring the weight.

It is a good practice to explain to the mother the importance of keeping the child still and calm.

Depending on the child's age and ability to stand independently, length or height is measured. Height which is measured in the standing upright position is 0.7 cm less than length, which is measured in the lying down position. It is important to make the necessary adjustments in length or height when recording in the growth chart. If a child is less than 2 years old and will not lie down for measurement of length, measure standing height and add 0.7 cm to convert it to length. However, if a child is aged 2 years or older but cannot stand, measure the recumbent length and subtract 0.7 cm to convert the measurement to height.

140 *The Link*: Pediatric History-Taking and Physical Examination

A stadiometer measures the height in an older child. A length board or infantometer measures the length or height in an infant.

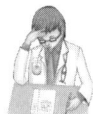

Plots of the weight, height and head circumference on the growth chart in a well-baby clinic is a benchmark for comparison, should the child fall ill. Crossing of percentiles is an indicator for urgent assessment and action. All vaccination visits provide this opportunity.

Height is measured in children aged 2 years or older and able to stand. The child should stand barefoot against a hard surface.

The recumbent length is measured in children below 2 years of age. The child is placed supine and length is measured roughly using a measuring tape or measuring board or an infantometer.

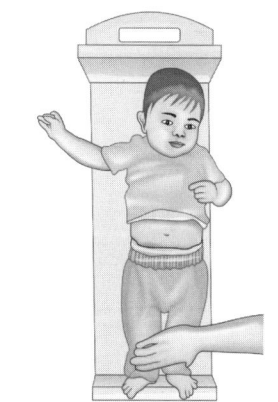

Recumbent length under 2 years.

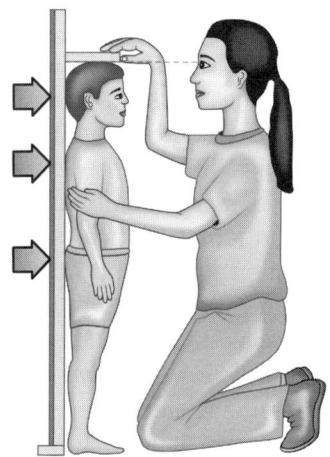

Height is measured when the child can stand independently. Measurements of height and weight in children are fundamental to the interpretation of subsequent physical findings.

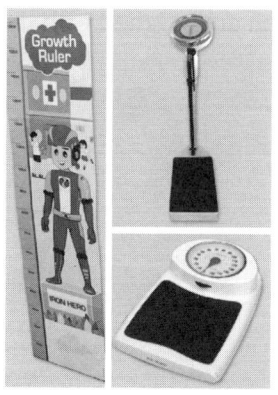

Normal trends in the increase of length and height[24,25,32,34,36,39,41]

Age	Length/height increase
0–12 months	25 cm (10 inches)
1 – 2 years	13 cm (5 inches)
At 3 years to puberty	Grows 5 cm/year (2 inches)

Head Circumference[20,24,25,32,34,36,39]

Brain growth is assessed by the head circumference. The head is measured at its greatest circumference; this is usually at the level of the supraorbital ridges and the mid-forehead anteriorly and the most prominent part of the occiput posteriorly.

The standard measurement is the occipitofrontal circumference (OFC) or circumference of head (COH) which is the largest circumference of the head after measuring three times. Sequential measurements are more useful than one-off measurements in the interpretation of head size. Head circumference measurements that progressively cross percentiles are a major concern. The commonest reason of a head that is growing but is large or small is a familial cause.

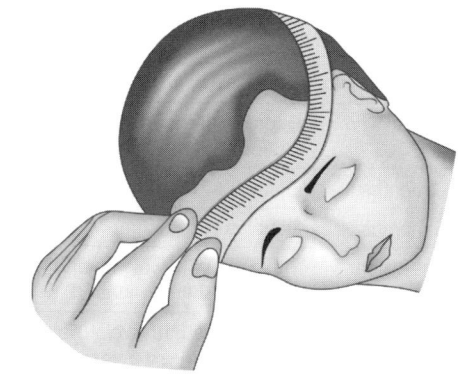

The COH or OFC is the occipitofrontal circumference

Pediatric Physical Examination 141

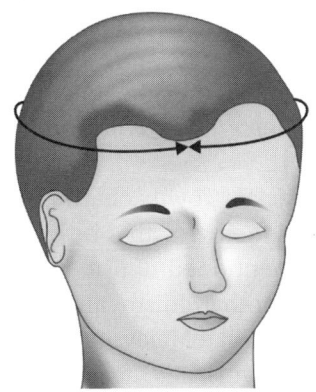

The largest of the three COH readings is taken.

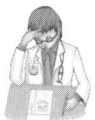

"So, I should measure the COH in all children under 2 years as this corresponds to the period of rapid brain growth. Yet, there are specific conditions, that must make me measure COH even after this age. In older children with abnormal weight and height measurements, it may give clues to the underlying pathophysiology. That's lateral thinking, isn't it?"

Specific indications for head circumference measurement in children over the age of 2 years[24,25,32,34,36,39]
History of seizures
Developmental delay
History suggestive of neurological diseases
Neurocutaneous stigmata
Cerebral palsy
Dysmorphism
Any deviation from normal in history or physical examination

Average measurements of head circumference[24,25,32,34,36,39]	
Age	Head circumference
At birth	35 cm
At 3 months	41 cm
At 6 months	43 cm
At 1 year	46 cm
At 2 years	49 cm

Three readings of the COH are taken for accuracy and the largest reading of the three is recorded (not the average!).

Normal trend in growth measured by head circumference[24,25,32,34,36,39]	
Age	Normal trend of increase in head circumference
At 0–3 months	Increases by 2 cm a month
At 4–6 months	Increases by 1 cm a month
At 6–12 months	Increases by half cm a month
At 1–2 years	Increases by 2 cm a year

Allowance should be made for prematurity. For growth, as it is for development, (Chapter 5), allowances for prematurity are made. If a child is born 8 weeks premature then 8 weeks must be deducted from the child's chronological age when plotting on the age and gender appropriate charts. Such correction is usually done for up to 2 years. The head circumference of a healthy premature infant increases rapidly in the first months of life which may be up to 1 cm per week. This rate is compared to the rate of head growth in the last trimester of pregnancy. Always remember the rate of growth is more important than head circumference at any single moment in time.

Growth Rates: General Guidelines[20,24,25,28,32,34,36,38,39]

Children have a range of normal values of the growth parameters. Refer to gender and age appropriate growth charts for accurate details. It is however useful to use these values as a rough guide to remember.

Growth Charts[24,25,28,32,34,36,38,39]

Growth charts which are actually a series of percentile curves that illustrate the distribution of selected body measurements in children are used to track the growth of infants, children, and adolescents.

Growth charts, which are gender and age-specific, show the average pattern of growth at various ages during childhood. In many countries, charts for different ethnic groups are available. There are also charts for special groups of children like for children with Down syndrome. In order to study the trend of growth of a child, height, weight and head circumference that are measured need to be plotted on a growth chart. It must be remembered that growth charts are tools that help form an overall clinical impression of the child's growth rate.

Standard growth charts have a range that is normally expressed percentiles at the 3rd, 25th, 50th, 75th, 90th, and 97th percentile (a range of normally expressed percentiles as the third, tenth, twenty fifth, fiftieth, seventy fifth, ninetieth, and ninety-seventh percentiles).

As mentioned earlier, a series of measurements demonstrating the trend in growth is more valuable than a single static measurement.

The child's growth should usually follow the curve of the percentile graph. Crossing the percentiles on the growth charts following repeated measurements is a cause for concern and an indication for medical intervention.

WHO growth standards can be plotted to monitor growth of infants and children from the age of 0–2 years. There are also growth charts for ages 2 years and older. The sample growth charts can be obtained at their websites.

The tenth percentile for height means that 10% of all normal children are shorter than this height at that particular age. As a guide, children who fall outside the area between the 10th and 90th percentiles should be reviewed with a detailed history and physical examination.

Children who fall outside the area between the 3rd and 97th percentiles will require appropriate investigations.

There are special growth charts for children with special needs and their growth is best interpreted along the percentiles mentioned above. Such examples are children with hypothyroidism and trisomy 21. In a multiethnic country like Malaysia, where people are of different genetic origins, it is ideal to plot growth charts of individuals belonging to their own ethnic groups, wherever possible. However, these are not always readily available.

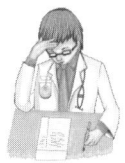

It is best to plot children with special problems on their specific growth charts. For example, there are specific growth charts for children with trisomy 21 and hypothyroidism.

Examples of Weight-for-age Appropriate Growth Charts[16,24,25,32,34,36,38,39]

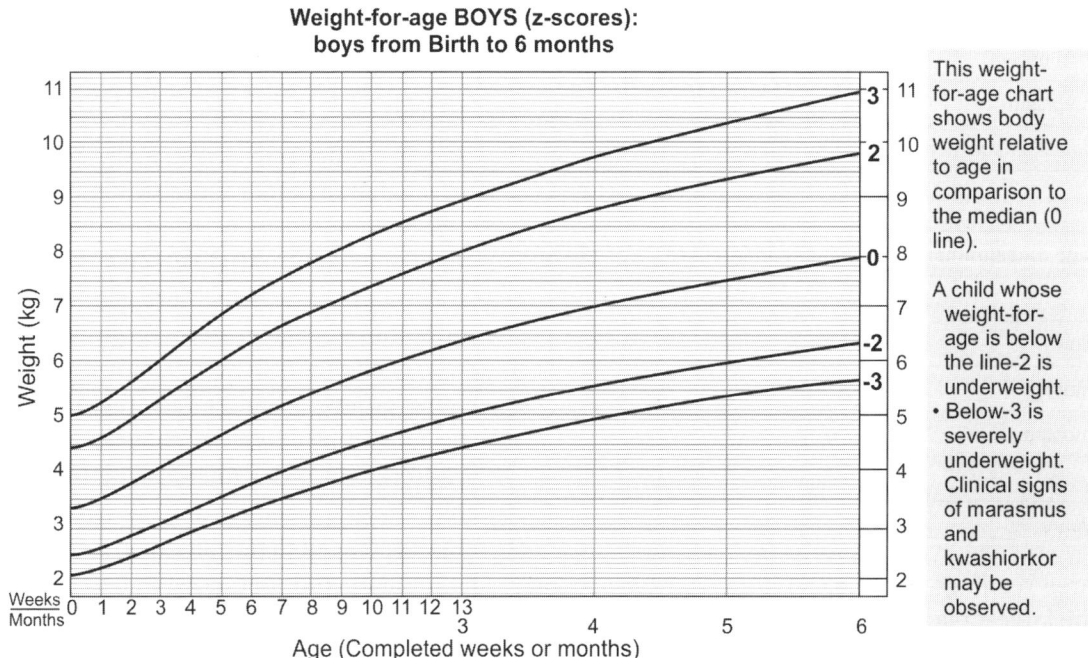

Pediatric Physical Examination 143

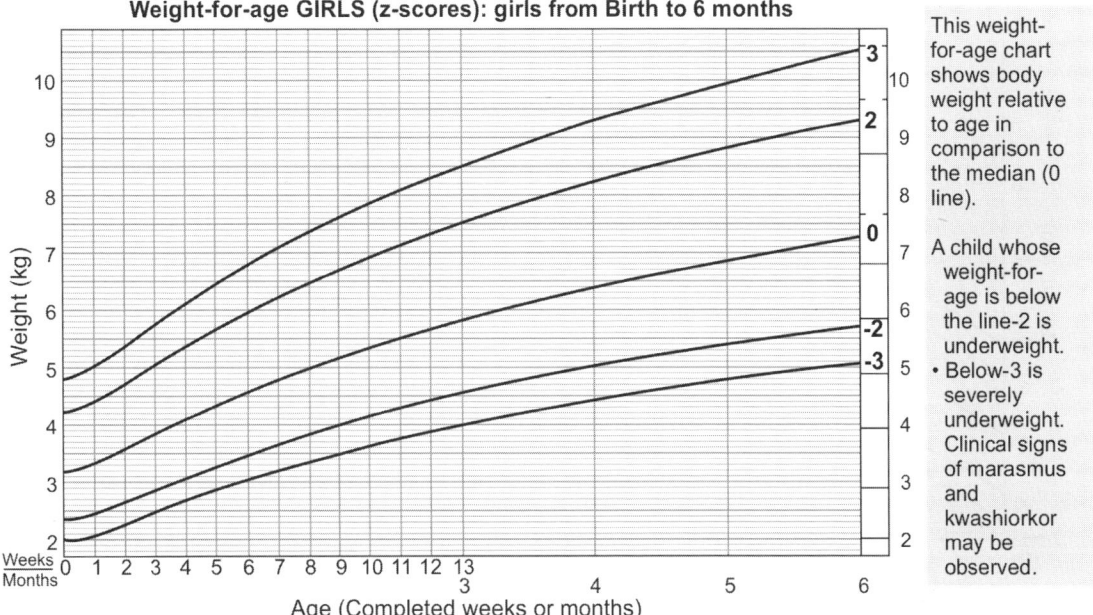

This weight-for-age chart shows body weight relative to age in comparison to the median (0 line).

A child whose weight-for-age is below the line-2 is underweight.
• Below-3 is severely underweight. Clinical signs of marasmus and kwashiorkor may be observed.

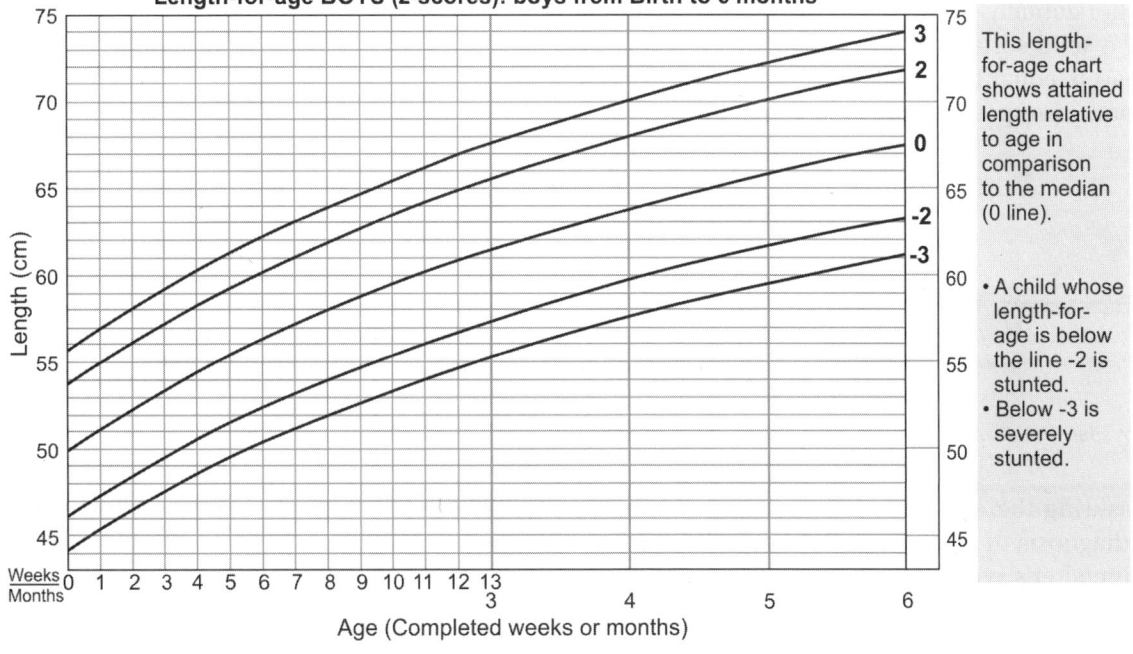

This length-for-age chart shows attained length relative to age in comparison to the median (0 line).

• A child whose length-for-age is below the line -2 is stunted.
• Below -3 is severely stunted.

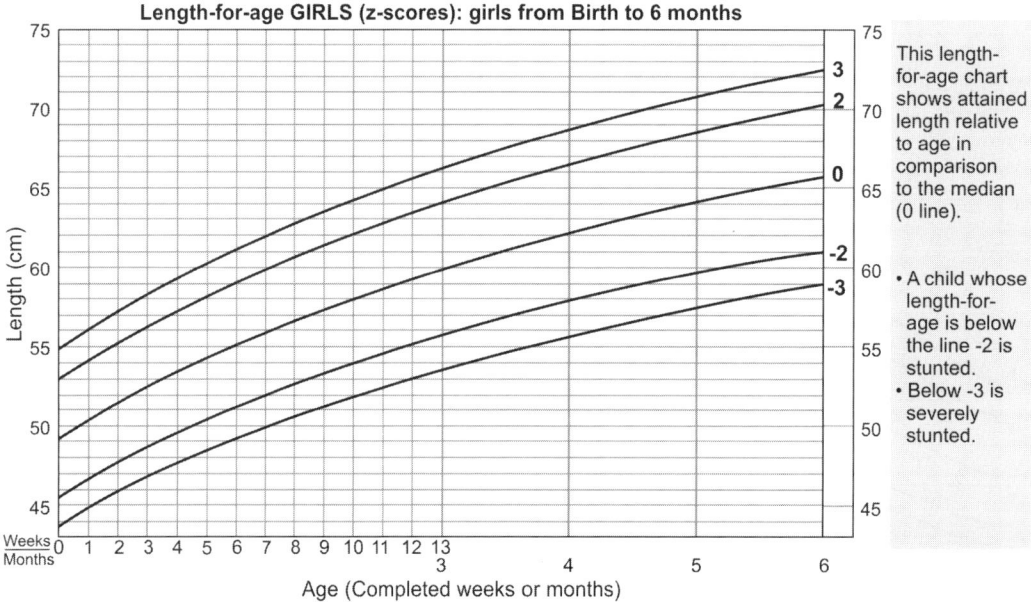

World Health Organization charts for Weight-for-age charts and Length-for-age charts (- z-scores: girls for Birth to 6 months, - z-scores: boys for Birth to 6 months, - z-scores: girls for Birth to 6 months and - z-scores: boys for Birth to 6 months).[38]

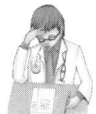

In a multiethnic country, individual growth charts based on ethnicity will be very useful for interpretation of growth as ethnic origins influence facets of growth.

Arm Span[20,24,25,32,34,36,39]

It is the distance between the tips of the middle fingers of the horizontally outstretched arms while standing against a solid surface. At the age of 10–11 years, the arm span is equal to the height of the child. In early childhood, arm span is slightly more than height.

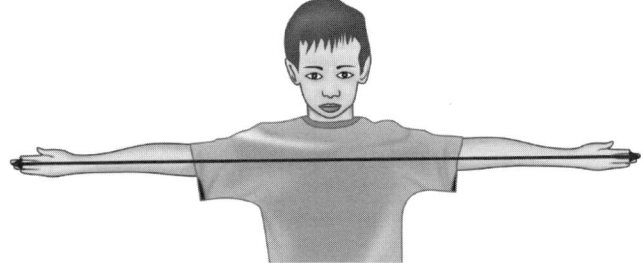

The arm span is measured as shown in the picture above from the furthest tip of one finger to the other.

Measuring the arm span is important as it helps in the diagnosis of diseases such Marfan's syndrome and Klinefelter's syndrome. For example, in Marfan's syndrome, arm span is significantly more than the height.

Mid-arm Circumference[20,24,25,32,34,36,39]

This measurement is useful to measure the nutritional status of a child.

It is measured using a measuring tape at midpoint between the acromion and the tip of the olecranon. Severe malnutrition is indicated by values below 80% of the normal. The mid-arm to head circumference ratio is useful in determining malnutrition.

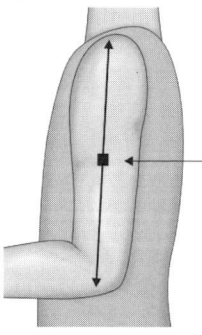

Mid-arm circumference is a useful measure of nutritional status in a child.

Torso Ratios[24,25,32,34,36,39]

The upper segment is measured from the head to the symphysis pubis and the lower segment is measured from the symphysis pubis to the toes. The upper-to-lower segment ratio is another useful tool to assess normal growth. High upper-to-lower segment ratios are seen in skeletal dysplasias, short limbed dwarfism and can be a sign of nutritional deficiencies affecting bones such as rickets. This ratio changes with age.

Normal upper–to–lower segment ratios	
Age	Normal upper–to–lower segment ratios
Infant	1.7
1 year old	1.4
10 years old	1.1

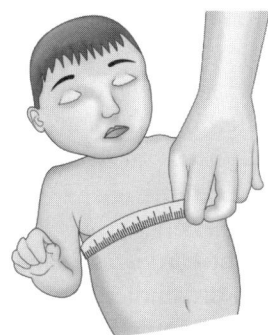

Chest circumference is measured at the level of the nipples in mid inspiration.

Chest Circumference[20,24,25,32,34,36,39]

It is measured at the nipples at the height of inspiration or in mid inspiration. At birth, a baby's head will look bigger than the chest because the head circumference is approximately 2.5 cm larger than the chest circumference (HC>CC). The chest circumference equals the head circumference by the time the child is 5-6 years of age.

Vital Signs[20,24,25,32,34,36,39]

- Blood pressure
- Pulse rate
- Respiratory rate
- Temperature.

Blood Pressure[20,24,25,32,34,36,39]
(Done at the End of the Physical Examination)

Blood pressure is best obtained after the main examination is over. The measurement of blood pressure is often distressing, hence kept to the end, and is vital in specific circumstances as in all cases of suspected cardiovascular or renal disease, or a relevant inherited, genetic or familial disorder from the history.

Measurements of blood pressure are done using the appropriate cuff available for the pediatric age group. The cuff should cover approximately 2/3rd of the length of the arm. The inflatable bag should be long enough to encircle the full circumference of the arm and should be of a width roughly half the length of the upper arm. Allow the child to familiarize himself or herself with the cuff and give some simple explanation of what is going on.

Measuring Blood Pressure[20,24,25,32,34,36,39]

- The best position for measuring blood pressure is in the sitting or lying position with the limb at the level of the heart.
- Use an appropriate sized cuff.
- The cuff size refers to the inner inflatable bladder and not the cloth covering.
- There should be enough space in the antecubital fossa to place the diaphragm of the stethoscope.
- The blood pressure should be recorded in all four limbs.
- Note that the blood pressure recorded in the lower limbs with the cuff technique is about 10 mm higher than in the arms due to direct transmission of pressure from the aorta to the larger descending aorta as compared to the narrow upper arm vessels.

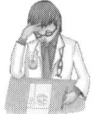

"I recall what I learnt in physiology-that the Korotkoff sounds represent arterial oscillations due to expansion of the arterial wall occurring with each cardiac impulse. This is as a result of partial occlusion of the brachial artery by the sphygmomanometer cuff. There are five phases. There is a clear tapping one, a soft murmur, a loud sound, an abrupt muffling sound and a phase where all sounds disappear"

The mercury sphygmomanometer should be read at eye level. Systolic blood pressure is the onset of a clear tapping sound corresponding to the 1st Korotkoff sound.

Diastolic blood pressure is at:
- Low pitched, muffling (4th Korotkoff sound) in children up to 12 years.
- Disappearance of all sounds (5th Korotkoff sound) for children above 12 years.

In small children and in infants, it may not be possible to determine the blood pressure by auscultation and the pulse can be palpated to obtain the systolic blood pressure. In babies, the flush method is used.

The flush method may be performed as follows: The arm is held up and tightly bandaged to exclude

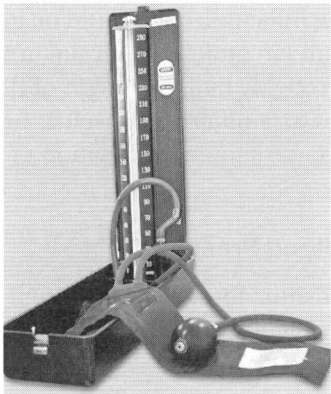

The width of the cuff is important in measuring the blood pressure.

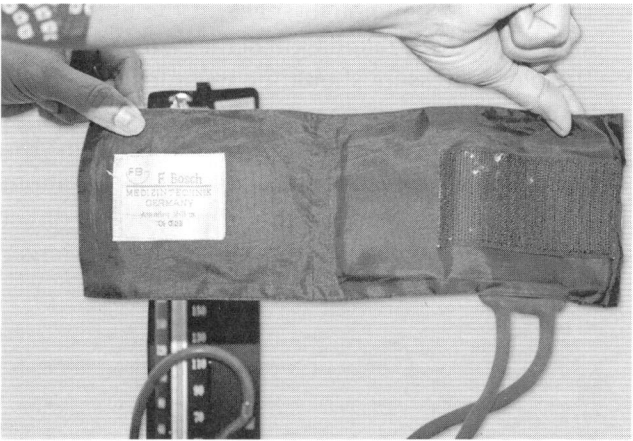

The width of the cuff and the length should be correct for the child's age.

The width of the cuff for different age groups is given below[20]	
Age group	Width of the cuff
Term and preterm neonates	3.5 cm
In the first year of life up to 2 years	4.5 cm
3–4 years	7 cm
5–9 years	10 cm
10–14 years	13 cm

the blood to the level of the cuff which is then inflated. The bandage is then removed to reveal a pale limb. The pressure in the cuff is gradually reduced. The point at which the skin regains color or flushes indicates the systolic pressure.

The average blood pressure in the arms is 80/50 mm Hg in the newborn, 85/60 mm Hg at 4 years, 95/65 mm Hg at 8 years, 100/70 mm Hg at 10 years and 110/75 mm Hg at 13 years.

The blood pressure in the legs must be taken in suspected cases of coarctation of the aorta. Hypertension is persistently elevated systolic or diastolic blood pressure at or above the 95th percentile taken at three readings.

Pulse Rate[20,24,25,32,34,36,38,39]

Assess the pulse when the child is at rest. Gently touch the child's hands; ensure that yours are warm.

Feel the radial and brachial pulses bilaterally. Palpate both right and left pulses simultaneously and note the rate, rhythm, volume and character. In young infants, the pulse is taken by palpation or auscultation of the chest. Auscultation at the apex is the apex beat. In older children, the pulse is taken at the wrist, palpating the radial arterial pulsations.

Arterial pulse assessment is vital in the general examination and in the cardiovascular examination. The radial artery is ordinarily studied but all other peripheral arteries must be examined. Do not omit the femoral pulses bilaterally.

Firstly, locating palpable pulses is important as mentioned below:

Radial: Medial and ventral side of wrist or styloid process of radius with gentle pressure.

Carotids: In the neck, just medial and below the angle of jaw. **Do not palpate both carotids simultaneously**.

Brachial: Just medial to biceps tendon.

Femoral: Inferior and medial to inguinal ligament. It is located midway between the anterior superior iliac spine and pubic tubercle.

Dorsalis pedis: With the foot slightly dorsiflexed on the medial side of dorsum of the foot, observe rate, rhythm, volume, character, tension and equality on both sides.

Rate and rhythm: When the child is at rest or asleep, count the pulse rate for one full minute. It is counted for a whole minute as sinus arrhythmia which occurs in children makes interpretation of the rate and rhythm more accurately defined when assessed for a minute. In neonates, periodic breathing where pauses can occur for up to 10 seconds, makes it necessary to assess the pulse for one full minute. Irregularities in rhythm must be appreciated and counted for at least one minute. Note whether the rate is normal, increased or decreased. A rise in pulse rate occurs in various conditions, including excitement, exercise, fever, physical distress, heart failure, thyrotoxicosis and due to certain drugs. Check the rhythm and assess whether it is regular or irregular.

If it is irregular further describe the irregularity. Is it regularly irregular or irregularly irregular?

Volume: It is the uplift produced by the arterial wall. It is a direct indicator of pulse pressure. When feeling the pulse volume, indicate if it is a weak pulse or a bounding pulse. A weak pulse is due to reduced cardiac output and narrow pulse pressure. A bounding pulse is due to increased cardiac output and increased peripheral resistance often felt in conditions associated with high stroke volume and high blood pressure.

Character: Differentiate the normal pulse character of a normal central aortic pulse wave, which is characterized by a rapid rise to a rounded peak.

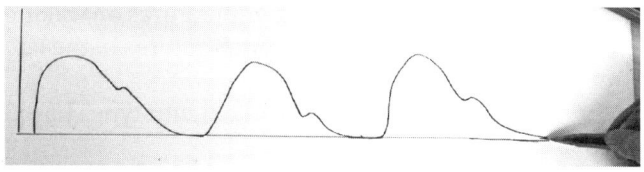

Sketch of the normal arterial pulse

Anacrotic or double beating pulses seen in significant aortic stenosis.

Bisferiens is an increased arterial pulse with a double systolic peak seen in mixed aortic valve disease as well as in hypertrophic obstructive cardiomyopathy.

Bifid or dicrotic pulse is seen in aortic stenosis.

Bigeminal pulse where there is a normal beat alternating with premature contraction may be seen in normal individuals after exercise or in cardiac tamponade and severe heart failure.

Pulses parvus et tardus is a weak and delayed pulse in aortic stenosis.

Pulsus alternans is a variation in pulse amplitude occurring with alternate beats. Pulsus alternans is seen in left ventricular failure—usually accompanied by S3 (a third heart sound). May be seen in patients with severe aortic regurgitation. Frequently precipitated by ectopic beats (bigeminal pulse).

Pulses paradoxus is seen in severe bronchial asthma (and in status asthmaticus), cardiac tamponade, in constrictive pericarditis and restrictive cardiomyopathy. Normally, systolic arterial pressure falls 8-12 mmHg during inspiration. If the pressure drops more than 20 mmHg during inspiration, this indicates pulses paradoxus. This is evaluated with a sphygmomanometer when the cuff is slowly released and the systolic pressure on expiration is first noted. The systolic pressure during inspiration can be detected when the pressure of the cuff is gradually reduced.

Bounding pulses are seen in patent ductus arteriosus, aortic regurgitation, large arteriovenous fistula, febrile states, hyperkinetic states, thyrotoxicosis, Gram negative sepsis, carbon dioxide retention, and anemia.

Collapsing pulses, Water-Hammer pulses or Corrigan pulse are seen in patent ductus arteriosus, aortic regurgitation, thyrotoxicosis and large arteriovenous fistulae. Here not only is the pulse of high volume, but the pulse is also felt as a tapping impulse through the forearm muscles when the arm is lifted up.

Relative bradycardia, though rarely used, is seen in typhoid fever, dengue fever and leptospirosis. Here a rise of 10 beats per minute of the normal pulse with a degree rise in temperature as would occur normally with fever, does not occur with every 1°C rise in temperature. Condition of the vessel wall is appreciated by gently rolling it against the underlying bone. In pediatrics, this may be important in the adolescent patient with familial hyperlipidemia or early onset of diabetes mellitus especially if uncorrected.

Equality: Usually 2 radial pulses are felt simultaneously and femoral pulses are felt 5 msec before the ipsilateral radial pulse. Compare radiofemoral pulses for the clinical diagnosis of co-arctation and radioradial pulses for radioradial delay in aneurysm of aorta, coarctation of aorta and supravalvular aortic stenosis.

The pulse rates vary at different age groups and have a range of the normal values.

Average pulse rates[24,25,32,34,36,39]	
0–3 months	100–150/minute
3–6 months	90–120/minute
6–12 months	80–120/minute
1–3 years	70–110/minute
3–6 years	65–110/minute

Respiratory Rate[20,24,25,32,36,38,39]

Assess when the child is at rest. The respiratory rates vary at different age groups and have a range of the normal values.

Average respiratory rates[24,25,32,34,36,39]	
Newborn	45/minute
Fifth month	40/minute
Second year	25/minute

A raised respiratory rate indicates respiratory or cardiovascular disease. It can also occur in anxiety and acidosis.

The **range** of respiratory rates and heart rates according to age groups are as follows:[24,25,32,34,36,39]

Age	Respiratory rate (breaths/minute)	Heart rate (beats/minute)
<2 months	<60	80–160
2–12 months	<50	<160
1–5 years	<40	<120
6–8 years	<30	<110
9–14 years	<20	<110

Temperature (Best Done at the End of Examination)[20,24,25,32,34,36,38,39]

Temperature taking may be done at the end of a routine examination of children. Use a thermometer with the gradations from 29°C to 43°C. In older children, oral temperature should be recorded. In younger children, axillary or groin temperature is recorded. Rectal temperature is not taken routinely except in the newborn.

Age	Site of temperature recording[24,25,32,34,36,39]
Newborn	Rectal temperature—measure core body temperature; also a means of diagnosing anal atresia
Infants	Rectal temperature
2–6 years	Axilla and groin
> 6 years	Oral temperature

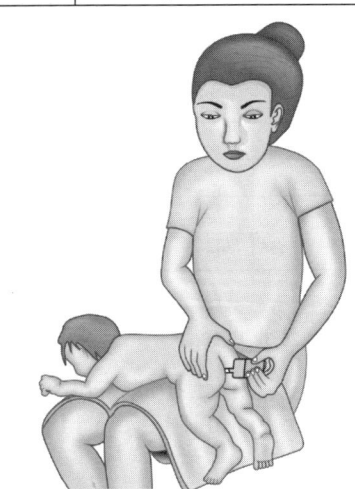

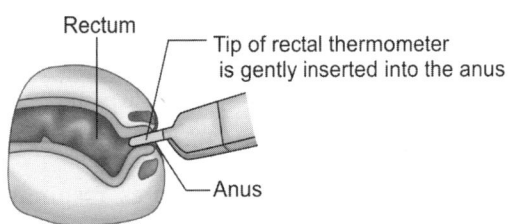

Mother can be taught to gently insert per rectal thermometer

Fever is very common and may be due to excitement, exercise, minor infections as well as to severe infections and other serious illnesses. Neonates and young infants often respond to infections with low temperatures. Hyperpyrexia is a rectal temperature above 41°C and hypothermia is a rectal temperature of less than 35°C. Rapid rises of temperature to 39.5°C or 40°C are sometimes associated with febrile convulsions in young children.

The temperature in the axilla or groin is about 0.5°C lower and in the rectum about 0.5°C higher than the oral temperature. The temperature of normal children varies between 36.5°C and 37.5°C and is about 1°C higher in infants than in older children. There is normal variation of 1°C with the lowest temperatures on waking in the morning and the highest temperatures in the late afternoon.

Fever can be clinically categorized into types based on following pattern:
- **Continued fever** does not fluctuate more than 1°C during a 24 hour period. It never touches baseline.
- **Remittent fever** fluctuates more than 2°C daily and does not touch baseline.
- **Intermittent fever** occurs only for a few hours a day and touches the baseline. When intermittent fever has a daily pattern, it is termed quotidian. When intermittent fever occurs in alternate days it is **tertian** and when 48 hours come between two episodes of fever it is **quartan**.
- **Step ladder fever** occurs classically in typhoid. Here the temperature rises gradually to a higher level with every fever spike.
- **Relapsing fever** has recurrent acute febrile episodes such as in Borreliosis.
- **Saddle back fever** is seen in dengue. Here the fever subsides for a day and returns.
- **Rigors or shivering** can occur in high fevers. It is due to a disturbance in heat regulation. When the temperature rises to higher and higher levels, constriction of the cutaneous vessels causes the surface of the body to feel cold causing shivering. Later vasodilation occurs making the body feel warm again with rising high pyrexia.

Physical Examination[20,24,25,32,34,36,38,39]

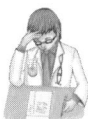

"I need to stand back and make an overall impression of the child, the parents and the surroundings and then concentrate on all the important observations involving the child himself or herself."

GENERAL OBSERVATION

Observation[20,24,25,32,34,36,38,39]

This may be further conveniently divided into distant observation and closer observation.

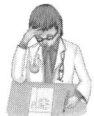

"Are there any clues to the diagnosis near and around the child? Is there any gadget the child uses that could help me link to the anatomical or etiological diagnosis?"

- Parameters like the breathing pattern of a child or how the child holds his bottle or reaches out for objects or interacts with his mother or the surroundings are best done from a distance when the child is not aware of your presence.
- The surroundings and other adjuncts used are observed from a distance.
- The interaction between the parents and the child can also be observed at this time.
- Gadgets and medication must all be observed in detail.
- Is there a nebulizer, an intravenous line (IV), or oxygen being administered to the patient?
- What is the nature of fluids being administered through the IV line?
- What sorts of medications are being given to the patient?
- Are there many soiled pampers around?
- Is the child being given oral rehydration solution?
- Is there a nasogastric tube in place?
- Is there a urinary catheter in place?
- Is the older child still in pampers?
- Is there a wheelchair or a walking aid of any kind?
- At this point, look at the parents or the siblings or the caregiver.
- Are there any specific, striking features? Short stature, tall stature, a big head, a small head. All of these observations must start with excluding familial causes first.
- Look at the interaction between the parent and the child. Is the mother duly concerned about the sick child?
- Specific odors like purulent odor of bacterial infections, the sweet smelling odor of maple syrup urine disease, the acetone odor in diabetic ketoacidosis or the uremic odor of renal failure are observations that a clinician can make using the sense of smell.

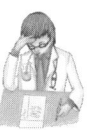

Important observations in pediatrics include observations such as short stature, tall stature, a big head and a small head. These observations must start with excluding familial causes first. Hence observation of the surroundings must importantly include looking at the parents and siblings too.

- You must use all your senses for observation.
- You may also listen to the cough or the cry of the infant to see if there are any peculiarities that can give clues to diagnosis.

Infant's Cry[8,20,24,25,32,34,36,39]

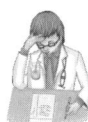

"How do the features of the cry help me link to the history? Is it of diagnostic importance?"

- Vigorous and lusty
  - Healthy, full-term infant
  - Healthy, premature infant
- Weak or feeble
  - Severe infection
  - Lethargy
  - Muscle weakness, such as myasthenia gravis and muscular dystrophy
- High pitched or shrill
  - In cerebral irritability (such as kernicterus and meningitis)
  - Abnormal central nervous system
  - Malnutrition especially marasmus
  - Cornelia de Lange syndrome
  - Cri-du-chat syndrome—a cry that sounds like a cat
- Grunting cry
  - Pneumonia
  - Sepsis
  - Pain
- Exasperation and agony
  - Pain – intense and long-lasting
  - Hungry, tired, cold – short duration
- Husky
  - Hypothyroidism
  - Trauma to the hypopharynx
  - Vocal cord paralysis
- Muffled
  - Epiglottitis

150 *The Link*: Pediatric History-Taking and Physical Examination

- Throaty, stridorous
  - Foreign body
  - Croup
  - Infection—abscesses, croup, epiglottitis
  - Laryngeal abnormalities
  - Oropharyngeal abnormalities
  - Tracheal abnormalities
  - Neoplasm.

General Observation (Closer)

Dysmorphism[20,24,25,32,34,36,39]

Note the presence of any gross congenital anomalies. Obvious congenital malformations are important observations to make in the general assessment of a child. Although they are rare in the general population, if they are recognized they give important clues to the underlying system to focus on during the physical examination. Some known causes of congenital malformations are drugs, chemicals, environmental factors and genetic factors.

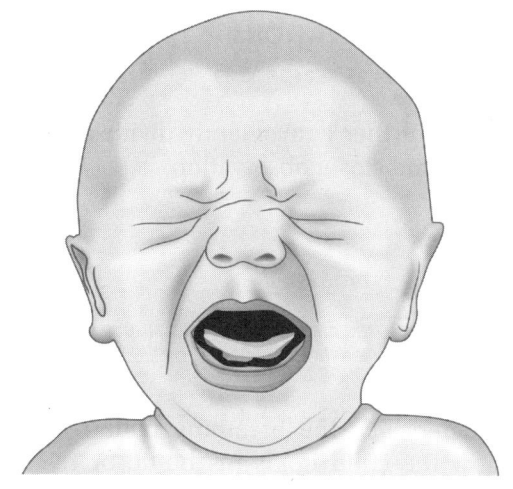

The cry of an infant can tell a lot about his or her health status. It reveals diagnostic clues, so listen carefully as observation involves looking, listening, touching and even at times, appreciating characteristic odors of important diseases or their etiological agents. Hence, it is very important that you sharpen your clinical acumen by astute observation.

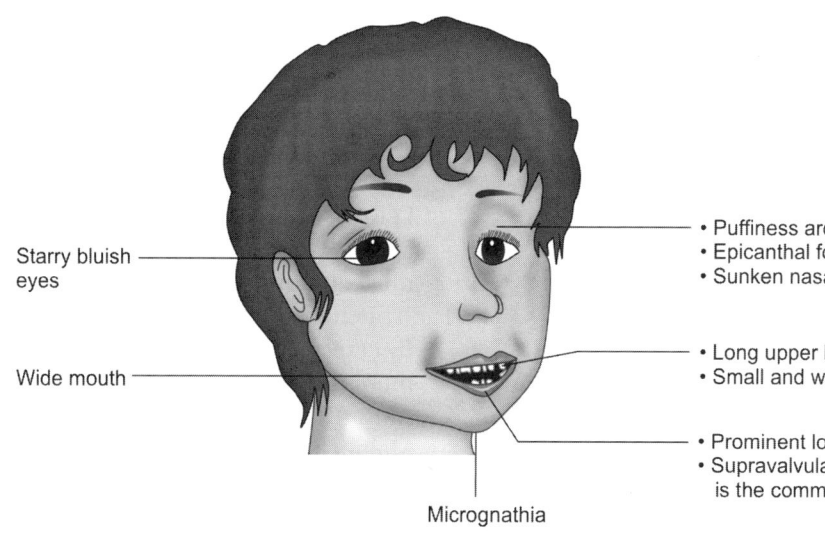

William syndrome

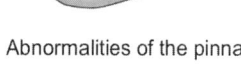

Observe the shape and other features of the ears

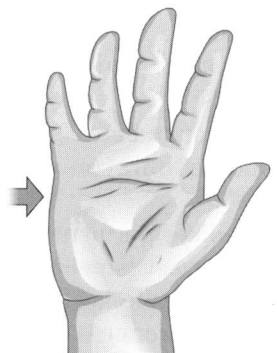

Simian crease in Down syndrome

Pediatric Physical Examination 151

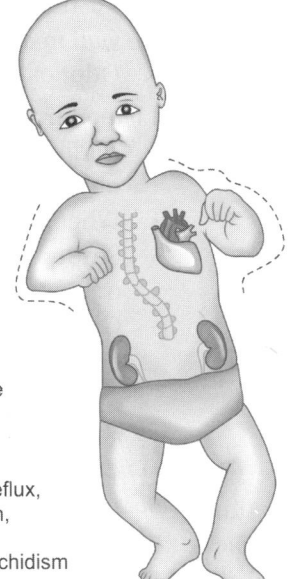

Macrosomia with excessive height and occipitofrontal circumference

Congenital cardiac defects such as such as septal defects and patent ductus arteriosus

Neonatal jaundice

Scoliosis and advanced bone age

Genitourinary anomalies such as such as bifid, duplex or absent kidneys, vesico-ureteric reflux, pelvo-ureteric junction obstruction, cystic kidneys, genital anomalies such as hypospadias and cryptorchidism

High forehead
Down slanting palpebral fissures

Pointed chin

Large hands and feet

Seizures and brisk tendon reflexes

Neonatal hypotonia and feeding difficulties

Solo Syndrome[3]

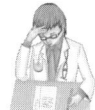

Some syndromes associated with dysmorphisms are "nice to know" as they give focus to the subsequent physical examination.

A dysmorphic child with an identifiable syndrome may have the typical features of Down syndrome, Turner syndrome in a girl, Noonan syndrome in a boy, Sotos syndrome, Williams syndrome or Russel-Silver syndrome. It is not mandatory that you know an exhaustive list of syndromes, although it is nice to know.

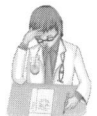

"Diseases of the endocrine system can involve any organ system. Hence, careful observation of growth parameters and a complete examination of all systems are the methods I would make use of to examine the endocrine system."

Many endocrine disorders can be clinically screened by attentive observation[24,25,32,34,36,39]

- Observe all features of the patient from head to toe.
- A child with short limbs may have achondroplasia.
- A child who is short and thin may have an associated chronic disease although psychosocial deprivation must also be considered if the history and other physical signs are suggestive.
- A child who is short and fat may have an endocrinopathy.

- Many other facets of the systemic examination like the vital signs, general examination of the neck, examination of the abdomen and genitalia must be done in considering an endocrinopathy.
- Among the observational differential diagnoses include (remember these are observational guidelines. Much more needs to be studied to make the diagnosis) the following:
  – A short fat child could have the following:
    - Panhypopituitarism
    - Hypothyroidism
    - Isolated growth hormone deficiency
    - Pseudohypoparathyroidism
    - Cushing's syndrome
    - Prader-Willi syndrome.
  – An unusually tall thin boy could have the following:
    - Marfan's syndrome
    - Klinefelter's syndrome
    - Homocystinuria
    - Growth hormone excess.

Comment on the following:

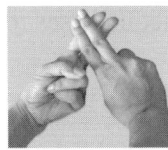

- Appearance of the child. You could do this from some distance and then again at a closer range.

152 The Link: Pediatric History-Taking and Physical Examination

- Take time to observe this with as much precision as possible. Do not wake up a sleeping child! Sleep positions can be varied in children.

In pediatrics, observation could be everything[24,25,32,34,36,39]

Assess the following:
- Well, ill or very ill
- Active, playful or uninterested
- Comfortable or uncomfortable
- Well-nourished or thin and emaciated
- Alert, dull, lethargic, delirious or comatose
- Irritable
- Slow or no response to things around
- A dusky color around the child's lips or with respiratory pauses when he or she stops breathing is a very ill child who requires immediate medical attention
- Striking pallor
- Mottling of the skin on the extremities in an inactive child is a sign of severe disease
- Dysmorphism with a recognizable syndrome
- Dysmorphism that does not characterize a syndrome but has some suggestive features
- Stature
- Disproportionate short stature
- Are the limbs unusually short?
- Is the child short and thin?
- Is the child short and fat?
- The general state of development; note the chronological and developmental age of the child by observing the overall size of the child and looking at all the things that he or she may be doing.
- Facies and expression
- Posture
- Rashes in children are usually due to minor infections and are not serious
- A rash that does not fade when pressure is applied may be a sign of meningococcal infection
- A toxic looking child with fever and lethargy can have sepsis or meningitis
- Sitting with posture of head and chin forward is characteristic of upper respiratory tract illnesses to ease upper respiratory obstruction
- Drooling of saliva is seen in acute epiglottitis
- Floppiness is seen in hypotonia
- Stiffness or jerky movements
- Photophobia
- Posture of neck retraction with arching back
- Gait in an older child
- Odor of breath, peculiar odor of urine.

Listen for (without stethoscope)[20,24,25,32,34,36,38,39]
- Audible breath sounds, which signify respiratory obstruction
- Wheeze
- Stridor. Listen. Is it inspiratory (common), expiratory or biphasic?
- Grunting.

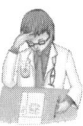

Does the chronological age tally with the development age of the child? Is the child "slow" because of illness?

Watching the child play allows an overall impression of the child's development. Comment on the general appearance. If unwell, comment on how sick the child is.

Comment on the General Appearance[20,24,25,32,34,36,38,39]

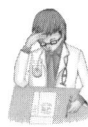

"I need to reiterate to myself that in pediatrics a large contribution to the diagnosis is by astute observation of the well-being and activity of the child."

Describe normal appearance and alertness using the following terms[24,25,32,34,36,39]
• Looking around the room
• Looking at the observer
• Eyes are shiny and bright
• Happily follows instructions (if age is correct)
• Sitting and moving arms and legs
• Swinging arms and legs on table
• Playing with toys
• Stacking up bricks

Describe playfulness and normal healthy vigor using the following terms[24,25,32,34,36,39]
• Vocalizing spontaneously
• Reaching for objects
• Squealing with excitement
• Vocalizing spontaneously
• Babbling
• Laughing aloud
• Smiling

Normal behavior patterns include[24,25,32,34,36,39]
• Consolabilty
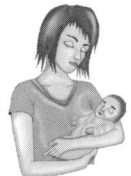
• Stops crying when held by mother
• Stranger anxiety in an older infant (at the appropriate developmental age)

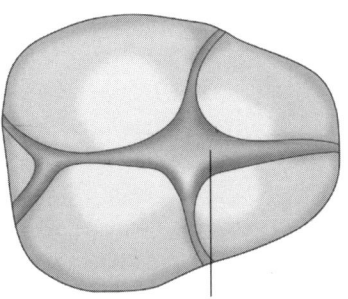

Diamond-shaped anterior fontanel

Signs of dehydration in an infant: sunken soft spot on top of head which is the anterior fontanel.

An ill child must be aptly described. Terms that are indicative of severe illness include the following:[24,25,32,34,36,39]

Staring vacantly or blankly into space
Inconsolable cry despite being held and comforted by mummy
Hydration Assessing hydration in a sick child is extremely important for diagnosis as well as for intervention. Examine for hydration status.
Signs of dehydration include the following: • Alertness—alert or lethargic • Sunken eyes • Dryness of mouth and tongue • Dyspnea • Depressed anterior fontanel • Skin turgor • Heart rate—tachycardia; also describe pulse volume • Respiratory rate—tachypnea (due to acidosis) in severe dehydration • Excessive thirst • Restlessness • Irritability • Oliguria with concentrated urine • Capillary refill time

As dehydration proceeds, the child becomes lethargic and stuporous[24,25,32,34,36,39]	
The degree of dehydration	
Mild	5%
Moderate	10%
Severe	15%
Examine the following for signs of dehydration[24,25,32,34,36,39]	
Pulse rate	Tachycardia (related to age) – absent or present
Palpable pulses	Present/present but weak/decreased
Blood pressure	Normal/orthostatic hypotension/hypotension
Cutaneous perfusion	Normal/reduced and mottled
Skin turgor	Normal/slightly reduced/reduced
Fontanel	If still patent, normal/slightly depressed/sunken
Mucous membrane	Moist/dry/very dry
Tears	Present/absent
Respirations	Normal/deep/deep and rapid
Urine output	Normal/oliguria/anuria

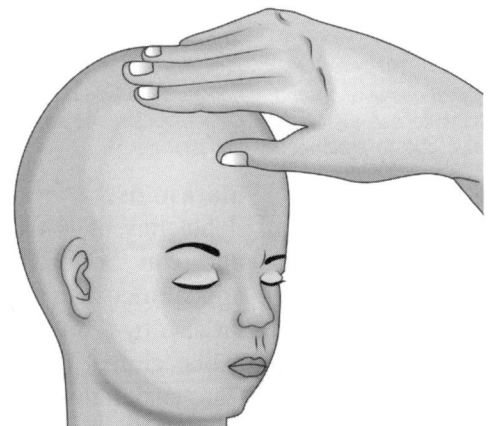

Palpate the anterior fontanel to see if it is sunken, normotensive, or bulging.

154 *The Link*: Pediatric History-Taking and Physical Examination

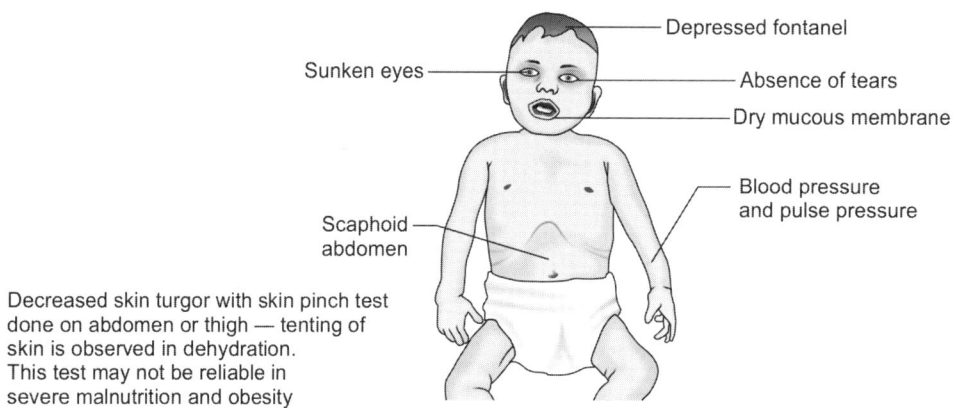

Some signs of dehydration in an infant—what else should you look for?

Observation of Nutritional Status in a Child[20,24,25,32,34,36,39]

In observation of the general appearance, the nutritional state of the pediatric patient must be noted. Some of the signs are mentioned elsewhere in the text under general and specific appearance. However, they are grouped together here under this heading on nutritional deficiencies to impress upon you that the pediatric general observation must take into account the nutritional status of the child. This is by taking anthropometric measurements, plotting them on age and gender appropriate charts as well as by looking for the signs of multinutrient deficiencies. A complete nutritional history will be an important tool to guide you to focus your examination on the signs of the more common nutritional deficiencies.

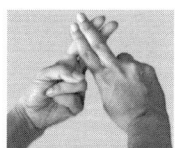

The nutritional link is pivotal in the general physical observation and examination of the pediatric patient as dietary intake can easily be compromised in the young child who is anorexic due to prolonged illness.

Although overt nutritional deficiencies are not as common in many parts of the world today, signs of nutritional deficiencies must be looked for and such deficiencies must also be considered in the differential diagnosis when the history is suggestive. In prolonged or recurrent infections or fevers, uncommon infections and in parasitic infestations (which may be cause or effect of poor nutrition), nutritional imbalances as possible contributors to the physical findings must not be overlooked. Non accidental injury in the form of nutritional deprivation can also cause nutritional deficiencies. Poverty and the sociocultural and environmental factors are also important in many parts of the world.

Dietary intake can easily be further compromised in the young child who is anorexic due to illness.

Hence the physical signs of nutritional deficiency states are important to know.

The weight, height and COH must be measured[20,24,25,32,34,36,39]

Wasting and edema must be noted[23-25,32,34,36,39]

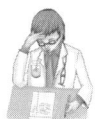

Children who suffer from malnutrition more commonly have a combination of deficient macronutrients and micronutrients such as marasmic-kwashiorkor and multivitamin deficiencies. "Hence, I must try to remember and link the spectrum of clinical manifestations of nutritional deficiency states by relating to physiology." For example, vitamin D deficiency is linked to calcium metabolism, iron deficiency to vitamin C metabolism and so on. This link is important to understand and rationalize.

Marasmus:[9,23-25,32,34,36,39] It is due to a total energy deficiency. It is usually seen before one year of age and can be prevented by breastfeeding. Wizened appearance with wrinkling of skin, loss of subcutaneous fat also by reduced skin turgor, loose skin folds under axilla, gluteal areas with muscle wasting, loss of fat from sucking pads of skin, distended or flat abdomen, atrophy of muscles and subnormal temperature. The child is usually irritable and has a voracious appetite.

Kwashiorkor:[9,23-25,32,34,36,39] The term kwashiorkor is derived from an African term which means 'first-second child'. This is because it usually affects children who are "weaned away" because of the birth of a second child. Inadequate protein intake with electrolyte disturbances like potassium deficiency and excess sodium and many other factors contribute to edema. It is usually seen during weaning after eighteen months of age. Pitting edema can be severe to progress to anasarca or generalized edema. Lethargy, apathy, irritability, loss of muscle tone, dermatitis, secondary skin infections, darkening of skin, dyspigmentation after desquamation, hepatomegaly, brittle and lusterless hair are part of the clinical picture. Parotid gland enlargement may be seen in any form of malnutrition.

The hair is sparse and thin, streaky red or gray in color (hypochromotrichia). Parasitic infestations are also seen.

Limited attention span, protuberant abdomen, delayed epiphyseal development, dental irregularities and delayed puberty are associated features.

In marasmic-kwashiorkor, a combination of the signs from marasmus and kwashiorkor occur. In both conditions, bacterial infections, dehydration (more difficult to assess) and circulatory disorders are important to search for as early management of these additional problems in the child can be lifesaving.

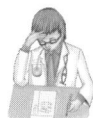

Pitting edema occurs in hypoproteinemic states as seen in kwashiorkor and in a child with nephrotic syndrome. It occurs in heart failure, liver failure and renal diseases. Lymphatic edema does not pit and is rarer in children.

Vitamin A deficiency[23-25,32,34,36,39]

- Night blindness, xerosis conjunctivae, xerosis cornea, wrinkling and cloudiness of cornea or keratomalacia
- Bitot's spots or dry gray plagues on bulbar conjunctivae, follicular hyperkeratosis, photophobia
- Pallor and other signs of anemia, hepatosplenomegaly
- Dry scaly skin, cornified vaginal epithelium, hematuria
- Hydrocephalus with or without cranial nerve palsies.

Vitamin B deficiency[23-25,32,34,36,39]

Thiamine deficiency[24,25,32,34,36,39]

- Undernourished and pale
- Apathy, irritability, poor concentration, depression, drowsiness
- Peripheral neuritis, decreased tendon reflexes
- Loss of vibration sense
- Hoarseness due to paralysis of the laryngeal nerve is typical
- Dry beriberi
- Nerve damage leading to a loss of muscle strength and muscle paralysis
- Wet beriberi
- Edema with dyspnea, hepatomegaly and signs of cardiac failure may develop.

Riboflavin deficiency[24,25,32,34,36,39]

- Cheilosis or perleche
- Glossitis
- Keratitis
- Conjunctivitis
- Photophobia
- Corneal vascularization
- Seborrheic dermatitis
- Pallor and other signs of anemia.

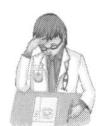

Hence anemia is seen in mineral and multivitamin deficiencies. What are the types of anemia that may manifest? "I know about microcytic, hypochromic anemia, macrocytic anemia and normocytic anemia. I must link the role of the micronutrient with the formation of the RBC to determine the type of anemia that occurs in the different types of nutritional deficiencies"

Niacin deficiency[24,25,32,34,36,39]

- Symmetrical erythema of the exposed surfaces that resemble sunburn
- Lesions on the hand or the pellagrous glove are sharply demarcated from the healthy skin
- Likewise the pellagrous boot is affected skin that is sharply demarcated from the healthy skin of the leg
- Casal necklace are lesions around the neck
- Vesicular lesions or bullous lesions can also be seen
- Stomatitis, glossitis
- Diarrhea, sometimes with constipation, dermatitis, and dementia are recognized.
- Pallor and other signs of anemia.

Pyridoxine deficiency[24,25,32,34,36,39]

- Convulsions of myoclonia or hypsarrhythmia
- Peripheral neuritis
- Dermatitis, cheilosis, glossitis, seborrhea around eyes, nose and mouth
- Anemia.

Vitamin C deficiency[23-25,32,34,36,39]

- Tenderness during diaper change or when infant is carried
- Pseudoparalysis or frog leg posture due to pain
- Edema and swelling of the legs
- Bluish spongy swellings of the mucous membranes of the gums
- Costochondral swellings and sternal depression
- Scorbutic beads are sharper than that seen in vitamin D deficiency
- Petechial hemorrhages, subdural hematomas, swollen joints
- Sicca syndrome characterized by xerostomia, keratoconjunctivitis and salivary gland enlargement
- Anemia—megaloblastic or iron deficiency due to bleeding.

Vitamin D deficiency[23-25,32,34,36,39]

- Craniotabes
- Delayed teeth eruption
- Harrison's groove, a horizontal depression along the lower chest border
- Enlargement of costochondral junctions
- Pectus carinatum
- Scoliosis
- Kyphosis
- Lumbar lordosis
- Narrowed pelvic entrance
- Epiphyseal enlargement of the wrists and ankles
- Bowlegs (more severe than expected for developmental age)
- Knock knees (more severe than expected for developmental age)
- Coxa vara
- Greenstick fractures affecting long bones
- Short stature or rachitic dwarfism
- Delayed motor developmental milestones.

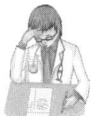

So deformities of the chest wall are seen in vitamin C and vitamin D deficiencies

Vitamin E deficiency[23-25,32,34,36,39]

- Malabsorption
- Anemia
- Premature infants may have hemolytic anemia.

Vitamin K deficiency[23-25,32,34,36,39]

- Hemorrhage.

SPECIFIC OBSERVATION AND EXAMINATION

Head[24,25,32,34,36,39]

Shape and Size of the Head

Some normal variations in the shape of the head are seen among infants; this is due to the patent fontanel and soft skull bones. The shape and size of the head should be noted.

Abnormal shape or size is due to premature fusion of the sutures or nonfusion of the sutures. Note if it is normal, big or small for the child's age.

Shape or size of the head[24,25,32,34,36,39]	Description[24,25,32,34,36,39]
Normal	Often asymmetrical in normal infants who tend to lie persistently on one side
Brachycephaly	The back of head is flattened
Scaphocephaly	Narrow bifrontal diameter
Acrocephaly	High and pointed with wide base
Oxycephaly	Elongated upward with pointed vertex
Plagiocephaly	Normal variation seen in many infants
Positional plagiocephaly	Occurs when the back or one side of an infant's head is flattened, often with hair growth affected in that area. Infants after put to lie on their backs may manifest this. May be associated with physical neglect in non-accidental injury.
Dolichocephaly	Elongated from the front to back
Trigonocephaly	Triangular head—small pointed forehead
Hydrocephalus	Round or globular shape
Microcephaly	May be a part of other abnormalities. May be caused by genetic causes, prenatal causes or due to postnatal causes that cause cerebral insults. In a jaundiced patient, microcephaly in the infant may suggest congenital infection
Prominence of the occiput	May signify Dandy–Walker syndrome
Macrocephaly	May be a part of other abnormalities
The scalp, skull, suture lines and fontanel Suture lines are not palpable after 6 months	There are the coronal, sagittal, lambdoid and metopic sutures
Fontanel	Time of closure
Anterior (diamond-shaped)	18th month (15th to 24th month)
Posterior (triangular)	2nd month (2nd to 3rd month)

Feel the fontanel gently with the child quite. The extent and feel of tension of the anterior fontanel is important; normally it pulsates and is in the same plane as the rest of the surrounding skull.

Auscultation of the skull for bruits over specific areas is useful. The globes, the temporal fossae, and retroauricular or mastoid areas should be listened to. Intracranial bruits are heard in many cases of angiomas, often accompanied by a palpable thrill. They can also be heard in anemia, thyrotoxicosis, and meningitis.

Transillumination of the skull is done with a torch light held against the head.

Craniotabes[24,25,32,34,36,39]

Pressing the scalp firmly just above and behind the ears and at the edges of the open fontanel causes a crackling sound.

Craniotabes is seen in:
- Normal full-term infants
- Normal premature infants
- Rickets
- Hydrocephalus
- Congenital syphilis.

Abnormalities in Suture Closure[24,25,32,34,36,39]

Abnormalities[24,25,32,34,36,39]	Etiology[24,25,32,34,36,39]
Delayed closure	• Protein-energy malnutrition • Rickets • Hydrocephalus • Down syndrome • Cretinism
Wide suture separation	• Hydrocephalus • Macewen (cracked pot) sign where sutures are separated, may indicate increased intracranial pressure
Early closure	• Craniosynostosis
Tense or bulging fontanel	• Normally tense when the child is crying • Sudden increase in intracranial tension (e.g. meningitis) • Intracranial tension • Subdural effusion
Depressed fontanel	• Severe dehydration • Marasmus
Pulsatile	• Normal (slight pulsations)

Anomalies on the scalp[24,25,32,34,36,39]	
Scalp anomalies	Cause
Swelling of the scalp	• Cephalhematoma (a tense collection of blood bounded by suture lines) • Caput (pitting edema of the scalp and can cross the suture lines) • Encephalocele • Secondaries from malignancies • Histiocytosis
Defect of the skull	• Histiocytosis • Secondaries from malignancies

Examination of the Hair[24,25,32,34,36,39]

Scalp hair is said to be our crowning glory. It can also reveal the state of our health.

Hair texture[24,25,32,34,36,39]	Disease[24,25,32,34,36,39]
Thin, sparse, brown Flag sign—intermittent bands of pigmentation and depigmentation Sparse and thin hair, streaky red or gray hair color or hypochromotrichia	• Kwashiorkor
Alopecia	• Alopecia areata • Fungal infection on the scalp • Trichotillomania or hair pulling
Generalized alopecia	• Cytotoxic therapy • Cranial irradiation • Ectodermal dysplasia: With dental hypoplasia and absent nails • Postmaturity
Posterior baldness	• Due to contact friction from bed clothes
Low hair line *These are nice to know*	• Turner's syndrome • Chromosomal aberration
Other abnormalities of hair	• White forelock of Waardenburg syndrome • Bushy eyebrows of Cornelia de Lange syndrome • Kinky hair in Menkes syndrome

Facial Appearance[24,25,32,34,36,39]

Describe the facial appearance of the child. A list of characteristic facies is given below. Observe the face for rashes on cheeks, note if flaring "alae nasi' is present, look out for cleft lip, dysmorphism and micrognathia. Note these anomalies and link other possible associated physical findings.

Abnormal facies[24,25,32,34,36,39]	Description[24,25,32,34,36,39]
Wizened facies	• Marasmus • Post maturity
Severe dehydration	• Weak cry • Sunken eyes • Lethargic gestures
Down syndrome	• Rounded face • Brachycephaly • Upward slant eyes • Epicanthic folds • Hypertelorism • Depressed nasal bridge • Brushfield spots • False macroglossia • Small mouth
Mental retardation	• May have a blank look • Open mouth • Drooling of saliva (especially with bulbar palsy)
Cretin	• Hoarse cry • Thick eye brows • Dull expression • Rough skin • Puffiness of eyelids
Micrognathia, Pierre Robin sequence and others	• Small mandible
Hurler syndrome	• Enlarged tongue • Hypertrophic gums • Hypertelorism
Chronic hemolytic anemia	• Unkindly called 'chipmunk facies' • Parietal and maxillary prominence • Malocclusion of jaw

Observation of the Eyes[24,25,32,34,36,39]

Be gentle. Ensure that your hands are warm. When examining the conjunctivae of a young child, use a toy so that the child looks upwards. When examining the sclerae, distract with a toy so that the infant looks downwards. Look for pallor of the conjunctivae and observe the sclera for jaundice. Look for Brushfield spots, which are gray-white areas of depigmentation of the iris seen in Down syndrome. Kayser-Fleischer rings seen in Wilson's disease are dark rings that appear to encircle the eye. Look for cataracts and conjunctivitis. The bulbar conjunctiva lines the eyeball and the palpebral conjunctiva covers the inner surface of the eyelids.

Short or slanted palpebral fissures must be noted. Is there extension of the eyebrows to the midline? You may see this in rare syndromes, such as Cornelia de Lange. Look for corneal clouding or lens opacity. Is the sclera blue? Blue sclerae are seen in osteogenesis imperfecta, Crouzon syndrome, Cornelia de Lange

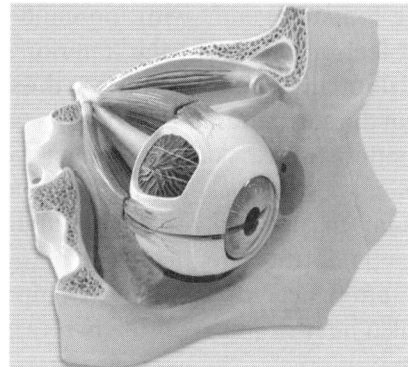

Model of an eye

syndrome, Ehlers-Danlos syndrome, Laron's syndrome, or Laron-type dwarfism, Marfan syndrome, pseudo-hypoparathyroidism and Turner syndrome. In infants, a squint may be detected by shining a light in front of the face. The light reflex should fall equidistant from the central nasal bridge at the same position on each cornea.

Check for ptosis of the eyelids and nystagmus. In older children, the lacrimal gland at the medial corner of the eyes are examined by asking the child to look downwards and inwards.

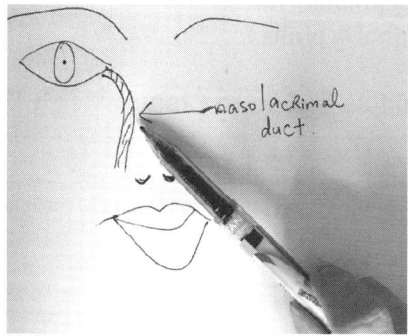

Position of the nasolacrimal duct is sketched

Check for periorbital or facial edema as dependent edema in the mornings in a child may occur in the face, different from an adult, due to the frequent habit of children sleeping with their faces down.

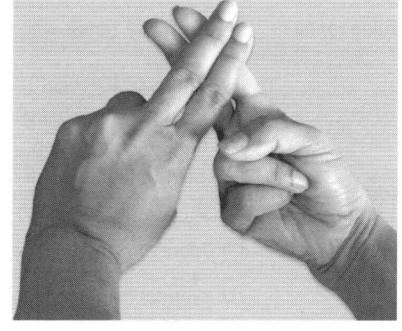

Pediatric Physical Examination

It is of practical relevance to consider facial edema in a young child who sleeps with his or her face down as this is dependent edema when a child sleeps in that position. Link possible physical findings to activities of daily living as obtained from the history.

Periorbital edema with decreased urine output is seen in nephrotic syndrome.

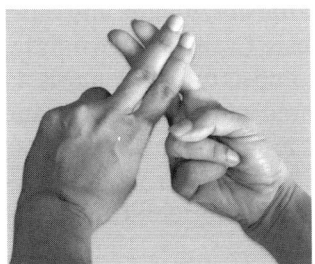

What are the physical links in a case of suspected nephrotic syndrome? Where else can edema fluid accumulate? What are the potential complications? How would assessing the blood pressure narrow the anatomical and pathological diagnosis?

Observe for allergic shiners which are bluish or purple discoloration below the lower eyelids.

The differential diagnosis of swollen eyes, conjunctival injection and Dennie-Morgan folds which are creases under the lower eyelids is atopy.

Abnormality[24,25,32,34,36,39]	Description[24,25,32,34,36,39]
Hypertelorism	Increased distance between pupils such that eyes are set widely apart (e.g. Down syndrome)
Yellow discoloration of the sclera	In a jaundiced patient, it is important to note if the patient is well- or ill-appearing as well as irritable or drowsy as both signs may indicate encephalopathy, infection or metabolic derangement
Posterior embryotoxon	A congenital defect of the eye with a ring-like deformity seen in some syndromes
Kayser-Fleischer rings	Dark ring around iris due to copper deposition in Wilson's disease

Look for signs of jaundice, avitaminosis, subconjuctival hemorrhage and congenital cataract	
Abnormality[24,25,32,34,36,39]	Found in the following conditions[24,25,32,34,36,39]
Cataract	• Congenital rubella syndrome • Down syndrome • Galactosemia • Retrolental fibroplasia • Diabetes mellitus • Long-term use of corticosteroids

Observation of the ears (ENT examination discussed later in this chapter)[24,25,32,34,36,39]

Low set ears are located below an imaginary line drawn from the lateral angle of the eye to the external occipital protuberance. Low set ears are seen in some congenital syndromes. Abnormalities of the pinna are linked to anomalies of the urinary tract.

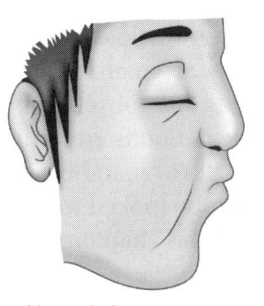 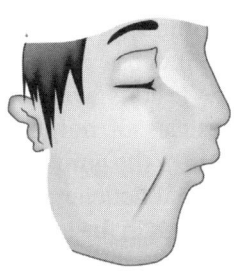

Normal pinna   Abnormal pinna

Anomalies of the external ear are visible on observation

General observation of the ear, nose and skin[24,25,32,34,36,39]	
Organ	Description
Ear	• Any discharge • Anomalies of the external ears • Preauricular sinuses and pits occur anterior to the pinna and are due to imperfect fusion of the first and second branchial arches
Nose	• Nasal congestion, discharge and block • Allergic salute is a transverse nasal crease found across the lower bridge of the nose
Skin	• Rashes – if this is obvious describe pertaining to distribution, color and morphology. • Subcutaneous bleeding • Bruises – multiple bruises of different ages in children under the age of 3 suggest the possibility of non-accidental injury • Skin turgor • Pitting edema • Pyoderma • Ichthyosis • Scabies • Erythema nodosum

Oral Cavity and Lips[24,25,32,34,36,39]

In an infant, observe for a unilateral or bilateral cleft lip which may be immediately apparent. In the older child, look carefully at the philtrum for an old scar of a repaired cleft lip.

Inspect the corners of the mouth for lesions suggestive of angular stomatitis.

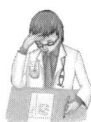

"The physical links in a child with a cleft palate include checking the ear for infections, checking the lungs to exclude aspiration, doing a complete physical examination as one anomaly can coexist with other anomalies. Growth, hearing and speech are important to assess. A CNS examination is also indicated. Can you tell me why?"

Aphthous ulcers can occur in the lower lip, tongue, buccal mucosa or palate. They are painful superficial yellow lesions with red margins. Observe the lips for vesicles of herpes simplex. Epulis describes any swelling in the gum of the maxilla or mandible. Signs of nutritional deficiencies have to be looked for here and are covered in the earlier part of this chapter. Look at the tongue for central cyanosis.

Inspection of the Tongue[24,25,32,34,36,39]

The tongue must be inspected for:

Color[24,25,32,34,36,39]

Central cyanosis is a bluish discoloration of the lips, tongue and mucous membranes of the mouth due to an increase in the amount of reduced hemoglobin in the blood. Cyanosis is dependent on the absolute amount of deoxygenated hemoglobin in the blood. It is due to the mixing of deoxygenated blood with oxygenated blood as can occur in intracardiac right-to-left shunts or intrapulmonary shunts. Cyanosis is visible by the naked eye with deoxygenated hemoglobin in mean capillary blood roughly equal to or more than 5 g% or 5 g/100 mL. This is a rough estimate and may be detected at lesser deoxygenated hemoglobin levels depending on the sampling of the type of blood (arterial venous versus peripheral blood). It is clinically detected when arterial oxygen saturation is about or less than 80%.

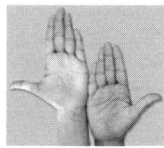

Link hemoglobin levels with the clinical detection of cyanosis

This discoloration may sometimes be more difficult to detect under some situations, such as in dark skinned individuals, and sometimes from bruising or ecchymosis. Remember that it is the tongue and mucous membranes of the mouth that must be inspected for central cyanosis.

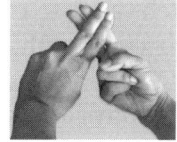

In bruising and ecchymosis, the skin will not blanch but in peripheral cyanosis, there is blanching of the skin.

Cyanosis of the lips, tongue and mucous membrane is central cyanosis. Cyanosis seen only in the extremities is peripheral cyanosis or acrocyanosis. Central cyanosis is often associated with peripheral cyanosis.

As cyanosis is dependent on the amount of absolute deoxygenated hemoglobin in the blood, it manifests earlier in a polycythemic child and is less easily evident in a very pale child.

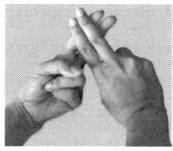

There is a link between central cyanosis and hemoglobin levels.

GOOD CLINICAL PRACTICE

Central cyanosis is seen in the following:[24,25,32,34,36,39]
- **Congenital cardiac diseases with right to left shunts in the heart** due to admixture of oxygenated and deoxygenated blood.
- Lung diseases that cause significant intrapulmonary shunts
- Severe pulmonary problems with ventilation perfusion inequality
- Impairment of diffusion within the alveoli
- Impaired transport of oxygen by hemoglobin
- Central nervous system causes that result in central hypoventilation
- Drugs that centrally depress respiration.

Peripheral Cyanosis[24,25,32,34,36,39]

When peripheral circulation is sluggish, peripheral cyanosis can result. Arterial blood oxygen content will be normal in peripheral cyanosis. All causes of central cyanosis can cause peripheral cyanosis. Additionally, peripheral cyanosis is likely to be seen with exposure to cold, where the cyanosed extremity is cold in polycythemia, and where there is decreased peripheral perfusion. When the extremity is cold, you must feel the peripheral pulses. It can also be the presenting sign in hypoglycemia and sepsis in infants. Any cause of arterial or venous obstruction can cause peripheral cyanosis as well.

Differential Cyanosis[24,25,32-34,36,39]

In differential cyanosis the upper part of the body is pink and lower part of the body remains cyanotic. This is seen in conditions in which there is right-to-left shunt from the pulmonary artery to the descending aorta through the patent ductus arteriosus (PDA).

Methemoglobinemia[24,25,27,32,34,36,39,40]

A condition in which the PO_2 may be normal but the individual may look cyanotic is methemoglobinemia. In these cases, the cyanosis is generalized and the cyanosed extremities are warm.

Normal methemoglobin level is less than 1%. Methemoglobin occurs as a result of oxidation of hemoglobin molecules from the normal ferrous to ferric state. This is maintained at the low level by the enzyme systems, methemoglobin reductase, found within the red blood cells but the activities of these enzymes are low in infants.

Fetal hemoglobin, which is more easily oxidized than the adult hemoglobin, makes infants more susceptible to methemoglobinemia.

Some identified risk factors for methemoglobinemia are the following:
- Topical anesthetics (prilocaine)
- Antibiotics (sulfonamides)
- Metoclopramide
- Products that contain nitrites and nitrates
- Inhaled nitric oxide
- Mutant hemoglobins with altered oxygen affinity give rise to cyanosis without respiratory distress
- In the newborn period
- In infants who have diarrhea, linked to nitrite-forming bacteria in the gut.

Inspect the tongue for state of hydration, deviation and size[24,25,32,34,36,39]

Macroglossia may be seen in hypothyroidism, Beckwith-Wiedemann syndrome, mucopolysaccharidosis and Pompe glycogen storage disease. Remember, that in Down syndrome there is no true macroglossia but the tongue seems large as the mouth is small.

Inspect the tongue for traumatic lingual ulcers. Nutritional deficiencies can also cause lingual ulcers. Many diseases of the gastrointestinal tract can cause oral ulcers and ulcers of the tongue.

The creamy white areas of oral thrush mimic small milk curds but milk curds can be easily detached. When patches of thrush are removed, there is a residual raw surface with pin point bleeding. Bottle feeding and poor bottle hygiene are a link to the etiology of oral thrush or monilial stomatitis caused by the fungus, *Candida ablicans*. If they extend to the tongue, buccal mucosae, gums and retrograde to the pharynx, it makes sucking and swallowing painful and difficult for the infant.

In scarlet fever or scarlatina, which is an acute contagious disease, the tongue is erythematous and coated which then evolves into the "strawberry red tongue". The strawberry red tongue is an important observation in a febrile child.

The "geographic tongue" or benign migratory glossitis is benign and can be seen in febrile children. In this condition, irregular, smooth, erythematous patches with white borders varying in size and shape in different parts of the tongue may be noted.

A smooth tongue due to the loss of lingual papillae is seen in iron deficiency anemia, pernicious anemia, sprue and many gastrointestinal disorders, and nutrient deficiency states including pellagra.

The sides and under surface of the tongue must be examined. A small ulcer in the frenulum is practically significant and is sometimes seen in whooping cough or any persistent cough.

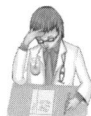

"Why does a frenulum ulcer develop in whooping cough? When the history is suggestive of a severe cough, I must look for the effects of friction of the tongue during repeated bouts of the cough. In the young infant, feeding and sucking will be difficult with such an ulcer. The ulcer must be immediately managed. I see how the history can lead me to a complete clinical examination as well as to a practical management"

Two types of cysts can be seen in the floor of the mouth:[14,22,24]
- A ranula is due to blockage of a duct of the mucous gland.
- A sublingual dermoid cyst, along the lines of embryological fusion of the mouth, is due to the presence of epidermal tissue beneath the skin.

The buccal mucosa is gently examined with a spatula. Koplik spots are seen in the catarrhal stage of measles and are small bluish white spots surrounded by a red area and seen opposite the molar teeth. When seen they are diagnostic.

The opening of the parotid duct is seen as a small swelling opposite the second molar tooth. This gland can enlarge in malnutrition.

The differential diagnosis of oral ulcers includes Crohn's disease in the older child. Oral pigmentation occurs in Peutz-Jeghers syndrome. Mucous membranes in a jaundiced infant are stained yellow.

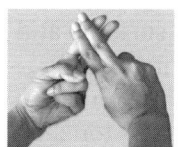

Yellow discoloration of the mucous membranes, the skin and sclerae are seen in jaundice. Link to the cause. Look at the age. Measure and plot the growth. Look for dysmorphism. Examine the abdomen. Inspect carefully. Look for signs of liver failure. Feel the liver, the spleen. Look at the color of the urine. Link to nutritional problems. Link to coagulopathies.

Gray pigmentation may be seen opposite the molar teeth in Addison's disease.

In an older child, check the teeth for caries. This is especially important in a child with underlying heart disease. Tetracyclines can stain the teeth with a yellowish color in children.

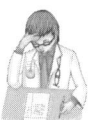

"Though pathognomonic, the patient who comes in the later stage of measles may not have Koplik spots; hence, I must also look for other typical features of a common infection so as not to miss the diagnosis".

Do not forget to look at the pharynx, the palate, tonsils and fauces for ulcers, erythema, and vesicles.

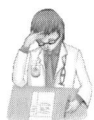

While knowledge of many abnormalities in the mouth and their possible etiologies will enrich my ability to make a logical list of differential diagnoses, I must not forget to exclude the simple things first. These include traumatic causes of ulcers in the mouth, a tooth with caries causing localized gum swelling and pain and so on.

While the mouth is open, quickly glance for petechiae on the palate which can be seen in thrombocytopenia and thrombasthenias (i.e. decreased platelet number or defective platelet function). Drug induced causes must be excluded. In the tropics and subtropics dengue hemorrhagic fever must be considered in a febrile child with oral or mucosal bleeding. Acute leukemias must be excluded where there is fever or signs of concern.

In infectious mononucleosis in the older patient, toxicity, sore throat, lymphadenopathy and palatine petechiae are noted. Petechiae involving the palate are seen in streptococcal tonsillitis and in rubella infections. Also link such petechiae to any cause of thrombocytopenia which is a cause of mucosal bleeding.

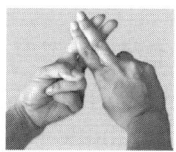

When Forchheimer spots on the soft palate are noticed, the physical links are to look for pharyngitis, suboccipital lymph nodes, conjunctivitis, and in the young teenage girl polyarthritis as these are seen in rubella.

Forchheimer spots which develop in a percentage of patients with rubella are rose colored spots on the soft palate.

The differential diagnosis of vesicles in the mouth in children include varicella zoster, herpes simplex gingivostomatitis and coxsackie infections, including hand-foot-mouth disease.

Examine the Gums[24,25,32,34,36,39]

Swollen gums are seen in scurvy, malignant infiltration as in acute myeloid leukemia and in children who are suffering from epilepsy on phenytoin.

Do not forget that localized gum swelling is associated with dental caries. Gum bleeding is seen in trauma, scurvy and any cause of thrombocytopenia. Accessory salivary tissue can be seen in the mouth, the hard palate being the most common site.

Examination of the Neck[14,22,24,25,32,34,36,39]

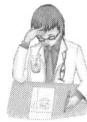

"This is a young child. I realize that the causes of a cyst in the neck can be different than from an adult. The first five branchial arches give rise to head and neck structures. Should I not consider a congenital anomaly as a cause of the neck swelling? I must review the embryological development of the branchial arches."

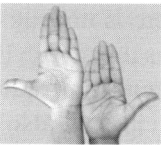

An abnormality must be examined in detail using the **The Cardinal Ten (Physical)**

- The neck must be inspected and examined. It is also a site to inspect for congenital anomalies, especially in the younger child.
- Look at the neck position for torticollis, opisthotonus, inability to support the head, mobility of head, sternocleidomastoid and any swelling or shortening. Observe for webbing of the neck.
- Observe for fistulae, sinuses and cysts.
- Look for a cystic hygroma, which is a benign lymphangioma. These are benign multicystic masses that are soft, easily compressible, transilluminant, and painless.

Branchial cleft cysts are noninflammatory lateral neck masses in children. Branchial cleft cysts comprise remnants from any of the first five branchial arches. These cysts may have different locations and features depending on the branchial cleft of origin. Most branchial cleft cysts are derived from the second branchial arch; a few from the first branchial arch while third and fourth branchial cleft cysts are rare.[14,22]

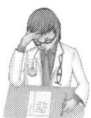

Most branchial cleft cysts are derived from the second branchial arch[14,22]

First branchial arch anomalies lie parallel to the external auditory canal in the preauricular area. They may be linked to a fistula or a sinus tract that may end in the middle ear or external auditory canal. They may also have an external opening leading to a cyst or sinus that has its passage through the parotid gland. Patients with first branchial anomalies may present with unilateral facial paralysis. First branchial anomalies may be associated with hemifacial microsomia.

Second branchial arch anomalies present as painless masses or dimples below the angle of the mandible. They may present as a tract ending in the tonsillar fossa or as a cyst.[14,22]

The rarer third and fourth branchial arch anomalies are close to the carotid artery or end near the piriform fossa.[14,22]

Hemangiomas, vascular malformations and lymphatic malformations of the head and neck are common congenital anomalies. Vascular tumors may be hemangiomas or vascular malformations. Hemangiomas are generally not present at birth and appear in the first few weeks of life. Hemangiomas tend to become larger in the first year of life then many involute and disappear by the age of 5–9 years.

Vascular malformations are present at birth although they may not be recognized. They tend to grow as the child grows.[14,22]

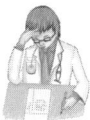

As vascular malformations grow proportionately with the child, they can increase in size with acute hemorrhage and infection. Puberty may also be associated with a sudden increase in the size of such malformations. Hemangiomas are firm while vascular malformations are easily compressible

Differentiate hemangiomas from vascular malformations as hemangiomas are firm and vascular malformations are easily compressible.

Lymphatic malformations include cystic hygromas and they present as painless subcutaneous swellings which can enlarge rapidly with infections.

Palpate the lymph nodes and differentiate lymphadenopathy from lymphadenitis.

Small lymph nodes can normally be felt in the anterior and posterior triangles of the neck, the maxillae and inguinal regions. Lymph nodes often enlarge in children due to local conditions such as tonsillitis or generalized diseases, such as rubella. The differential diagnosis of such reactive cervical lymphadenopathy must include local causes, even head lice (pediculosis capitis) and ear infections.

Check the thyroid gland. Describe it in terms of size, contour, bruit, isthmus, nodules and tenderness. Check the tracheal location; feel for centrality (refer section on respiratory system). Hyperthyroidism in Graves' disease produces a diffuse toxic goiter.[14,22]

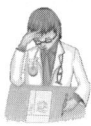

In the teenage girl with a diffuse thyroid swelling, the physical links include warm and moist skin, sinus tacychardia, lid lag, lid retraction, proptosis, muscle weakness, proximal muscle wasting and onycholysis. The historical links are fatigue, heat intolerance, weight loss with increased appetite, palpitations, diplopia, eye pain, diarrhea or insomnia. Difficulty in concentrating, emotional lability and menstrual irregularities must be asked for.

A thyroglossal duct cyst which moves with tongue protrusion is a midline swelling. Other midline swellings are dermoid cysts and lipomas. Thyroglossal duct cysts are midline masses appearing anywhere between the base of the tongue and the thyroid gland. Dermoid cysts are usually found in the submental area. Lipomas may appear anywhere as soft, painless masses.[14,22]

164 The Link: Pediatric History-Taking and Physical Examination

Deformity[14,22,24,25,32,34,36,39]	Description[14,22,24,25,32,34,36,39]
Link neck masses in young children to your knowledge of embryology	
Klippel–Feil syndrome	Failure of the separation of the cervical vertebra results in a short neck
Turner syndrome	Short neck, webbing
Torticollis	Muscle spasm causes stiffness of the neck with inability to turn the head (congenital or acquired)
Bull's neck	Massive lymphadenopathy or subcutaneous emphysema causes significant swelling of the neck
Fistulae, sinuses and cysts	Branchial arch anomalies
Hemangioma and vascular malformations	Capillary, arteriovenous fistulae or malformations
Lymphangioma or cystic hygroma	Cystic masses that transilluminate 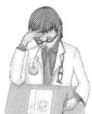 *Why are they transilluminant?*
Asymptomatic neck masses	Thymic masses
Thyroglossal cysts and fistulae	Seen in the midline of the neck and may extend to the base of the tongue. The cysts may contain aberrant thyroid tissue
Thyroid masses	Describe the lobes, the isthmus, contour and presence or absence of bruit
Laxity of the skin around the neck	Down syndrome, pseudoxanthoma elasticum, Ehlers– Danlos syndrome

Examination of the Shape of the Chest and Abdomen[12,22,24,25,32,34,36,39]

When inspecting the chest inspect anteriorly, posteriorly and from both sides.
Look at the shape of the chest, look at the movement and compare both sides, look for any scars.

When inspecting the abdomen look from the anterior aspect and squat down so that your eyes are at the level of the umbilicus and astutely observe abdominal movements. If visible peristalsis is present, spend some time to observe its nature and direction.

Look at the shape of the abdomen, looking for distension and if distended, note areas or quadrants of distension. Look at the overall movement of the abdomen during respiration, remembering that the abdomen is more protuberant in young children than in adults.

Examination of the Arms and Legs[24,25,32,34,36,39]

- Confirm the existence of the BCG scar. It is usually seen on the left upper arm.

If the child has a chronic cough, would a well-defined BCG scar make the diagnosis of tuberculosis unlikely?

- Look for muscle wasting of the arms. Loss of turgor, especially of the calf muscles and skin over the abdomen, is evidence of dehydration. Look at any obvious deformities of the legs.
- Look for ankle edema. Demonstrate pitting edema by applying pressure with one finger on the pretibial area.
- Observe the posture of body and limbs.

Examination of the Hands and Nails[24,25,32,34,36,39]

Check peripheral perfusion by capillary refill which is normally less than 2 seconds. Confirm the absence or presence of clubbing of fingers. In finger clubbing, the tissues at the base of the nail are thickened; the angle between the nail base and the adjacent skin of the finger is obliterated. The nail itself loses its longitudinal ridges and becomes convex. In the last stage of clubbing, the drumstick appearance of the fingers is called hypertrophic pulmonary osteoarthropathy.

GOOD CLINICAL PRACTICE

It is good clinical practice to ask yourself why these nail changes occur. When do these changes occur? How do they occur? When you see such changes, what is the anatomical diagnosis? What is the etiological diagnosis? What is the pathophysiological reason? Read widely; then look for the physical links.

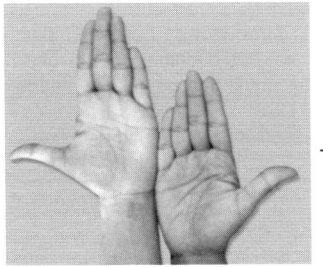 +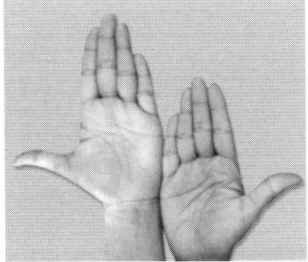

Most likely Hypothesis of Clubbing[24,25,32,34,36,39]

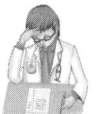

A hypothesis must be further tested by a scientist.

There are many hypotheses for the clinical signs of clubbing. One is that megakaryocytes are normally fragmented into platelets in the lungs. Processes that interfere with the normal pulmonary circulation, such as chronic lung inflammation, or intracardiac right-to-left shunts, may allow whole megakaryocytes to enter the systemic circulation. When their large size causes them to become impacted in the fingertip circulation, megakaryocytes and megakaryocyte fragments are activated to release platelet-derived growth factor (PDGF). PDGF encourages growth, permeability of the vessel and neutrophil chemotaxis. This leads to the accumulation of many vascular smooth muscle cells and fibroblasts; these are found in the pathology of clubbing. Extrapulmonary conditions that cause clubbing are associated with arteriovenous fistulae which result in a similar process.

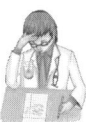

"In a patient with clubbing, from the history and my knowledge of the causes of clubbing I must link my physical signs, both the positive and negative ones to make a diagnosis. I must certainly keep the age in mind when considering the differentials."

Some childhood conditions associated with clubbing[24,25,32,34,36,39]
• Familial or hereditary
• Cyanotic congenital heart disease
• Cystic fibrosis
• Empyema
• Biliary atresia
• Biliary cirrhosis
• Bronchiectasis
• Celiac disease
• Cirrhosis
• Inflammatory bowel disease
• Severe interstitial pneumonitis

Clubbing is seen in severe chronic cyanosis, congenital heart diseases, suppurative lung diseases, inflammatory bowel diseases and cirrhosis.

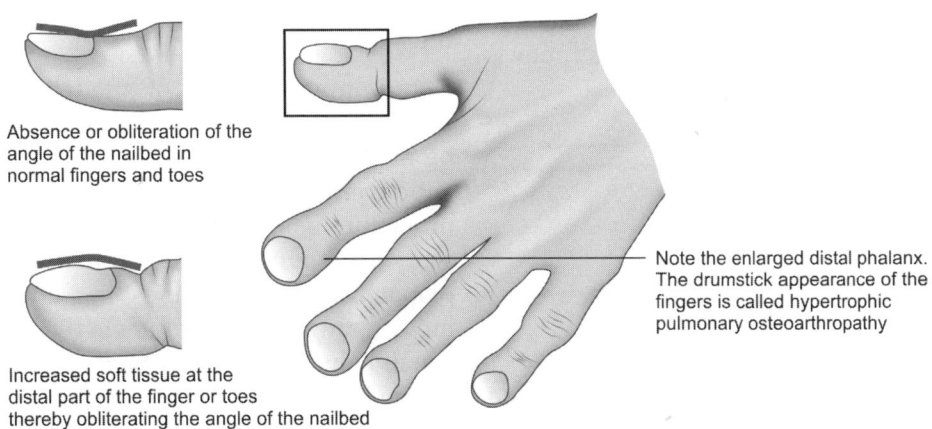

The shape of the fingers when clubbed

Nail Changes[24,25,32,34,36,39]

The shape of the nails can be influenced by the health status of the child. One nail deformity is koilonychia, which is the softening and thinning of the nails, making them brittle and concave.

Other deformities to look for are as follows:[24,25,32,34,36,39]	
Part of the hand	Description
Finger tips	Osler nodes
Palms	• Janeway lesions • Palmar erythema • Single transverse palmar crease • Carotenemia – this yellow pigmentation is usually most prominent over the palms and soles and around the nose, and spares the conjunctiva
Fingers	• Brachydactyly (short fingers) • Campylodactyly (contracture of the fingers) • Clinodactyly (curved fifth finger) • Polydactyly (more than five fingers on either hand) • Syndactyly (two or more fingers fused by soft tissue or bone) • Arachnodactyly (long spider like fingers)
Nails	• Splinter hemorrhages • Koilonychia • Leukonychia • Constant nail biting—psychological disturbances • Cyanosis (peripheral) • Clubbing

Examination of the Legs and Feet[24,25,32,34,36,39]

Check for ankle and leg edema. Also look for deformities of the foot such as the following:

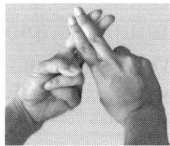

- Talipes equinovarus or rocker bottom feet linked to spina bifida cystica, peroneal muscular dystrophy
- Talipes equinovalgus
- Talipes calcaneovalgus
- Talipes calcaneovarus

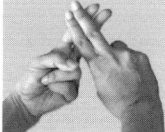

- Pes planus or flat foot
- Pes cavus or a high arched foot linked to spina bifida occulta, Friedrich's ataxia, diastematomyelia, peroneal muscular dystrophy.

In trisomy 21, deformities of the foot include a wide gap between the 1st and 2nd toes (sandal gap deformity), a plantar furrow extending backwards on the foot and wide, short dorsiflexed big toes. Hands and feet show characteristic dermatoglyphics in trisomy 21.

Examination of the Spine and Back[24,25,32,34,36,39]

Deformities of the head and brain	Description
Anencephaly	• Forebrain, upper brainstem and skull does not develop • The majority are stillborn. Others die in the neonatal period
Myelomeningocele	• A defect in the overlying bone and skin. There is an outpouching at the back covered by meninges containing neural tissue and CSF • This is associated with hydrocephalus and Arnold-Chiari malformation
Cranial meningocele	• A meningeal sac protrudes through a defect in the skull
Spinal meningocele	• A swollen fluctuant mass covered with skin or as a thin walled, transilluminant membranous lesion. It does not contain any neural element and neurological symptoms are absent
Encephalocele	• A midline defect of the skull with outpouching of the brain and meninges. Linked to hydrocephalus or other brain defects
Spina bifida occult	• This is due to failure of fusion of the vertebral arches. There may be dermal hyperpigmentation, hemangioma, a patch of hair, a lump or a dermal sinus • Spinal dysraphism or failure of fusion of the vertebral arches and malformation of the spinal cord
Sacral edema	• Is dependent edema in a recumbent patient

Inspection of the Genitalia, the Nappy area and the Anal Orifice[24,25,31,32,34,36,39]

Determining the sex of the child is done when screening the newborn. Examination of this area can be done when the child is lying down or when the child is sitting on the mother's lap. Always explain the procedure before you proceed further. Ascertain the size of the penis and scrotum. The testis should be palpated with warm hands, in a downward direction moving towards the scrotum in the line of the inguinal canal. Palpate normal hernial orifices. In girls, check the vulva for discharge, fusion of the labia and enlargement of the clitoris. In ambiguous genitalia, it is difficult to discern the gender accurately. Accurate determination of gender is important to allay parental anxiety, for further management and for future proper psychological development of the child.

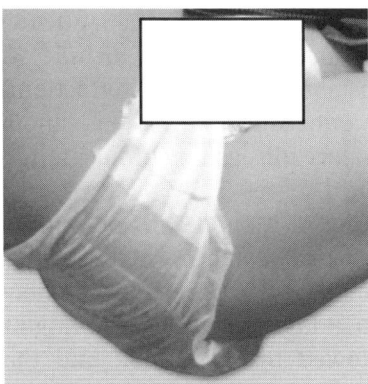

Do not forget to open the diaper or napkin for a complete physical examination (do not forget to "stick" it back when your examination is complete, either!).

Nappy Area for Diaper Dermatitis[24,25,31,32,34,36,39]

The nappy area (after requesting mother's permission) should be exposed to look for rashes and excoriations. Skin rashes in this area, known as diaper dermatitis may be due to irritation of the skin by the diaper material or due to causes other than the diaper. Specific irritant dermatitis due to laundry products that are used to wash napkins can occur.

Irritant diaper dermatitis from contact with feces or urine can be infected with fungi or bacteria. Diaper dermatitis due to *Candida albicans* has satellite nodules at the edges of the area of erythema. Secondary bacterial infections are also seen and these must be identified and treated. Bacterial diaper rash associated with Staphylococcal infections occur with large pus filled bullae, pustules or honey colored crusted lesions.

Diaper dermatitis, can be due to seborrhea where oily yellowish scales are seen in the inguinal area and the scalp as well. Atopic eczema is also seen in the diaper area, is itchy and lesions may appear elsewhere. In atopic eczema, there will be scratching so during diaper change look for evidence of scratch marks. Acute, generalized pruritic dermatitis of scabies can also affect the diaper area where a family history of a pruritic rash may be obtained. Perianal excoriation is seen in lactose intolerance which usually occurs secondary to severe diarrhea in infants. Acrodermatitis enteropathica is an inherited disorder of zinc and involves lesions in the perianal and perioral areas. Langerhans cell histiocytosis and congenital syphilis can also manifest in the nappy area.

Abnormality of penis/testes[24,25,32,34,36,39]	Description[24,25,32,34,36,39]
Retractile testes	• Testes retract into the inguinal canal; this happens due to an exaggerated cremasteric reflex • Cremasteric reflex is weak or absent at birth • Testis is palpable at birth, but if it becomes impalpable later, this is suggestive of retractile testes • Can be brought down by careful palpation when child is relaxed in a warm room. A retractile testis is normal
Micropenis	• Normal length of the penis is greater than 2.5 cm and the stretched penile length averages about 2.8 cm in the full-term newborn • Associated with hypothalamic hypo-pituitary disorder and some syndromes (e.g. septo-optic dysplasia, Kallmann syndrome, Prader–Willi syndrome)
Undescended testes	• Failure of descent into scrotum
Congenital hydrocele	• Congenital hydrocele is due to accumulation of peritoneal fluid in the patent processus vaginalis which usually resolves as the baby grows

Inspection of the anal orifice[24,25,31,32,34,36,39]

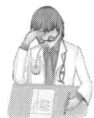

What causes such conditions in children? How are they different in adults?

Examine the anus by gently separating the buttocks.

Look for:
- Fissures
- Sinuses
- Anal tags
- Polyps
- Visible hemorrhoids
- Rectal prolapse.

Perianal excoriation is seen in lactose intolerance which usually occurs secondary to severe diarrhea in infants. Infections like perianal abscesses can occur in children and must be excluded in any child with fever where a focus cannot be found. Children with immunodeficiencies can present in this way.

Perianal streptococcal lesions are seen in infancy and childhood. Sometimes a family history of recent streptococcal disease may be obtained. Perianal viral lesions like molluscum contagiosum may be rarely seen due to autoinoculation. Anogenital warts may be seen in children. Such unusual infective lesions, tears or injuries in this area in children must make one suspect non-accidental injuries in children. Sexual abuse can take many forms; hence, a high index of suspicion is necessary, if the history or physical examination is suggestive.

Per rectal examination is not usually done. It is done only when indicated, such as to look for blood and mucus in a case of suspected intussusception. This is done gently with the little finger so as not to cause undue pain or induce an iatrogenic anal fissure! (Examination of the genital and anal area is part of the abdominal examination. Refer to the appropriate section).

SYSTEMIC EXAMINATION

General observation is very important and has been described[24,25,32,34,36,39]

Specific systemic observation and examination of the respiratory system must then be done.

Specific observation is observation of signs pertaining to the system that is clinically assessed to be the system involved in the disease process. Signs may be positive if present and negative if absent.

THORAX[24,25,31,32,34,39]

Inspection is the most important part of the examination in children. On inspection, observe the respiratory rate and look for chest recessions in a quiet child. This is a pivotal step as it provides important information. It is important to know the standards for the different pediatric age groups before making conclusions on the rate. Bear in mind that children are mainly abdominal breathers.

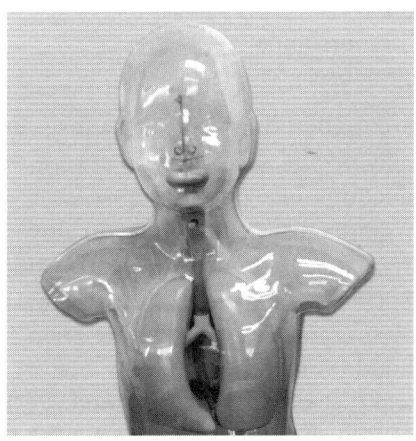

Model of a child's lungs.

Inspection of the Thorax[24,25,32,34,36,39]

- Tachypnea (respiratory rates vary with age).
- Nasal flaring, grunting and respiratory retractions. These are indicative of respiratory distress:
  - Respiratory retractions include suprasternal, subcostal and intercostal retractions. Intercostal and subcostal recession indicate acute respiratory diseases, chronic lung diseases or cardiac diseases.
  - Grunting in a child with pneumonia is due to the reversal of the normal respiratory rhythm. It occurs when the child breathes against a closed glottis. Generally, grunting on expiration is followed by inspiration and then a pause. It occurs in respiratory diseases and as a nonspecific sign in a very ill child with high fever or metabolic acidosis.
  - Stridor in an infant or young child is a harsh high pitched sound of turbulent airflow in upper airway obstruction.
  - Inspiratory stridor is heard as a result of supraglottic obstruction.
  - Biphasic stridor is heard as a result of glottis or subglottic obstruction.
  - Expiratory stridor is heard as a result of tracheal or large bronchial compression.
  - Stertor in an infant or child is a low pitched snoring sound as a result of partial nasal obstruction or due to nasopharyngeal obstruction or as a result of hypopharyngeal obstruction.
  - Wheezing is a continuous whistling high pitched sound on expiration as a result of constriction of the bronchioles.

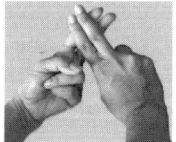

Use the physical links

Listen to types of cough:
- A dry or hacking cough of a viral infection.
- A brassy cough is heard in croup.
- A whoop in the cough is heard in pertussis.
- A staccato cough appreciable in chlamydial infections.
- A paroxysmal cough may suggest foreign body aspiration, pertussis or chlamydia.
- A "honking" cough may suggest psychogenic cough.

- A "chesty" cough or a wet cough in bronchitis and in lower respiratory infections like pneumonia. A recurrent cough worse on lying down in postnasal drip, or the cough of cardiac failure. Nocturnal cough is seen in bronchial asthma. A habitual or psychogenic cough disappears when lying down.

Transmitted sounds are usually from the upper airway due to secretions or nasal obstruction.

Inspection[24,25,32,34,36,39]

- Harrison's sulcus
- Deformities of the chest wall
- Hyperinflation of the chest
- Asymmetry of chest movements
- Pectus excavatum or pectus carinatum
- Kyphosis
- Kyphoscoliosis
- Thickening of the costochondral junctions or rachitic rosary (can be seen and felt) and occurs in rickets
- Absent clavicles
- Absent pectoralis
- Scars of sternotomy, thoracotomy, previous chest drains
- Compare both sides and observe movement closely.

Auscultating the Thorax[24,25,32,34,36,39]

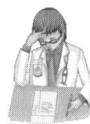

"I must be sensible in my approach to how I examine the young child."

The examination of the chest is adjusted to the age of the child[24,25,32,34,36,39]

In the infant and young child, auscultation of the chest is best done immediately after observation. This is so because the chest sounds are best heard when the infant is fully cooperative. Performing palpation and percussion before auscultation is risky as the level of cooperation may not be the same after that or restlessness and impatience may make the child cry making appreciation of the chest sounds difficult. General auscultation of a child's chest can be carried out using a stethoscope with a small bell chest piece. In the older more cooperative child, you may perform palpation and percussion before auscultation as you would in an adult.

- Breath sounds[24,25,32,34,36,39]
  - The normal breath sounds may be vesicular or bronchovesicular, depending on the site of auscultation. Tracheal breath sounds are heard over the trachea and are harsh sounds.
  - Bronchial breath sounds are normally appreciated over major airways in the anterior chest near the second and third intercostal spaces. Bronchial breath sounds are more tubular and hollow than vesicular sounds, but not as harsh as tracheal breath sounds. Bronchial sounds are loud with a short pause between inspiration and expiration, which are more or less of equal length.
  - Vesicular and bronchovesicular sounds have an inspiratory phase that is longer than the expiratory phase. In children, the thin wall makes the breath sounds louder and sound more like bronchial breathing. Remember that bronchovesicular breath sounds are commonly heard in children.
  - Vesicular sounds have an inspiratory phase that is longer than the expiratory phase. Vesicular breathing is low pitched, breezy and rustling in character.
  - Bronchovesicular breath sounds have an expiratory sound that is harsher and more of a bronchial character than vesicular breath sounds.

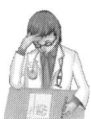

So the normal findings on auscultation include loud, bronchial breath sounds over the large airways in the anterior chest near the second and third intercostal spaces, bronchovesicular sounds over the mainstream bronchi, between the scapulae, and below the clavicles and soft, breezy, low-pitched vesicular breath sounds over the peripheral lung fields.

- Transmitted sounds[24,25,32,34,36,39]
  - Upper respiratory infections usually result in loud coarse sounds, which may be transmitted down the trachea and main bronchi. Auscultation over the lower chest will indicate that transmitted sounds are louder over the trachea as they are from the upper airway. You may also perform the condensation test. If a small metal piece placed at the nostrils does not condense when the patient breathes, it indicates that one or both nostrils are blocked.
  - Additionally, adventitious sounds originating from the upper airway can be differentiated if one places the stethoscope over the mouth and

mentally subtracts the sounds heard by this route from the sounds heard through the chest wall. This could be used to differentiate transmitted sounds from intrathoracic sounds.
- In the event that the breath sounds do not come under these two categories, they are perceived as abnormal.

Abnormalities in breath sounds and adventitious sounds[24,25,29,32,34,36,39]	
Type	Description
Reduced or absent breath sounds	In collapse of the lung or parts of the lung, fibrosis, pneumothorax and pleural effusions.
Prolonged length of expiratory phase	Expiratory phase is heard longer than inspiratory phase
Bronchial breath sounds	The expiratory phase is equal to or longer than the inspiratory phase with a gap in between; the quality is harsh. This is normally heard when you auscultate along the large airways
Adventitious breath sounds	Sounds conducted from the upper airways that are common in children. These are also heard without the stethoscope. Using the stethoscope, it is possible to differentiate it from sounds originating in the lower airway as they are louder when the neck is auscultated
Rhonchi	High pitched sounds usually heard during expiration
Crackles or crepitations	May either be coarse and low pitched or fine and high pitched

Bronchovesicular breath sounds are mainly heard in:
- Anterior auscultation:
  - At the roots of the lung, in the upper midline
  - At the right apex for a few centimeters below the clavicle
- Posterior auscultation:
  - Above the spine of the scapula near the midline.

Abnormal Breath Sounds[24,25,29,32,34,36,39]

Breath sounds in infants and children are more intense and more bronchial in character due to the thin chest wall than in adults. In addition, most of a young child's respiratory movement is produced by abdominal movement and very little movement is produced by the intercostal motion.

In infants, congenital lesions of the airways must also be thought of as a differential diagnosis when abnormal breath sounds are heard.

The tables below summarize the various pathological conditions in which abnormal and added breath sounds may be heard.

Abnormal breath sounds and its pathological causes[24,25,29,32,34,36,39]	
Abnormal breath sounds	Likely pathological condition
Reduced or absent	Link to collapse of the lung or parts of the lung and consider fibrosis, pneumothorax, pleural thickening and pleural effusion
Prolonged expiration	Link to bronchial or pulmonary diseases such as congenital or acquired emphysema, bronchial asthma and bronchiolitis. In these diseases, the act of expiration is performed more slowly than in healthy individuals
Prolonged inspiration	Linked to laryngeal or tracheal diseases
Bronchial breath sounds	Link to consolidation, presence of a large cavity and over a pleural effusion. The expiratory sound is more intense than the inspiratory sound, higher pitched, as long as or longer than the inspiratory sound. The quality of the expiratory sound is characteristic and a gap exists between inspiration and expiration

Added breath sounds and its pathological causes[24,25,29,32,34,36,39]	
Added breath sounds	Likely pathological condition
Transmitted sounds	• Sounds conducted from the upper airways are commonly heard in children. Many of these are also heard without a stethoscope; using a stethoscope, it is distinguished from lower airway sounds as it is louder on auscultation of the neck
Rhonchi	• Heard commonly in airway diseases of children due to the smaller diameter of the airways; the younger the infant, the greater the risk of airway obstruction • Prolonged uninterrupted noise heard in the bronchi due to partial obstruction of their lumen, by mucosal swelling, viscid secretion, or by bronchoconstriction. High pitched rhonchi are known as sibilant. Low pitched rhonchi are called sonorous and may sometimes be palpable. • Heard in bronchiolitis, bronchitis and bronchial asthma. Also heard in foreign body aspiration where they may be localized
Crackles or crepitations	• Crushing paper or bubbly sounds produced in the alveoli, bronchi, and in the cavities • May be coarse and low pitched or fine and high pitched • Fine crepitations are due to the presence of fluid in the alveoli in heart failure or in the early stages of pneumonia. Recall the pathological stages of lobar pneumonia including congestion, red hepatization, gray hepatization and resolution. When consolidation occurs, bronchial breathing is heard. In pediatrics, fine crepitations are heard all over the chest in bronchiolitis whereas coarse crepitations are heard in bronchitis and bronchiectasis • Post-tussive crepitations are crepitations that are persistent or amplified after a cough and are heard in tuberculosis
Pleural rub	• Heard in early stages of pleurisy and may be fine or coarse • A rubbing sound that is heard in the corresponding part of inspiration and expiration
Stridor	• This is usually an inspiratory sound heard without the stethoscope. Heard in laryngomalacia and viral croup, epiglottitis, tracheitis and foreign body inhalation

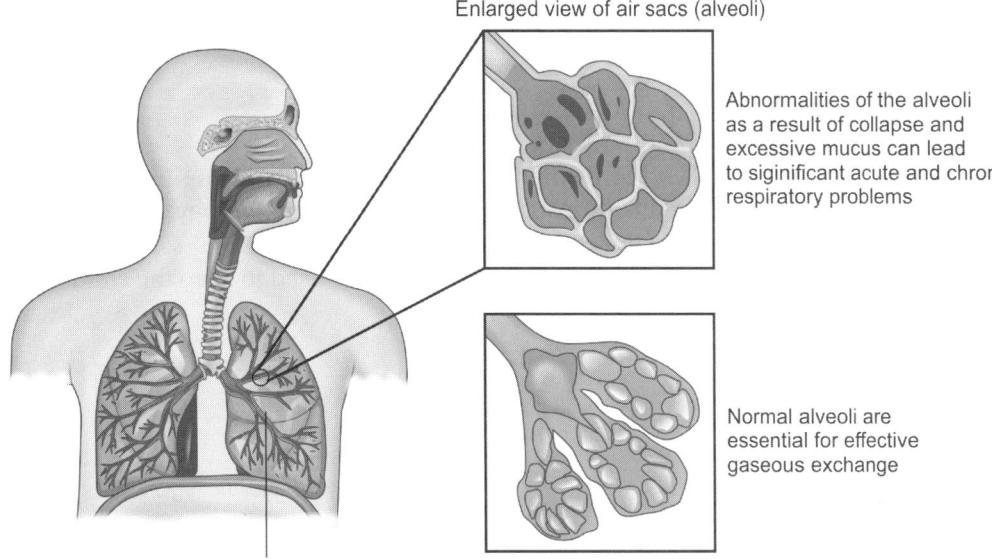

Enlarged view of air sacs (alveoli)

Abnormalities of the alveoli as a result of collapse and excessive mucus can lead to siginificant acute and chronic respiratory problems

Normal alveoli are essential for effective gaseous exchange

Bronchiolar constriction can be caused by mucus, inflammation or intraluminal obstruction
Partial obstruction of the lumen of bronchiole due to excess mucus

Palpation of the Thorax[24,25,32,34,36,39]

- Put your hand gently on the chest especially if there are obvious masses or if the patient says there is pain in any area or if the mother perceives that there is an area of pain. Avoid touching the area of pain first. The nature of any swelling should be determined. Fluctuation occurs when an abscess has formed in the chest wall and is uncommon in children.
- Palpation of tracheal centrality is difficult to do and interpret in an infant as the neck is short. In bigger children with a longer neck (as opposed to infants) feel for the trachea in the suprasternal notch and the insertion of the sternocleidomastoids. Also feel for the position of the cardiac impulse.

> - Conditions that **pull the trachea and apex** to the same side of the lesion include collapse or fibrosis of the lung. Conditions that **push the trachea and apex** away from the site of the lesion include pneumothorax and pleural effusion
> - Displacement of the trachea alone is suggestive of pathology involving only the upper lobe
> - The **cardiac apex** is on the right side in dextrocardia (situs solitus involves only the heart, situs inversus involves the heart and abdominal viscera)
> - The **cardiac apex alone** can be displaced in abnormalities, such as the following:
>   - Cardiomegaly
>   - Kyphoscoliosis
>   - Pectus excavatum
>   - Scoliosis

- Vibrations may be palpable. Low pitched rhonchi can be felt as a purring sensation under the palms of the hands.
- In older children, vibrations may be palpable by asking the child to say one, one, one (ninety-nine if older). This must be compared to the corresponding areas of the chest on both sides.

COMPARE, CONTRAST, CAPTURE AND CONSOLIDATE (CCCC) YOUR FINDINGS[24,25,32,34,36,39]

Vocal fremitus is only done in older children. Vocal fremitus is not very significant in young children and furthermore it is difficult to make the younger child fully cooperate to perform it. It is increased when the lung is consolidated or when there is a large cavity near the surface.

> *When the vocal fremitus is done in the older child remember that it is absent over a pleural effusion, increased with or without whispering pectoriloquy over consolidation, decreased over collapse and decreased over a pneumothorax. Vocal resonance – (auscultated over the chest wall while the patient speaks or vocalizes). It is reduced in bronchiolitis, absent in pneumothorax and in pleural effusion and collapse.*

Percussion of the thorax[24,25,32,34,36,39]

Percussion is rarely informative in the young child and, as such is not routinely done in a child who is less than 2 years. In older children, percussion of the chest should be light and in small children can be directly carried out i.e. the chest wall is tapped directly without the use of the pleximeter finger. The chest is found to be much more resonant in children than in adults.

> When percussion is done in the older child, remember that the percussion note is stony dull over a pleural effusion, dull over consolidation, dull in collapse and fibrosis of the lung and resonant over a pneumothorax.

ABDOMEN[12,24,25,32,34,36,39]

The abdomen is divided into 9 regions for convenience of description. In young infants, observation of the abdomen during the feeding provides useful clinical clues to underlying pathology. Look around for any used nappies with stool which gives some clue of the child's digestive system.

In young children innovative techniques of palpation may have to be used to keep the child at ease.

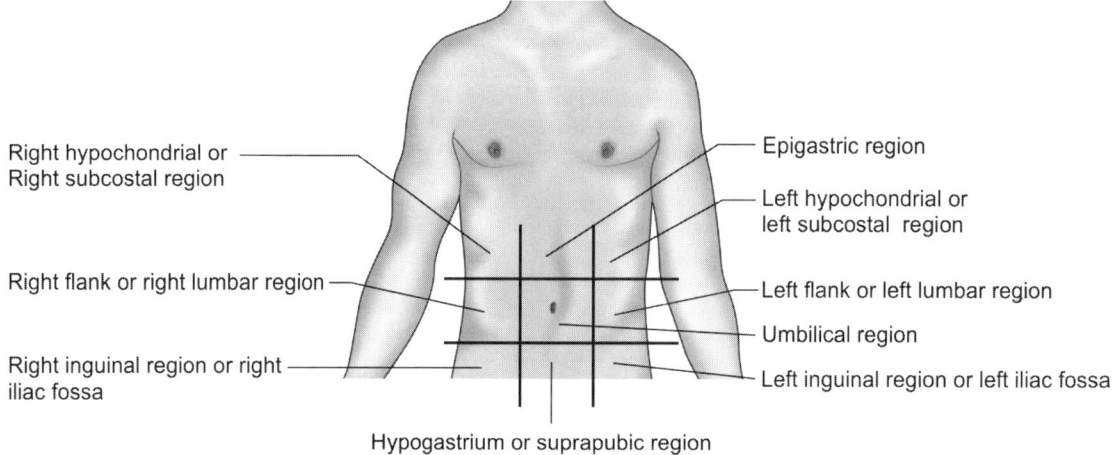

The 9 areas (anatomical) of the anterior abdominal wall.[6]

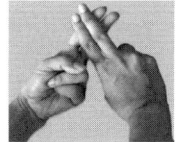

Link general observation and specific observation for a better clinical picture of the underlying condition

General observation must be done. This has already been described.

Specific observation must focus on the following:[12,24,25,32,34,36,39]

Inspection of the Abdomen.

Again this can be done from a little far off and then at a close distance.

Remember to squat down to observe the quadrants carefully, if necessary.

- Inspect the abdomen for movement of all regions of the abdomen.
- Bear in mind that children normally have a protuberant or prominent abdomen.
- Observe how the child is lying down.
- Observe if the child is in pain.
- Observe if there is intermittent colicky abdominal pain.
- Look out for any masses or swellings.
- Look for visible organomegaly.
- Observe for visible peristaltic movements. This is seen in pyloric stenosis especially during feeding.
- Observe the shape of umbilicus and hernias and swellings from within and around the umbilicus.
- Umbilical hernias are common in some normal children, prematurity, hypothyroidism, Down syndrome and in mucopolysaccharidosis.
- Examine the lower abdomen for a distended bladder.
- Observe for dilated veins; these are seen in severe malnutrition, portal hypertension and inferior vena cava obstruction. Enlarged veins are seen in severe malnutrition where they are more prominent than normal due to loss of subcutaneous fat. In portal hypertension, the umbilical vein forms collaterals with the veins of the abdominal wall as they function

as portal outflow tracts, hence, the caput medusa that is diagnostic of portal hypertension. The direction of blood flow in these veins in portal hypertension is normal, which is upward, in those above the umbilicus and downward in those below because the blood is flowing from the portal system to the systemic system. The veins of the abdominal wall may be dilated due to obstruction of the inferior vena cava. Here, the direction of blood flow will be reversed below the umbilicus as the blood flows from the femoral vein to the superior vena cava.

- Look out for operative scars, their site and size. Operative scars are initially raised and red; they fade to pink and by 6 months are flat and skin colored or gray. Wounds that heal without infection, by first intention are thin and regular, infected wounds heal by secondary intention and are wider and irregular.
- Observe the gluteal area for rashes and muscle wasting, Wasting of the buttocks is typically seen in celiac disease.
- Look for an unusual number of pampers and if seen observe its contents.
- Inspect the stools in the pampers whenever you have a chance.
- See if the child is on an intravenous drip; if on one look at the type of fluid being given.
- Observe the feeding mode, i.e. whether breastfeeding or bottle feeding.
- Be sensitive to any peculiar or characteristic odors.
- See if the child is on any special diet or milk formula.
- Look at the input-output chart and study it.
- Look for jaundice, spider nevi or palmar erythema seen in chronic liver disease.
- Inspect for abdominal distention and remember that fat, feces, flatus and fluid cause abdominal distension.
- Fecal distention is seen in constipation and Hirschsprung disease.
- Flatus is present in malabsorption, lactose intolerance and celiac disease. It can also be due to swallowing of air. Intestinal obstruction can cause significant obstruction and is a cause of abdominal distension in an ill-looking child.
- Fluid may be due to any cause of ascites, exudation or transudation of free fluid within the abdominal cavity, due to hypoproteinemic states like nephrotic syndrome.

Palpation of the Abdomen[12,24,25,32,34,36,39]

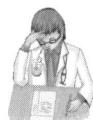

"Think of how you could palpate the abdomen thoroughly with minimal discomfort to the child. Young infants can be given a feed to stop them crying. In children from 1 to 3 years, the abdomen can be palpated from behind when the child is standing over the mother's lap and looking over her shoulder; or maybe you could first palpate by putting your hand gently on top of his or hers in a young child."

Adapt the examination of the abdomen to the age of the child[24,25,32,34,36,39]

The abdomen cannot be palpated satisfactorily in a child who is crying or resisting the procedure. Small infants can be given a feed to stop them crying. Children from 1 to 3 years may not allow you to examine them lying down. However, in this age group, the abdomen can be palpated from behind when the child is standing over the mother's lap and looking over her shoulder.

Alternatively, in infants you may flex their knees with one hand then palpate the abdomen with the other to relax the abdominal muscles. In the toddler and young child you may put your hand over the child's hands and palpate the abdomen first. Later when some confidence and cooperation is achieved you may palpate the abdomen with your hands while the child puts his or her hands on yours.

Another method to examine the abdomen is for the child to lie on his mother's lap with the head on her lap and the child's feet on your knees.

- Ensure that your hands are warm.
- Palpation should be gentle and light. Abdominal tenderness is sensed by watching the child's facial expression during palpation. Palpate first with his or her hand or by putting your hand on top of his or hers in a young child to gain cooperation.

Inspect for the liver from the right iliac fossa. The liver edge can be felt quite easily and in young children it normally extends down to 2 cm below the right costal margin.

Palpation of the Liver[24,25,32,34,36,39]

It starts from the right iliac fossa towards the right hypochondrium in the **mid-clavicular line, i.e. not crossing the lateral border of rectus**.

Measure the liver below the right costal margin in the mid-clavicular line. Feel whether the surface is smooth, granular or nodular, border (round or sharp) consistency (soft, firm, hard) whether tender or pulsatile.

Palpation of the Spleen[24,25,32,34,36,39]

- Examine for the spleen from the right iliac fossa with the left hand splinting the lower rib cage posteriorly. In the event that the spleen is not definitely palpable, lay the child on his or her right side and palpate again while he or she is taking deep breaths. The spleen, when enlarged, can be felt below the left costal margin, describe the spleen if palpable. Slight enlargement of the spleen is usual and occurs in many infections. Tenderness or hardness over the spleen or below the left costal margin is important to describe.
- It starts from the right iliac fossa towards the left hypochondrium
- Feel for the notch to differentiate it from a renal mass
- Measure the size below the left costal margin
- Feel for the consistency. Is it soft, firm or hard?
- In some neonates and in young children it may be just felt. But if more than the tip of the spleen is appreciably palpable (more than about a finger breadth or about 2 cm) then splenomegaly is present.

Features clinically differentiating the spleen from the kidney[24,25,34]
• One can get above a kidney but not a spleen
• The spleen enlarges in a diagonal fashion from left to right along the line of the ninth rib
• A splenic notch may be felt on its medial margin
• The percussion note is resonant over the kidney due to bowel gas but it is found to be dull over the spleen
• Splenic percussion is done on the Traube's space (see text) and if dull is indicative of an enlarged spleen
• The spleen moves with respiration whereas the kidney does not
• The kidney is ballottable and palpable bimanually but the spleen is not
• The splenic notch is palpable in gross splenomegaly

Examination of the Kidneys[12,24,25,32,34,36,39]

In infants you may flex knees with one hand then palpate the abdomen with the other to relax the abdominal muscles and the iliopsoas posteriorly. Both the kidneys can be balloted and the bladder is often palpable. In the toddler and young child, you may put your hand over the child's hands and palpate the abdomen first. Later when some confidence and cooperation is achieved you may palpate the abdomen with your hands while the child puts his or her hand on yours.

- The kidneys are sometimes normally felt by ballottement (bimanual palpation). The left kidney needs to be differentiated from the spleen. The tip of the left kidney and a part of the right kidney may be palpable in the young child. In the adolescent, the left kidney is higher than the right kidney and is not palpable. The lower part of the right kidney is occasionally palpable per abdomen.
- Remember to palpate and later, percuss for the urinary bladder. The bladder is usually palpable per abdomen in the infant. A full bladder presents as a firm mass arising out of the pelvis. Differentiate fecal masses which can be felt in children who are constipated. Fecal masses are indentable on abdominal palpation.
- Ascites is tested by shifting dullness or the fluid thrill.

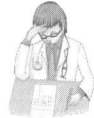

When would you use the fluid thrill? How much fluid must there be? Would it be useful if there is only minimal ascites? Why?

When an abdominal mass is palpable, differentiate it from a normal structure based on your knowledge of basic anatomy[12,24,25,32,34,36,39]

A visible or palpable mass or swelling must be defined using the important questions:
- Site
- Size
- Shape
- Edge
- Tenderness
- Surface
- Contour
- Consistency
- Mobility
- Ability to get above the swelling
- Pulsatility (pulsatile or not)
- Maneuvers to define exact location and nature, e.g. intra-or extra-abdominal, transilluminability
- Comparison with other masses, if present, e.g. on other limb
- Percussion note over the swelling (done over nontender masses to differentiate cystic from solid)
- Auscultation.

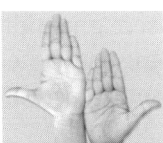

Examine thoroughly all features of a palpable mass using
The Cardinal Ten (Physical)

Some descriptive features of an abdominal mass[24,25,32,34,36,39]	
Site	• If the mass disappears or becomes less noticeable when the patient tries to sit up, it is within the peritoneal cavity. On the other hand, if it remains the same size it is within the layers of the abdomen
Size and shape of organs of origin	• The larger the swelling arising from the stomach, small or large intestines, pancreas or peritoneum the more it alters the anatomical delineation of the organs of origin
Surface, edge and consistency	• A solid ill-defined tender mass is mostly due to inflammation while if hard and nodular may be malignant
Mobility and attachments	• Swellings occurring in the liver, spleen, kidneys, gallbladder, and distal stomach move downward during inspiration due to diaphragmatic contraction • Swellings that are bimanually palpable are usually renal in origin
Tenderness and rebound tenderness	• If palpating or touching an area causes pain it is tender • If gentle pressure is exerted over a painful area and if this pressure is gradually increased then suddenly lifted or released and if release of pressure worsens the pain, there is rebound tenderness and is a sign of acute appendicitis
Pulsations	• Place two fingers on the swelling and observe what happens to them in systole • In the event that the fingers remain parallel, then the pulsation is transmitted, however, if the fingers tend to separate, true expansile pulsation is present
	• Abdominal masses can be malignant or benign. Some typically are likely to cross the midline and this feature helps in the differential diagnosis • Congenital and acquired abdominal masses include hydronephrosis, polycystic kidney disease and congenital duplication of the gut • Non-infectious inflammatory masses include renal vein thrombosis • Neoplastic masses include Wilms' tumor, which is less likely to cross the midline, neuroblastoma, more likely to cross the midline, lymphomas, hepatoblastomas, rhabdomyosarcoms and the benign ganglioneuroma

A Jaundiced Child[24,25,32,34,36,39]

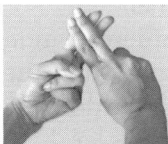

Use the physical links to guide you towards a complete examination:
- In a child who is jaundiced, look for hepatomegaly
- A small liver may indicate cirrhosis and end-stage liver disease
- The presence of a palpable spleen, ascites and caput medusa suggest portal hypertension and chronic liver disease
- In an infant, the diaper must be checked for pale stools and dark urine
- The presence of ataxia and asterixis warrant urgent investigation.

Percussion of the Abdomen[24,25,32,34,36,39]

Percussion delineates abdominal organs and abdominal masses.

Liver

- Define the upper and lower borders of the right lobe of the liver.
  - Start anteriorly at the 4th intercostal space where the percussion note is resonant over the lung.
  - In the normal liver, the upper border is at the 5th intercostal space.

Spleen

If splenomegaly is suspected, dullness to percussion over an enlarged spleen confirms the findings detected on palpation. Percuss the Traube's space, which is an area marked superiorly by the left sixth rib, laterally by the left anterior axillary line, and inferiorly by the left costal margin.
- If the Traube's space is dull, it is a sign that the spleen is enlarged. This sign is easier to elicit in thin patients.

Bladder

- The dullness indicates that the swelling is cystic or solid and not gaseous: Percuss to define its superior and lateral margins.

Other Masses[12,24,25,32,34,36,39]

- The dullness of a solid or cystic mass distinguishes the mass from adjacent bowel loops.

- Examine for ascites: The presence of free fluid can be confirmed by percussing the abdomen.
  - For shifting dullness, there is a line of demarcation from the umbilicus towards the flanks where the resonance of the bowel gas becomes the dullness of the free fluid. Keep your finger at this level.
  - Roll the child onto his or her side without moving the finger that has demarcated the earlier point of dullness. The fluid moves to the lower flank and the line of demarcation between dullness and resonance shifts. Percuss the same areas now and the dull area becomes resonant because the fluid has shifted. This test is positive even when there is minimal ascites.
  - The fluid thrill is another clinical test for free fluid in the abdomen. This test is positive with a greater amount of free fluid than for shifting dullness and is less often done in the child. As a rule, the fluid thrill is present only where large amount of ascites is present under tension, and therefore is not a sensitive indicator of the presence of minimal to moderate amounts of abdominal fluid.

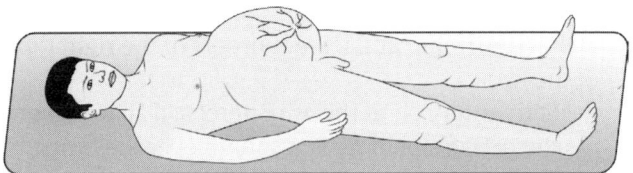

Diagrammatic representation of ascites with portal vein thrombosis. When the abdomen is markedly distended, observe for distended collateral veins and eversion of the umbilicus. Portal hypertension with associated emaciation due to malnutrition makes the abdominal veins very prominent. Inferior vena caval obstruction is a less common cause in the pediatric age group. If the marked distension is due to fluid, the fluid thrill is positive.

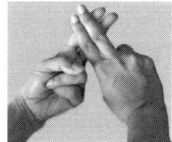

Use the physical links, then think and conduct a good physical examination.

The physical links to suspecting the presence of ascites are:
- A distended abdomen
- An everted umbilicus
- Dilated abdominal veins with distension
- Flank fullness
- Apparent edema in any other part of the body
- The presence of hepatomegaly
- Signs of liver disease, e.g. jaundice, palmar erythema, spider nevi, clubbing, jaundice
- Signs of renal disease, e.g. oliguria or periorbital edema
- Signs of cardiac failure, e.g. tachypnea, tachycardia, cardiomegaly, fine basal crackles in the lung
- Signs of fever suggestive of an infective disease like dengue hemorrhagic fever where pathology is due to transudation of fluid due to leakage of capillaries
- Signs of nutritional deficiencies like kwashiorkor.

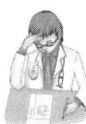

"Physical links help me complete my physical examination in a focused and clinically meaningful manner."

Auscultation of the Abdomen[24,25,32,34,36,39]

- Listen for bowel sounds slightly to the right of the periumbilical area and always ensure that you auscultate over any visible swelling
- The bowel sounds are particularly important to determine in cases where the abdomen is distended or the child has a nasogastric tube
- It is important in states linked to electrolyte imbalances as hypokalemia can cause paralytic ileus
- In simple acute mechanical obstruction of the small bowel, the bowel sounds are markedly increased
- It is also carefully listened to in the patient recovering from abdominal surgery
- Borborygmi are frequent low pitched gurgling noises
- In an obstructed loop of bowel, when strangulation and gangrene supervene, the bowel sounds become less frequent and may then be absent
- In generalized peritonitis, there is no bowel activity and paralytic ileus ensues
- In lactose intolerance usually secondary to a severe gastroenteritis there may be hyperactive bowel sounds
- Rubs and bruits are also noted by auscultation.

Remember that the rectal and genital examination is an important part of the abdominal examination.

Rectal Examination[24,25,32,34,36,39]

- Inspection is important. However, per rectal examination is usually not routinely done in children
- Examine for perianal rash and stools for red currant jelly appearance in intussusceptions

- Inspect for perianal fissure. Anal fissures can occur in constipation and with large impacted stools as occur in some children with constipation, and inflammatory bowel diseases
- Fissures and tears are sometimes seen in non-accidental injuries
- Rectal prolapse occurs in heavy parasite burdens of *Trichuris trichiura* (whip worm) and in severe malnutrition
- Perianal abscesses occur in leukemia, congenital or acquired immunodeficiency syndromes and fevers of unknown origin
- Perianal skin tags are rarely of significance
- Taking the rectal temperatures in the newborn is one way of detecting anal atresia. Perianal redness and excoriation occur in lactose intolerance.

Genital Region[24,25,32,34,36,39]

- The genital area is examined routinely in all children.
- Meticulous inspection must be done.

Inspection of the Genital Region[12,24,25,32,34,36,39]

Male Child Inspection

- Check the size of the penis and testes, scrotum development and look out for any pubertal changes.
- Check for circumcision, meatal opening, hypospadias, phimosis, adherent foreskin, cryptorchidism, hydrocele and look for any hernia.
- Check for swellings that increase in size when the child cries or coughs which imply the presence of a hernia and a positive cry or cough impulse. When the infant cries or when the older child coughs there is an increase in intra-abdominal pressure. This causes hernias to increase in size.

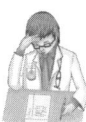

Obstruction of an inguinal hernia could be a cause of a symptom like vomiting. You may not have found anything abnormal in the abdominal examination. Do not forget the importance of the genital and inguinal examination in a case of vomiting.

- Look for perineal rash. Nappy rashes or diaper dermatitis have been described earlier.

Palpation

- In the genital examination in the male child, palpate for the testicles before the child has fully undressed in order not to stimulate the cremasteric reflex.
- In a young patient who is more comfortable examined in the sitting position, one may choose to examine while sitting in a chair holding his knees with his heels on the seat; the increased intra-abdominal pressure may push the testes into the scrotum.
- Ensure that the testes are palpable. Feel for the testes in the scrotum but remember that an active cremasteric reflex which is fairly common in children may retract them into the abdomen.
- Thus one must gently milk the testes down into the scrotum to feel them.
- Observe for scrotal hydroceles and if present confirm by transillumination.
- The examination for cryptorchidism starts above the inguinal canal, then slowly, downward to prevent pushing the testes up into the canal or abdomen.
- In the obese patient, the pubic pad of fat may make the penis appear abnormally small. In most cases, if this fat is pushed back, a penis of normal size is usually seen.

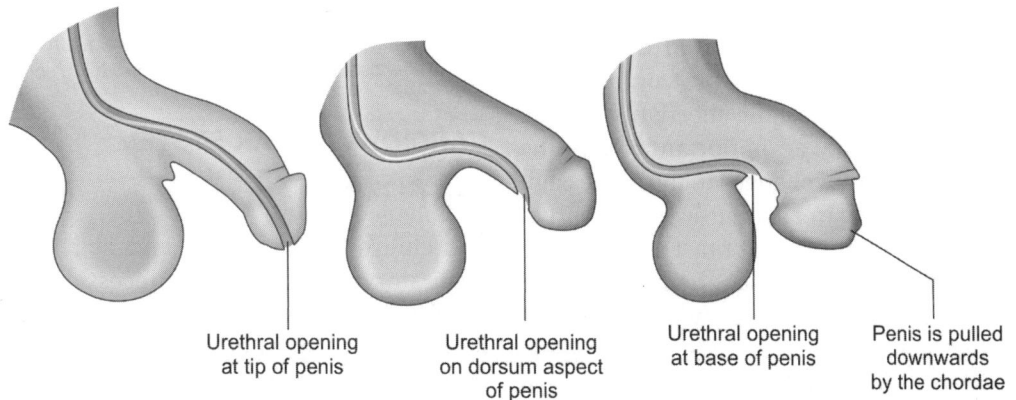

Hypospadias—a congenital anomaly due to incomplete embryological development of the anterior urethra and corpus spongiosum. It is usually diagnosed immediately at birth upon initial examination.

- Examine the ventral surface of the penis for hypospadias which is a congenital anomaly where the external urethral meatus opens not at the tip of the glans penis but on its ventral surface in the midline. This could be anywhere from the glans to the shaft and in severe cases the opening could even be in the perineum.

Epispadias is where the external urethral meatus opens on the dorsal surface of the penis.

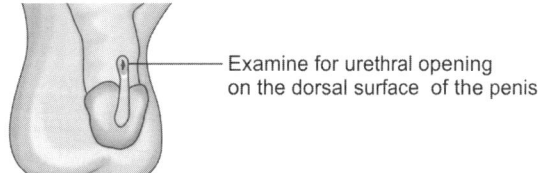

Examine for urethral opening on the dorsal surface of the penis

Epispadias

Female Child

- In the female child, inspect the vagina for imperforate hymen, discharge, adhesions and hypertrophy of the clitoris.
- Pubertal changes in the genitalia in the adolescent must be noted.
- In the child with ambiguous genitalia:
  - Remember to have examined the child on the whole first; look in particular for dysmorphisms
  - Look for increased pigmentation of the skin, the areolae, nipples, skin creases and genitalia. These may be due to increased adrenocorticotrophic hormone (ACTH) seen in congenital adrenal hyperplasia (CAH)
  - Look for increased hair growth over the body, pubic area, and axillae.

Pubertal Assessment[24,25,32,34,36,39]

Tactfully approach the overt and covert changes in this age group. Many physiological, emotional and functional changes occur at this time in the lives of human beings. Many such changes are controlled by a shift in the internal homeostatic mechanisms. The function of sex steroids play an important role in the phenotype features. Pubertal changes in the adolescent must be assessed routinely in all adolescents as part of a complete physical examination. It must also be done in specific situations where the assessment of pubertal changes are important. In suspected endocrinopathies or diseases that can affect the endocrine system, pubertal staging must be done. An example is a case of thalassemia major on blood transfusion. Here growth and endocrine assessment are important as iron overload can affect endocrine organs.

Tanner Staging of Breast and Pubic Hair[24,25,32,34,36,39]

Stage 1→Stage 5

The Tanner staging of puberty spans from breast development where the elevation of papilla is the prepubertal stage followed by the elevation of breast and papilla as a mound.

Development of the breast continues to advance until stage 5 where recession of areola to contour of the breast occurs. Likewise pubic hair development is noted in the staging where stage 1 refers to no pubic hair and stage 5 refers to the adult type hair extending on to the medial thigh.

The onset of puberty is with breast enlargement in girls and testicular enlargement in boys. The mean age of puberty is slightly earlier in girls than in boys. The timing of the growth spurt occurs earlier in girls than in boys. In girls, breast development in stage 2 is the projection of areola and papilla to form a secondary mound above the level of the breast. This must occur for the onset of menstruation.

Clinically approach them as friends and they will respond by mutual understanding and cooperation with you.

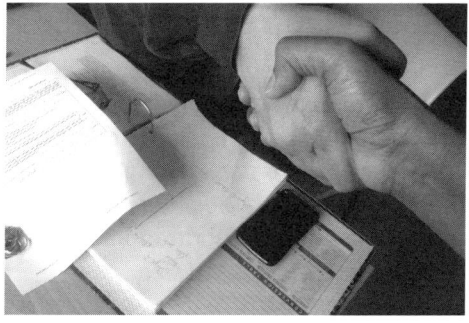

"A firm handshake and a warm smile gains confidence and cooperation from the adolescent patient—A tactful approach to the overt and covert changes in this vulnerable age group is required."

CARDIOVASCULAR SYSTEM[2,24,25,32,34,36,39]

Heart[24,25,32,34,36,39]

The child's growth, color and activity are vital. The respiratory rate and chest recessions are important observations. As mentioned in the general observation, dysmorphisms must be looked for. In pediatrics, certain dysmorphisms must make your search for specific cardiac lesions. Some examples are Down syndrome, Turner syndrome, some craniofacial anomalies, Vater syndrome, Noonan syndrome, Marfan's syndrome.

Pediatric Physical Examination

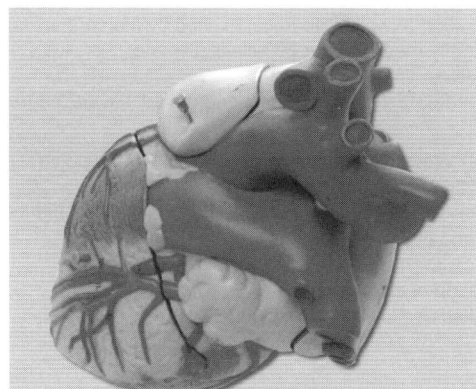

Model of the heart.

Examine for VSD, ASD, AVSD and endocardial cushion defects. Examine the lungs and the liver to look for signs of heart failure and link the history to the examination as a guide to links in other systems, e.g. if nutritional history is indicative of poor appetite examine growth, search for all nutritional deficiencies. Conduct detailed abdominal examination if the history is suggestive of vomiting or constipation, the ENT if history reveals recurrent ear infections and so on.

Link the history and the physical examination to make the differential diagnosis and provisional diagnosis.

In Williams syndrome, there is a higher incidence of supravalvular aortic stenosis.

Knowing this, in a child who has Down syndrome, the links in the physical examination include examination of the heart. To examine the heart completely and in detail, know that there is a higher incidence of anomalies.

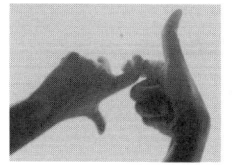 +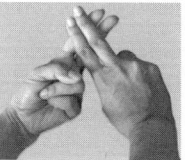

General observation must be done as mentioned. Specific observation and examination must then follow.

Specific Examination of the Cardiovascular System[2,24,25,32,34,36,39]

Criteria[2,24,25,32,34,36,39]	Characteristics[2,24,25,32,34,36,39]
Inspection	• Observe the tongue for central cyanosis • Examine for clubbing seen in congenital cyanotic heart diseases • Splinter hemorrhages and Osler's nodes are seen in infective endocarditis • What are the underlying cardiac lesions in a child with infective endocarditis? Should these lesions occur in high pressure chambers of the heart where there is a high jet flow across the defect? What are the factors that put a child at risk of this condition?
	• Tuberous and tendon xanthomas are seen over the elbows in familial hypercholesterolemia "When tuberous and tendon xanthomas are seen, what else must I look for? What are the suggestive features to elicit in the history, using open ended and closed ended questioning?" • Blood pressure measurements are meticulously taken in the upper limb and lower limb in the cardiovascular examination • Feel the pulse for rate, rhythm, volume and character and palpate both radials and femorals • Tachypnea (differs at different age groups) • Chest recessions • Precordial bulge • Ventricular impulse or apex beat • Operative scars • Look for chest deformity, asymmetry, and precordial bulge. Examine for scars over the chest, subscapular and axillary areas as well as posteriorly. The site of the scar reveals whether an open cardiac surgery has been performed. A central thoracotomy scar has a different significance from a subscapular scar of a Blalock-Taussig shunt • In a thin child, the cardiac pulsations on the chest wall can be observed

180 *The Link*: Pediatric History-Taking and Physical Examination

Palpation	• Localize the apex beat which is the furthest lateral and inferior position at which the finger is lifted by the cardiac impulse • In infants and young children, it is on the 4th intercostal space slightly medial to the mid-clavicular line. • In older children, it is on the 5th intercostal space on the mid-clavicular line • Feel for thrills at all the auscultatory areas, the left sternal edge and parasternal heaves along the left sternal edge. The left parasternal heave signifies right ventricular hypertrophy
Auscultation	• In the infant and young child, it is best to auscultate immediately after observation to obtain maximum cooperation when listening to the heart. In older children, auscultation may be performed after palpation • Listen to the apex, the left lower sternal edge at the 4th intercostal space, the left upper sternal edge at the 2nd intercostal space, the right upper sternal edge at the 2nd intercostal space, and over both carotids • The normal splitting of the second heart sound is easily heard in children • The second heart sound is important to determine in the examination of a child's heart • If it is normal in intensity and splits normally, many important cardiac conditions are excluded

Defining features of a cardiac murmur are summarized as follows:

Defining features of a cardiac murmur[2,24,25,32,34,36,39]	
Feature	Description
1. When it occurs or its timing	• Murmurs are longer in duration upon auscultation than heart sounds • Heart sounds can be easily appreciated. Palpation of the carotid arterial pulse while listening to the heart sounds may be useful • The murmur may be systolic, diastolic or continuous
2. Its auditory features	• Palpation of the carotids during auscultation can further help you to appreciate if the murmur is systolic or diastolic • Increases in intensity as you listen • Decreases in intensity as you listen • Increases and then decreases in intensity as you listen • Same intensity throughout the auditory phase
3. Where it is maximally heard	• Is determined by the site of origin of the murmur • State whether it is at the aortic, pulmonary, tricuspid, or mitral auscultatory areas
4. Other areas that the murmur can also be heard or its radiation	• Reflects the intensity of the murmur. Indicates the direction of blood flow. Murmurs may radiate to the axilla, to the carotids or to the back

5. How loud it is or its Intensity	• Measured by a 6-point scale where:
	  - Grade 1 = Inaudible or very soft
	  - Grade 2 = Just appreciable
	  - Grade 3 = Moderately loud
	  - Grade 4 = Loud and palpable (thrill)
	  - Grade 5 = Heard with stethoscope a little off the chest with a thrill
	  - Grade 6 = Audible without a stethoscope needed accompanied by a thrill
	
	• The loudness of the murmur may not necessarily indicate the size of a defect as a small VSD could cause a loud murmur due to greater resistance to blood flow across a smaller defect

6. Pitch or tone	• High, medium, low
7. Nature	• Blowing, harsh, rumbling (a resonant, deep sound), and musical
8. Other associated features	i. Variation with respiration. In most of the cases the right-sided murmurs change more than left-sided ones ii. Alters with position of the patient iii. Changes with special maneuvers like bending forward, breathing in or out, turning to the left side, lifting legs up if venous hum
9. Functional murmurs	• It is also known as a flow murmur, benign murmur, vibratory murmur, hemic murmur or an innocent murmur • Venous hums and functional systolic murmurs or an innocent murmur are often heard in normal children

Summary of the auscultatory areas for common pediatric heart murmurs.

Regions for auscultation for common pediatric heart murmurs[2,24,25,32,34,36,39]	
Area auscultated	Murmur heard
Upper sternal border, right side	Aortic stenosis, venous hum
Upper sternal edge, left side	Pulmonary flow murmurs, pulmonary stenosis, atrial septal defect, patent ductus arteriosus
Lower left sternal edge	Ventricular septal defect, Still's murmur, tricuspid valve regurgitation, hypertrophic cardiomyopathy, subaortic stenosis
Apical area	Mitral valve regurgitation

The 10 links beginning with "S" of a physiological murmur[34]
Safe and symptom free
Surely systolic (musical and ejection systolic)
Simply short
Soft and sweet (audible only if carefully listened to by a stethoscope)
Small area (heard over)
Split 2nd sound (physiological split)
Sitting or standing (varies with position)
Sternal depression (chest cage deformities such as kyphoscoliosis or pectus excavatum)
Sans (without) abnormal signs
Specific tests are normal (CXR, ECG, ECHO)

An innocent murmur may be heard in normal children during:
- Fever
- Exercise
- Excitement.

Additional Note on Functional and Pathologic Murmurs[24,25,32,34,36,39]

Positional Changes—an example of the application of cardiovascular physiology to the clinical signs in the disease.[2]

The vibratory functional murmur heard in a young child (Still's murmur) decreases in intensity when the patient stands. As for most pathologic murmurs, they do not change significantly with standing. One important exception is the murmur of hypertrophic cardiomyopathy—a rare potentially life-threatening condition and an important cause of sudden death in athletes. This murmur increases in intensity when the patient stands.

Sinus arrhythmia is observed in many children. In order to determine its effect on the rhythm, the child should be asked to take a deep breath. Extrasystoles are not uncommon in childhood.

> Note:
> - Pathophysiology of the murmur of hypertrophic cardiomyopathy
> - In the upright position, venous return to the heart is reduced, resulting in a decrease in the left ventricular end diastolic volume. As left ventricular size decreases, systolic outflow obstruction increases due to narrowing of the ventricular outflow tract. This narrowing increases the intensity of the murmur

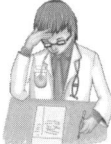

"The pathophysiological changes that occur to venous return and the volume of blood in the left ventricle, is how cardiovascular hemodynamics when standing, can influence the intensity of the murmur. Therefore I see how my knowledge of cardiac physiology is applied to the patient clinically."

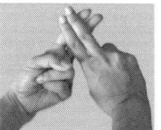

Using this example, think of the pathological processes that occur in the abnormal heart and link to site, nature and intensity of murmur

NERVOUS SYSTEM[24,25,32,34,36,39]

Nervous System and the Neurodevelopmental System

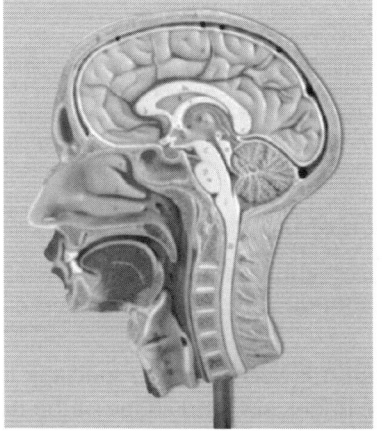

Model of a cross-section of brain and spinal cord

What is the age of the child?
What is the level of cooperation to reasonably expect of the child?
How do I approach the examination?

GOOD CLINICAL PRACTICE

In young children, the neurological examination depends mainly on two factors—their age and cooperation. In older children, examination of the nervous system can be done in the usual manner, as it is carried out in the adult. Cranial nerve examination in the infant and young child who cannot obey instructions has often to be creative. Cranial nerve examination in the older child follows the format as for the adult. As cooperation can be unpredictable from the infant and young child, the neurological examination can be done together with the developmental assessment as the combined neurodevelopmental assessment. This will give you a lot of information, by observation and inference in the overall neurological assessment of the young child.

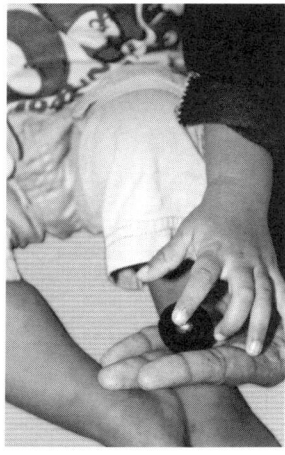

The pincer grip is an example of how the developmental assessment can give much information on a number of neurological functions, by inference; information that the child can see and that the use of the muscles of the thumb and index finger in adduction is normal. Hence, you may use the developmental assessment as a tool to roughly assess many neurological functions in the young child, when used together is called the neurodevelopmental assessment.

Observation of the Nervous System[24,25,32,34,36,39]

General observations must be done as already mentioned. Specific observation of the nervous system is important.

Observation is very crucial, especially in the young child. In the infant, size and shape of the head must be observed. Plotting the occipitofrontal circumference (OFC) is part of the pediatric neurological examination at all ages. The measurements of head circumference from both parents may be relevant as familial macrocephaly and microcephaly are common and must be first excluded.

To obtain the child's cooperation, it is useful to measure the circumference of head (COH) of the parents first. In infants or toddlers, leave the assessment until the end of the examination. Special charts are available for OFC. Plot the circumference of head (COH) on an age and gender appropriate chart.

Sequential measurements are more useful than one-off measurements in the interpretation of head size. Measurements of head circumference that progressively cross percentiles are more worrying than a large or small head from birth which is growing along the same percentile.

Hypo- or hypertelorism of the eyes is based on the interpupillary distance which has age specific charts. Look for epicanthal folds, palpebral fissures, ptosis, corneal clouding, lens opacities, blue sclera and iris colobomata. Observe for abnormalities of the pinna of the ears; are the ears low set? Is there a cleft lip or palate?

Observe if macroglossia is present. Also observe for facial dysmorphisms including shape of the face, low nasal bridge and micrognathia or prognathia. Malar or maxillary hypoplasia is seen in some dysmorphic syndromes. Observe the head size and shape and assess if the occiput is flat or prominent. Do any of these relate to the clinical history?

Think of physical links and proceed to a focused physical examination. What do you know of macroglossia? Knowledge is necessary to improve your linkage ability. Do not worry, this will come with time and reading. Train yourself to think broadly (lateral thinking) and deeply (in depth) when a positive link is elicited.

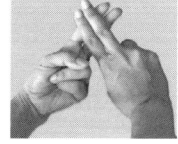 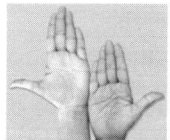

Lateral thinking is made easier with the physical links

Think in depth with **The Cardinal Ten (Physical)**

For example, a history of obstinate constipation and macroglossia will make you examine all other signs of hypothyroidism whereas a history of macroglossia with parental consanguinity may make you think of mucopolysaccharidosis. If Beckwith–Wiedemann syndrome is considered complete abdominal examination is a must. Dysmorphism with macroglossia must make you think of chromosomal abnormalities.

Observe the head posture. Abnormal head postures may be due to torticollis, strabismus or hemianopia.

Also look out for abnormal trunk postures like scoliosis, kyphosis and lordosis. Look for the frog leg posture of hypotonia.

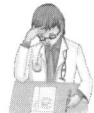

Think of cause and effect of abnormal head postures. Why should a child with uncorrected torticollis develop a squint? What are the physical links? What are the historical links? Do you need to go back to the history to ask about something more?

Look for dilated veins on the scalp and down turning of the eyes or the sunset sign of hydrocephalus.

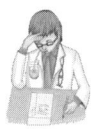

The skin is often a window to problems involving the brain just as the eyes are. The skin is an organ directly accessible to observation whereas pathologies of the brain have to be inferred by studying the physical signs produced. Hence, neurocutaneous stigmata if recognized, are useful to make a diagnosis.

Inspect the skin for neurocutaneous stigmata. Although not commonly seen, some **neurocutaneous stigmata** that are useful to remember include café au lait spots and neurofibromas of neurofibromatosis, adenoma sebaceum and depigmented macules of tuberous sclerosis and facial hemangiomata of Sturge–Weber syndrome. In patients with fair complexion, achromic spots may only be visible with a Wood's lamp.

Look at the pulsations of the anterior fontanel before palpating to appreciate its tension. The diagnosis of a lethargic infant with fever and a bulging anterior fontanel is meningitis.

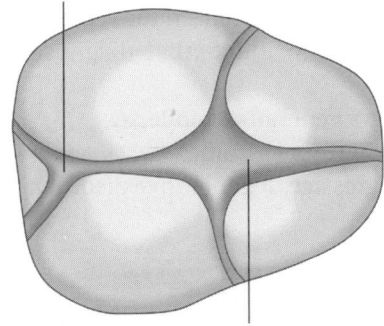

Anterior and posterior fontanel.

Meningitis is suggested by:
- Bulging anterior fontanel (up to 2 years)
- Irritability
- Lethargy
- Drowsiness
- High fever
- Somnolence
- Delirium
- Fits
- Neck stiffness: Passive flexion of the neck will normally allow the chin to touch the chest. Neck muscle spasm or pain in the neck limits this movement. Such limitation is seen in meningitis.
- A positive Kernig's sign in the older child: Extension of knee with hip fully flexed causes pain in the hamstrings. This is seen in meningitis.

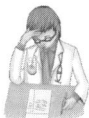

"I need to look at the patient as a whole before doing the CNS examination. Clues of cause and effect of diseases can be critically analyzed by astute general observation."

- In **meningitis, associated physical signs** can be links to the etiological diagnosis.
- Enteroviral infection is suggested by the presence of exanthems, conjunctivitis, herpangina, and hand-foot-mouth disease.

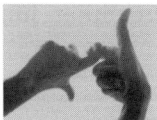

In meningitis, physical signs outside the CNS can be links to the etiological diagnosis.

- Viral meningitis may be suggested by a morbilliform rash with pharyngitis and lymphadenopathy.
- Evolving skin lesions like macules that become purpuric in nature suggest meningococcemia.
- Herpes zoster virus is suggested by vesicles distributed along a dermatome.
- Genital vesicles suggest HSV-2 meningitis.
- Ear discharge, otitis or tenderness of the sinuses suggests direct extension into the meninges, usually due *S. pneumoniae* or, less often, *H. influenzae*.
- Rhinorrhea or otorrhea suggest a cerebrospinal fluid (CSF) leak that occurs as a result of basal skull fracture. Here, if meningitis occurs, it is most commonly caused by *S. pneumoniae*.

- Hepatosplenomegaly and lymphadenopathy suggest a systemic disease, such as cytomegalo-virus, Epstein–Barr virus and human immunodeficiency virus.
- Further, link your physical findings with known pathophysiology of these diseases to make an anatomical and etiological diagnosis. A heart murmur suggests infective endocarditis with secondary bacterial seeding of the meninges.

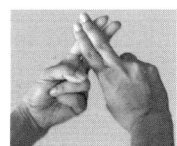

Examine the **arms and legs for posture, deformity** and **muscle bulk**. See if an adducted shoulder, flexed elbow, wrist and clenched fist is present as these suggest a pyramidal tract problem, usually cerebral palsy.

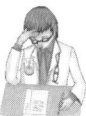

What are the suggestive historical links of these conditions?

Look out closely for the waiter's tip of Erb's palsy which is due to shoulder dystocia at birth; other odd postures to look out for are the claw hand of a lower brachial plexus injury and a radial nerve injury or arthrogryposis where other joints are involved as well.

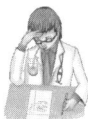

What are the links in the posture of the child that can tell me if the wasting is due to upper or lower motor neuron pathology?

In the lower limbs, observe for generalized bilateral wasting as seen in spina bifida or spinal muscular atrophy.

Take note of any **abnormal movements** or **dyskinesias**. Chorea is rapid involuntary rhythmical movements and athetoid movements refer to slow, involuntary, writhing movements.

Choreiform movements:[24,25,32,34,36,39]
- Jerky nonsuppressive movements
- Involuntary purposeless movements
- Affecting distal muscles and face.

Tics[24,25,32,34,36,39]
- Habit spasms
- Repeated identical movements
- Recurring and sustained.

Tremors[24,25,32,34,36,39]
- Involuntary repeated movements.

Titubations[24,25,32,34,36,39]
- Tremors involving the head and the neck.

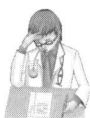

"When I see abnormal movements in a child, I try to analyze these movements to see if they fit into categories that I know about. I then think of the possible differential diagnoses including drug-induced side effects, rheumatic heart disease, Wilson's disease, or choreoathetoid cerebral palsy, if the clinical picture is suggestive. I need to link all categories of the history which will guide me, then the physical examination of which observation is crucial, and arrive at a clinical diagnosis."

Athetosis[24,25,32,34,36,39]
- Slow involuntary semi purposeful writhing movements
- Affects arms and legs.
- Hemiballismus[24,25,32,34,36,39]
- Unilateral rapid non rhythmic
- Nonsuppressive
- Flinging movements
- Affects proximal arm or leg.

Dystonia[24,25,32,34,36,39]
- Sustained irregular involuntary muscle spasms
- Last longer than chorea
- Distort the body or limb.

Hemiplegic dystonia is an example.

Myoclonus[24,25,32,34,36,39]
- Brief muscle jerks
- There are distinct pauses between each movement
- Repetitive jerks occur in the same muscle.

In children, the differential diagnosis of myoclonus include:
- Primary generalized epilepsy
- An epilepsy syndrome
- A progressive degenerative disorder.

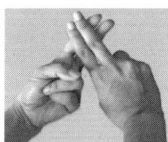

Link the observations of motor function and gait with the age of the child.

Watch how the active child walks, jumps, hops, stands up from lying and sitting positions, dresses and undresses. If the child can walk, look for abnormalities of gait, including wide based gaits, waddling gaits, hemiplegic gaits, or the scissoring of spastic diplegia and the presence of a limp or ataxia. The causes of a waddling gait include myopathies, muscular dystrophies, and bilateral developmental dysplasia of the hip (DDH).

Note: A limp is a gait where the time for weight bearing is less on one leg as compared to the other.

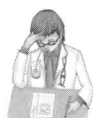

How do you obtain maximum information of posture or its dysfunction? How would you arrive at the anatomical diagnosis of the child's problem?

While engaging in a ball game with the child, elicit evidence of dysfunction in posture and movement. Observe gait, power and coordination as the ball is caught, thrown or kicked.

Toe-walking may suggest lower-limb muscle weakness with or without spasticity.

Impaired walking on the heels indicates foot dorsiflexion weakness, whereas difficulty hopping, standing from a squat or climbing stairs are suggestive of weakness in the muscles of the pelvic girdle.

In the presence of macrocephaly, the transillumination test can be done. A strong light source (or a torch) is held close to the back of the skull, preferably in a dark room.

A diffuse increase in transillumination occurs in hydranencephaly and severe hydrocephalus. A focal increase may occur in subdural effusions and porencephaly. Meningeal irritation or spasm of the spinal muscles is confirmed by resistance to passive flexion or neck stiffness.

CORRELATE, COMPARE, CAPTURE AND CONFIRM (CCCC)[24,25,32,34,36,39]

Muscle Tone[24,25,32,34,36,39]

Comparison on both sides is important.

Hold both the child's wrists and shake them loosely and fast. Observe how freely they move; compare the difference between the two sides. As for the legs, lightly lift each leg and try to flex it at the knee and the hips repeatedly. Try to abduct each hip with the knee flexed while keeping the pelvis fixed with one hand. The infant with hypotonia will feel like a 'rag doll' when held under the axillae. Head control may be poor resulting in abnormal head lag on pulling to sit and this is also a sign of hypotonia. Central hypotonia affects the trunk with normal muscle power and increased or normal tendon reflexes.

Peripheral hypotonia affects the limbs and is associated with decreased muscle power and hyporeflexia.

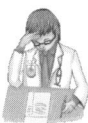

"I must ask myself if hypotonia is associated with significant muscle weakness."

Scissoring of the legs due to spasticity is a sign of hypertonia. This is a sign of upper motor neuron pathology as seen in spastic diplegia.

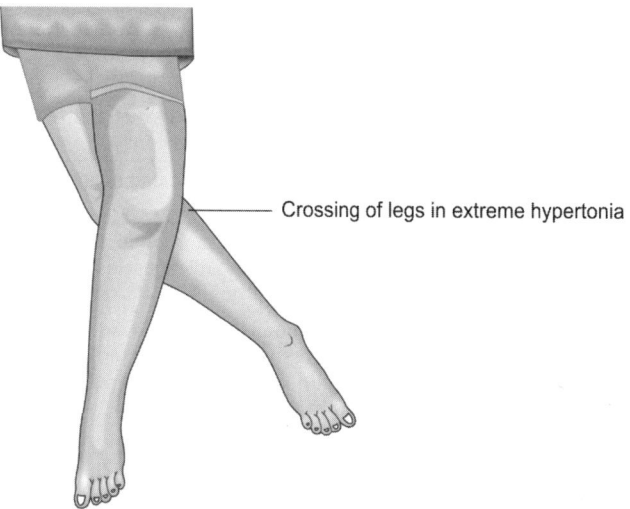

Scissoring of legs is observed in hypertonia such as in spastic diplegia

Elucidate the upper motor neuron lesion pertaining to site and etiology by utilizing the historical and physical links.

Dysfunction of the corticospinal or pyramidal tracts occurring at any point from the cerebral cortex to the spinal cord is indicated by:

The presence of pyramidal signs with the finding of increased tone, and greater weakness involving the extensor muscles of the upper limb and the flexor muscles of the lower limb. The tendon reflexes are observed to be brisk with an extensor plantar response.

Link the History and the Physical Examination[24,25,32,34,36,39]

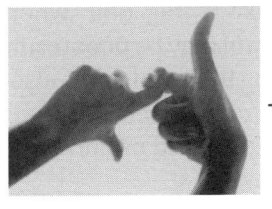 +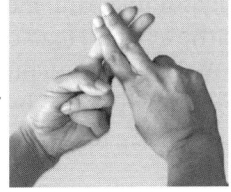

Muscle Power CCCC[24,25,32,34,36,39]

Correlation of pathophysiology, comparison with the other limb, accurate description following standard grading of muscle power and confirmation by additional tests, if required, are important when examining muscles. Each movement during the assessment of muscle power is tested by comparison either with the examiner's own strength or by comparison with what is judged to be normal in a person of comparable age and stature to the patient. The table shows the assessment of power in the different parts of the body.

Assessment of power in the different parts of the body[24,25,32,34,36,39]	
Body part involved	Assessment of power
Arms	The infant with normal power will flex at the elbows opposing your pull when this is done gently
Hands	The strength with which the child grips your hand reveals power in the hands
Legs and pelvic girdle	Ability to stand from the sitting position tests power of both lower legs and the pelvic girdle muscles
Legs	Independent walking normally is achieved at 10–18 months. Passively flex the legs as for examining tone and observe how hard the infant pushes you; power of the legs is also assessed by the gait

Grading of muscle power is carried out using the following criteria[24,25,32,34,36,39]	
Grade 0:	Complete paralysis without any visible muscular contraction
Grade 1:	A flicker of contraction only hence, without movement
Grade 2:	Power detectable only when gravity is removed or eliminated by appropriate postural adjustment
Grade 3:	The limb can be held against the force of gravity, but not against the examiner's resistance
Grade 4:	There is a certain degree of weakness, usually described as poor, fair or moderate strength
Grade 5:	Normal power

Reflexes CCCC[24,25,32,34,36,39]

Reflexes in young children may seem difficult to elicit. Distract them by a toy or by mother's familiar voice.

In younger children, reflexes are most easily examined with the child sitting on the parent's or carer's lap resting his or her legs in the examiner's lap. The parent or carer restrains one arm while reflexes are elicited in the other. Give the child a toy to play. This helps during examination of lower-limb reflexes. Percuss the tendons gently; this is best done with a pediatric tendon hammer.

Reflex[24,25,32,34,36,39]	Nerve root involved[24,25,32,34,36,39]
Knee jerk	Spinal segments lumbar 2, 3 and 4
Ankle jerk	Sacral segments 1 and 2
Triceps jerk	Cervical segments 6 and 7
Biceps jerk	Cervical segments 5 and 6
Supinator jerk	Cervical segment 5 and 6

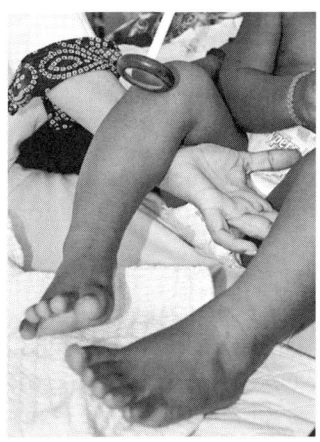

Reflexes in young children may seem difficult to elicit. Distract them by a toy or by mother's familiar voice.

Clonus[24,25,32,34,36,39]

Grasp the foot with one hand and dorsiflex the foot while bending the patient's knee. Repeated contraction alternating with relaxation is clonus. Sustained clonus is clinically significant and occurs when contraction and relaxation occur more than five times.

Interpretation[24,25,32,34,36,39]

Sustained clonus is evidence of upper motor neuron lesions.

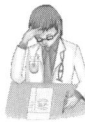

In the neonate and young infant, clonus is normally elicited. It is not sustained. Myelination of the nerves are incomplete at this age. This is the cause.

Plantar Reflex[24,25,32,34,36,39]

Plantar responses are best left until last. The plantar responses are elicited by running a blunt object (e.g. a key) along the outer edge of the sole of the foot from the heel to the toe. The plantar response is extensor in normal infants up to the age of one year. Babinski sign is a sign of pyramidal tract dysfunction. The Babinski sign is dorsiflexion of the great toe and fanning of the toes. This is normal up to 1 year of age so symmetry is the important feature to look at below 1 year.

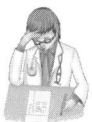

Incomplete myelination of the nerves is why the plantars are upgoing in the infant: Also known as a positive Babinski sign. Therefore, this sign must be interpreted at this age in the context of other neurological findings. A symetrical Babinski sign is feature to note in infants less than a year.

Interpretation[24,25,32,34,36,39]

The persistence of an extensor response after the age of two years suggests an upper motor neuron lesion.

Grading the reflexes[24,25,32,34,36,39]
Absent
Present
Brisk
Very brisk
Clonus

Abnormal Reflexes[24,25,32,34,36,39]

The following characteristics increase the likelihood that a reflex is abnormal[24,25,32,34,36,39]	The 4Cs – Correlate, Compare, Capture, Confirm[24,25,32,34,36,39]
They are asymmetrical	Compare with other limb and with all other reflexes
They are exaggerated in amplitude	Correlate with normal reflexes
There is a wide afferent field meaning that the reflex can be elicited away from the usual point of stimulus	Capture and confirm
There are crossed responses	Compare upper and lower limbs
There is an extensor plantar response (Interpretation: abnormal if child is older than one year)	Correlate with age
If there is associated muscle wasting (Capture by observation the muscle wasting)	Correlate with other physical findings

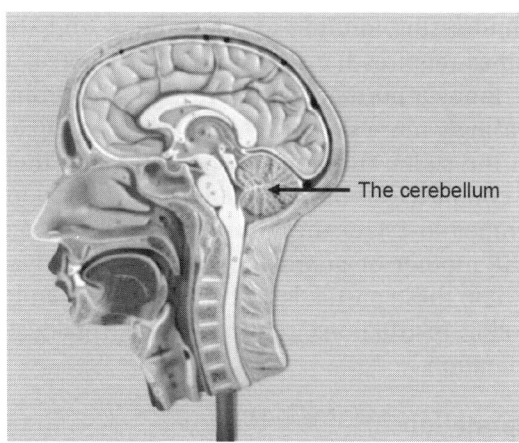

Cerebellar Signs[24,25,32,34,36,39]

When the cerebellum is affected by disease, muscular hypotonia, incoordination and ataxia result. Truncal ataxia is associated with difficulty in sitting up or standing and can be tested by asking the patient who is at an age to understand simple instructions, to do these things.

Ataxia is the incoordination of movement which is not due to the following:
- Weakness
- Loss of postural sense
- Involuntary movements
- Changes in muscle tone.

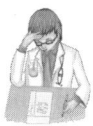

So much useful information can be obtained by watching a child at play.

Coordination[24,25,32,34,36,39]

Coordination is assessed by modification of the finger-to-nose test; the child is instructed to reach out to touch a toy that is held in the examiner's hand. It can also be simply tested by observing the child play. In general, coordination may appear impaired by poor visual acuity or a squint. In a young child, observe the movement of the limbs.

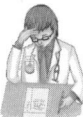

Coordination is linked to age. Doing and interpreting test of coordination must be logical.

As for the upper limb, reaching out for objects, feeding himself or herself, buttoning shirts or dressing and undressing, putting toys into holes and stacking up cubes requires hand coordination, whereas in the lower limbs a normal gait implies good coordination; increasingly more sensitive tests include going up and down the stairs, running and hopping; and these are more complex tests of coordination. However, you must remember to relate these interpretations to age and ask the mother or guardian when the child was first able to do these particular tasks. In an older child who can follow instructions, continue with formal testing of coordination.

Interpretation[24,25,32,34,36,39]

If a child is not used to stacking up cubes, he or she may appear clumsy when demonstrating this. Here the age, previous experience, and the developmental maturity have to be considered in the observation and interpretation.

Upper Limbs Incoordination[24,25,32,34,36,39]

Ask patient to touch the point of his nose first, then the examiner's forefinger with his index finger. Do this ensuring the patient's hands are outstretched and that the patient touches the examiner's forefinger in an arc. The finger-to-nose test is a test of coordination of the upper limbs. If this is done smoothly, no incoordination of the upper limb is present.

Sense of Position[24,25,32,34,36,39]

The patient is then instructed to carry out the same action with his or her eyes closed. This tests the disturbance of sense of position.

Lower Limbs[24,25,32,34,36,39]

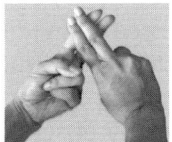

Link physical findings of coordination to the age of the patient.

Incoordination and Sense of Position[24,25,32,34,36,39]

The child must be at an age to understand simple instructions. If the patient is able to walk, ask the patient to walk along a straight line. If the patient is not able to walk with both eyes open, instruct him or her to lift one leg and place the heel of this leg on the opposite knee and then to slide the heel down the shin towards the ankle. Tandem walking and heel-to-shin test are tests of lower limb coordination.

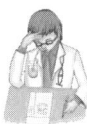

"I can only do specific tests of coordination in the older child. I must know the developmental milestones before I ask a young child to do this. For example, I can only ask a child to walk heel to toe at the age of 5 years or above as that is when most children are able to do this."

Dysdiadochokinesia[24,25,32,34,36,39]

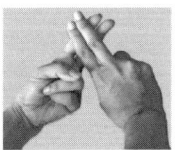

At what age can you ask the pediatric patient to do this for a meaningful interpretation? The patient is asked to flex his or her elbow to a right angle then alternately supinate and pronate the forearm. In the normal state of health, this can be done very quickly; however, in dysdiadochokinesia, there is difficulty in performing this action. How a child reaches for and manipulates toys can check for coordination. Rapid tapping of the foot can assess for dysdiadochokinesia.

Romberg's Test[24,25,32,34,36,39]

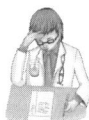

"I need to link to the developmental age before I sensibly do and interpret this. One must not cause undue anxiety to the parents by doing it without age relation."

Romberg's test is a test to assess the loss of position sense in the legs. The patient is asked to stand with feet close together. If he or she is able to do this then he or she is asked to close his or her eyes. In the event that the Romberg's test is positive, as soon as the eyes are closed the patient sways or falls. When asking an unsteady child to close his/her eyes, one must stand behind him/her to prevent from falling. The Romberg's sign is positive in sensory ataxia.

Sensation[24,25,32,34,36,39]

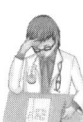

"Sensory testing is difficult in the young child. Hence, I must observe and infer sensibly based on the things that he or she can do according to the age."

Objective testing is difficult in the younger child. Good coordination of the hands and feet require normal sensation. In the older child, a cotton wool can be used to lightly touch the area to be tested.

Forms of sensation that are assessed in the older child[24,25,32,34,36,39]
Awareness of touch
Position sense
Recognition of the size, shape, weight and form of objects
Vibration sense
Pain
Temperature

Sensory[24,25,32,34,36,39]
- Pinprick, light touch, position, and vibration sense.
- Object discrimination, which tests for higher cortical functions, can be done using coins, paper clips, or rubber bands.

Cranial Nerves[4-7,18,24-27,30,32,34,36,39]

Cranial nerve examination, examination of craniospinal tracts and somatosensory tracts can localize lesions in the brainstem.

The cranial nerves are tested for their normal function. Their function also gives an idea of the function of the midbrain, (as in cranial nerves 3 and 4), the pons (as in cranial nerves 5,6,7,8) and the medulla (as in cranial nerves 9,10,11,12). Only the fourth cranial nerve fibers decussate before leaving the midbrain.

In the older child, as in the adult, formal testing of the cranial nerves is done as instructions that are given, can be followed by the older child. However, in the young child and infant, close observation and innovation are both used in conducting and interpreting the examination of the cranial nerves as shown below.

The Cranial Nerves—their Functions and Procedure for Testing in Young Children and in Older Children[4-7,18,24-27,30,32,33,36,39]

The cranial nerves—their functions and procedure for testing[18,24,25,32,34,36,39]			
Cranial nerve testing in infants and young children[18] (please also cross refer cranial nerve testing in the older child)			
Cranial nerve	*Function*	*Test*	*Difficulties that one has to overcome*
I – Olfactory nerve The olfactory nerves go through the cribriform plate and enter the olfactory bulb connected to the olfactory area of the cerebral cortex		Not routinely tested in children	
II – Optic nerve The nerves take origin from the ganglionic layer of the retina, forming the optic chiasma, the optic tracts and the optic radiation. They terminate in the visual cortex of the cerebral hemisphere	Visual acuity Get the young infant or the young child to fix on a bright object Visual field Show a toy at the periphery of the visual field **standing at arm's distance** and notice if the child sights the toy Examination of the fundi is done by appreciating the optic disc, the macula and the retina.	Optokinetic nystagmus give some indication that cortical vision, visual fields and function of the frontal and parietal lobes are normal. Optokinetic nystagmus can be elicited starting at 4 to 6 months of age This test is done by moving a strip of cloth with black and white squares in front of the eyes. The eyes will follow a moving object up to a point and then quickly move back to fixate on a new object.	Since infants are unable to fix their gaze, this test is difficult to do

One has to wait with the ophthalmoscope, appreciate the red reflex and obtain quick glances of the optic disc |
| **III, IV, VI – Oculomotor, trochlear, abducens** Cranial nerve III and IV must be tested for their function; additionally they also offer a view of the midbrain Cranial nerve VI must be tested for function and its testing also offers a view of the pons | These nerves are responsible for normal extraocular movements of the eye. | Capture the infant's interest and make him or her follow a bright object moving in various directions including lateral, medial, up and down and closely simulate the H points. Intently observe the movements of the eyes | Inference mainly made by observation |

Contd...

Contd...

Cranial nerve	Function	Test	Difficulties that one has to overcome
Cranial nerves III, IV and VI work together for conjugate eye movements. The medial longitudinal fasciculus (MLF) is the prime central connection for cranial nerve III, IV and VI. It connects the vestibular nuclei and cranial nerve III, IV and VI. It also connects the vestibular nuclei with the cervical motor neurons on the same side. Cranial nerve III–Supplies the levator palpebrae superioris, superior rectus, medial rectus, inferior rectus and inferior oblique muscles			
The parasympathetic fibers supply the constrictor pupillae of the iris and the ciliary muscles		Shine a torch into the eye. Pupillary constriction is by the parasympathetic fibers of the IIIrd nerve	Ensure that the child is comfortably seated on the mother's lap or close to her
The superior oblique muscle is supplied by the trochlear nerve		The downward and inward motion of the eye is by this nerve	Ensure the child is comfortably seated on the mother's lap or that the mother is closeby
The abducent nerve (CN VI) is purely motor and supplies the retractor bulbi and lateral rectus muscle		Abduction of the eye is by this nerve	A happy child with the parents nearby or helping with the toy that is used to test eye movements, ensures maximum cooperation
V—Trigeminal Cranial nerve V must be tested. Lesions of the pons may also affect its function.	Involved in sensory supply to the face and motor supply to the muscles of mastication The masseter, the temporalis, the medial pterygoid and the lateral pterygoid are the muscles of mastication	The ability of the young child to bite a wooden spatula and resist your attempts at removing it, implies that the power is intact in the muscles supplied by the 5th nerve	
The mandibular division of the trigeminal nerve supplies the muscles of mastication and the tensor tympani and veli palatini		To check for sensation in the older child, touch the forehead, cheek and chin with a cotton wisp while the child indicates if he or she feels it	
VII—The facial nerve has three components namely the motor, sensory and parasympathetic fibers. The facial nerve supplies the muscles of facial expression. The anterior two third of the tongue and palate are supplied by the sensory fibers of the facial nerve. The tear gland, mandibular and sublingual salivary glands are supplied by the parasympathetic component	The upper part of the face including the forehead is innervated bilaterally, sparing the upper part of the face in UMN involvement—link this to your knowledge of neuroanatomy	Astute observation is crucial here. Check for the symmetry of the nasolabial folds, downward deviation of the corner of the mouth, and drooling of saliva Assessment of the motor nerve is done by making the child smile The entire ipsilateral side of the face is affected in lower motor neuron lesions (LMNL) In upper motor neuron lesions (UMNL), there is facial weakness but the movement of the eyelid, eyebrow and forehead are spared due to bilateral innervation	Make the child laugh and observe the nasolabial folds, make the child look up to a bright light or an interesting toy so that you can observe the forehead creases. In a crying child, observe the deviation of the angle of the mouth

Contd...

Contd...

Cranial nerve	Function	Test	Difficulties that one has to overcome
VIII—This nerve has two distinct functions. The vestibular part of the vestibulocochlear nerve is involved in eye and body position, adaptation with respect to head movement and the cochlear component is involved in hearing	It has two parts and is responsible for transmitting sound and information on equilibrium from the inner ear to the brain Noting the eye movements after turning the infant several times in a clockwise and counterclockwise direction can check vestibular function	Hearing is tested in the developmental assessment by a rattle or the distraction test. The test is done based on the knowledge that the young child at this developmental stage will turn to and locate a sound of interest presented at ear level outside the visual field. Any facial expression that indicates that the child has heard the sound must also be recognized by the occupier	Must be done in a quiet room (refer below)
IX, X—Glossopharyngeal and Vagus Both cranial nerves share sensory and motor nuclei. Glossopharyngeal nerve innervates palatine and pharyngeal structures, posterior 1/3rd of tongue and pharyngeal mucosa. The parotid and zygomatic salivary gland is innervated by the parasympathetic components of both the nerves. The parasympathetic branch goes to the mucous glands of the larynx, pharynx, thorax, organs in the neck, and abdomen. The nerve supplies the laryngeal and pharyngeal skeletal muscles. The sensory component of the external auditory meatus and tympanic membrane is supplied by the vagus. Information from the thoracic and abdominal viscera, aortic body and aortic arch is sent through the vagus. The vagus nerve transmits taste from the mouth and the larynx	The glossopharyngeal nerve (CNIX) provides sensory supply to the palate The vagus nerve (CNX) provides motor supply to the pharynx	Observing the ability to suck and swallow tells you about the 9th and 10th cranial nerve. The gag reflex tests parts of IX and X where IX is the afferent sensory limb to the posterior aspect of the pharynx and the X controls the muscles of the pharynx and elevation of the palate	Inference mainly made by observation
XI—Accessory This nerve supplies the sternocleidomastoid and trapezius	Allows movement of the sternocleidomastoid and trapezius muscles. Turning the head to look for the sound of the rattle, gives you information regarding the 8th and 11th nerve	The shrugging of shoulder or turning of the head to the direction of the toy or a familiar face gives some information on the 11th nerve	Inference by observation
XII—Hypoglossal gives branches to intrinsic and extrinsic muscles of the tongue and the geniohyoideus.	The movement of the tongue reveals information on the 12th nerve	Fasciculation of the tongue while resting in the mouth and unilateral atrophy of the tongue and deviation to the affected side gives information on the 12th nerve	Inference mainly made by observation

Cranial nerve testing in older children[4-7,18,24-27,30,32,34,36,39]

Cranial assessment in older children is carried out as summarized below:

Cranial nerve anatomy	Link anatomical knowledge with test of function
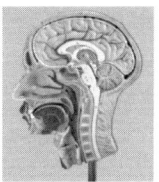	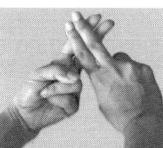
I–Olfactory nerve Olfaction is a sensory input, which does not go through the thalamus. It has direct access to the cerebral cortex. The olfactory tracts project to the uncus of the temporal lobes	• Tests smell (not routinely tested and of limited value) • Assess using aromas of coffee or peppermint • Hyposmia or reduction of the sense of smell, anosmia or loss of the sense of smell, parosmia or the altered perception of odors that are pleasant to become unpleasant and olfactory hallucinations are abnormalities involving this nerve or its pathways. ENT problems and head injuries can cause such alterations in smell. Olfactory hallucinations may occur in focal temporal lobe seizures
II—Optic nerve The visual pathway involves 3 neurons: • Consists of the bipolar and retinal ganglion cells • The lateral geniculate nucleus lies in the diencephalon • The optic radiation is an extension of axons. The visual pathway consists of the retina, optic chiasm, optic tracts, lateral geniculate bodies, optic radiations and visual cortex 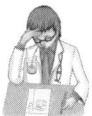 *The unique pathway of the optic nerve is useful in localizing lesions because of its "X" shaped course from the eye to the occipital cortex.*	• **Visual acuity**—the Snellen chart is used to assess visual acuity which should be tested both with and without wearing spectacles or contact lenses • **Color**—the Ishihara plates are used to test color vision in an older child. This test identifies patients who are color blind • **Fields**—request the patient to look directly at you. Then wiggle one of your fingers in each of the four quadrants. Ask the patient to identify which finger is moving. The pattern of a visual field deficit indicates if the anatomical lesion is pre- or postchiasmal at optic tract, optic radiation or calcarine cortex. Visual inattention can be assessed by moving both fingers at the same time and checking whether the patient identifies this • **Pupillary light reflex**—the patient stares into the distance as the examiner shines the penlight obliquely into each pupil, looking for pupillary constriction. The neural pathway of the light reflex involves the optic chiasm, optic tracts and its fibers that travel into the superior colliculus. These fibers terminate in the parasympathetic nucleus of the Edinger-Westphal. The efferent fibers end in the ciliary ganglion which via the short ciliary nerves supply the iris sphincter. **Direct response**—pupillary constriction is seen in the eye where the light is shone **Consensual response**—pupillary response is seen in the opposite eye **The swinging flashlight test:** Swing the light between the two pupils. Direct and consensual responses are seen by shining the torch in one eye. As you shine the light from one eye to another, there is a moment of pupil dilatation in both eyes. Think of the possible physical links if the light reflex is abnormal and conduct a focused physical examination. The anatomical pathway of this reflex involves the optic afferent and the efferent is the parasympathetic fibers in the oculomotor nerve. Hence remember that the light reflex can be normal in cortical blindness, as the reflex does not involve the visual cortex. Hence, in visual blindness, pupillary light reflex is affected but in cortical blindness it is not. Cortical blindness occurs in perinatal ischemic injury to the brain, meningitis, encephalitis and congenital lesions of the brain
	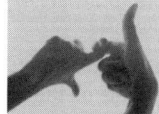 When cranial nerve examination is abnormal, link with your knowledge of the anatomical site of the nerve pathway and its nucleus **Funduscopy**—check both fundi. In raised intracranial pressure, papilledema is usually seen in children with closed cranial sutures and fontanels

Contd...

Contd...

III, IV, VI—Oculomotor, trochlear, abducens • The abducens (VI nerve) has the longest intracranial tract and is responsible for "false localizing signs" of the abducen 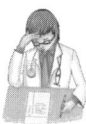 *The trochlear supplies the superior oblique muscle, which is important in looking down and in or towards the midline. This downward movement of the globe when the eye is adducted as when one climbs down stairs is of practical importance and can affect daily living activities* • The abducens supplies the lateral rectus which abducts the eye	These nerves control the six extraocular muscles controlling movements of the eye, and also affect pupillary size. The IIIrd nerve innervates the superior, medial and inferior recti and the levator palpebrae superioris. The superior rectus and inferior oblique move the globe of the eye upwards, the inferior rectus moves it downward, and the medial rectus moves it medially. The sphincter muscles of the iris is innervated by parasympathetic fibers of the Edinger-Westphal nucleus causing constriction of the pupil. The ciliary muscle which is responsible for changes in the lens for near vision is supplied by parasympathetic fibers by way of the ciliary nerves. • Inspect for ptosis, eye position and nystagmus • Note shape and asymmetry of the pupils (PERRLA – an abbreviation that refers to pupils' equal, round and reactive to light and accommodation) • Shine the light from the side to study the pupil's light reaction. • Direct and consensual light reflexes should be assessed. • Assess the afferent pathway by moving the torch in an arc from pupil to pupil. Alternatively, you may ask the cooperative patient to place a hand extending vertically from his face, between his eyes to test one eye at a time. • "Hold your head still and follow my finger with your eyes only." Muscle palsy and nystagmus may be noted
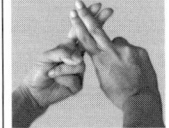	• Accommodation is tested by looking at a distant object. A finger moved centrally towards the nose tests convergence
V – Trigeminal nerve	This nerve gives sensory supply to the face including mouth and part of the dura and motor supply to the muscles of mastication. It is important to test the corneal reflex in appropriate cases as it is innervated by the trigeminal nerve. • Corneal reflex is rarely done in pediatric patients and may find some use in the comatose child. Patient looks up and away. Check that both eyes blink, when you lightly touch the lateral part of the cornea with a small piece of damp cotton wool. CCCC, Compare findings on the other side of the face. • The sensation of the face is tested by lightly touching with a cotton wool on the forehead, cheek and jawline. Feel the temporal, masseter muscles when clenched. Trigeminal neuralgia is sensory affection with severe lancinating pain involving the nerve causing facial numbness and pain. Involvement of the opthalmic division of the trigeminal nerve during the reactivation of herpes zoster is common. The corneal reflex can be lost in lesions of the cavernous sinus with cutaneous sensory loss. Motor affection affecting the muscles of mastication may occur in myasthenia gravis. • Test jaw jerk in an older child. The jaw jerk is brisk in pseudobulbar palsy. The examining finger is gently tapped with a patellar hammer whereby a normal response is slight closing of the mouth. If exaggerated, link to upper motor neuron pathology.
VII—Facial nerve 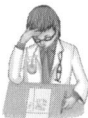 *Observation of the pattern of facial asymmetry in the young infant and older child reveals the type of VIIth nerve involvement. A peripheral VII nerve lesion causes all of the muscles ipsilateral to the affected nerve to be weak whereas with a central VII nerve lesion, only the muscles of the lower part of the face contralateral to the lesion will be weak as the part of the VII nerve nucleus that supplies the upper face receives bilateral corticobulbar or UMN input*	Facial expression, lacrimation, salivation and taste are functions of this nerve. This nerve is motor to the muscles of facial expression. It delivers parasympathetic secretomotor fibers to the lacrimal, submandibular and sublingual salivary gland. It receives taste sensation from the anterior two-thirds of the tongue through the chorda tympani. Assessment of this nerve can be carried out by doing the following: • Inspect both sides of the face for asymmetry. CCCC • The muscles of facial expression are tested clinically by asking the patient to look up and by observing the wrinkles on the forehead. Feel muscle strength by pushing down on each side. In unilateral upper motor neuron lesions, the wrinkles of the forehead are preserved because of bilateral innervations of the forehead. There is marked weakness of the lower facial muscles. The nasolabial folds are flattened and the corner of the mouth droop but eye closure is usually preserved. Bilateral facial palsies are not common but can occur in Guillain-Barre, Lyme disease and HIV infections.[6] • With an intact facial nerve, it would be difficult to open each eye that is tightly shut. If the shut eye can be opened easily, there is weakness of the 7th nerve • CCCC. Compare nasolabial folds on each side when the patient smiles • If the 7th cranial nerve is intact, the patient will be able to perform many actions such as to frown, smile showing teeth and blow out his or her cheeks • The efferent pathway for the corneal reflex is the facial nerve but this reflex is seldom done in a child • Clinical testing of the facial nerve can be picked up by careful observation. It causes facial asymmetry due to unilateral weakness with indistinct facial creases, resulting in typical 'facial drooping'

Contd...

Contd...

	• A typical facial asymmetry is seen in lower motor neuron weakness. In unilateral lower motor neuron weakness, there are no forehead creases and there is widening of the palpebral fissures with incomplete eye closure, Bell's phenomenon, decreased nasolabial creases and retraction of the corners of the mouth. Bell's phenomenon is the presence of superolateral eye deviation when blinking. The observed facial asymmetry is much less obvious in upper motor neuron weakness. In unilateral upper motor neuron lesion, weakness is marked in the lower facial muscles and upper face is spared. This is different from Bell's palsy involving the lower motor neuron where there is weakness of the upper and lower facial muscles. This condition is commonly preceded by mastoid pain. Other causes of lower motor neuron VII nerve paralysis are cerebello-pontine tumors, trauma and parotid tumors[6]
VIII—Vestibulocochlear nerve (auditory or acoustic nerve)	This nerve is the eighth of twelve cranial nerve. It helps in the transmission of sound and equilibrium or balance from the inner ear to the brain. • CCCC. Check the external auditory canals and eardrums • CCCC. Check both ears of the patient • Whisper into the ear or rub two fingers to produce a noise. Do it on both sides • Ask the patient in which ear he or she hears the whisper or the rub Increase the intensity of the sound observing for abnormality **Weber's test: Lateralization** • Use a 512 Hz tuning fork. Place the vibrating 512 Hz fork on top of patients head or forehead • Ask the patient in which ear he or she can appreciate the sound better 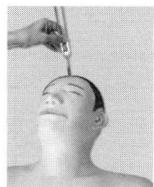 • If hearing is normal, the sound is heard best at the center of the forehead. **Rinne's test: Air vs. Bone Conduction** • Use a 512 Hz tuning fork. Place the vibrating fork on the mastoid process behind each ear. When the patient stops hearing it, ask him or her to tell you so. Then move the tuning fork next to the external auditory meatus • When patient stops hearing it, move the tuning fork to the patient's ear so patient can hear it • Normally air conduction is better than bone conduction • The tuning fork is used in the Weber and Rinne tests 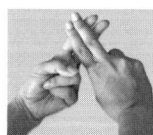 *Link clinical testing of nerve with function.* The vestibular component is clinically tested with the oculocephalic reflex (Doll's eye maneuver) and oculovestibular reflex (ice water caloric test)
IX, X—Glossopharyngeal nerve and vagus • Vagus contains motor, sensory and parasympathetic fibers. The vagus nerve supplies the upper pharyngeal and laryngeal muscles. It courses into the thorax within the carotid sheath and gives origin to the pharyngeal and recurrent laryngeal branches which are motor to the pharyngeal and laryngeal muscles. CNIX has both motor and sensory fibers and autonomic fibers. It is the nerve of ordinary sensation to the mucous membrane of the pharynx, fauces, and palatine tonsil, as well as supplies the sensation of taste from the posterior third of tongue. The sympathetic efferents supply the parotid gland	The Glossopharyngeal nerve (CN IX) provides sensory innervations to the palate; the vagus nerve (CN X) provides motor supply to the pharynx. Damage to the recurrent laryngeal nerve produces a bovine cough and dysphonia while bilateral lesions produce dysphagia and dysarthria 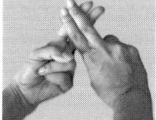 *Link nature of cough to nerve palsy*

Contd...

Contd...

	• The palate is examined for uvular displacement • Ask the older child who can follow instructions to say "Ah"; symmetrical soft palate movement must be noted. Unilateral X nerve damage causes ipsilateral upward movement of the soft palate which makes the uvula deviate away from the side of the lesion when patient says "Ah". **Gag reflex (sensory IX, motor X):** • Gently touch the back of the throat each side (make sure the child has not just had his or her meal). There is gagging each time this is done. This is not usually done in routine testing in children unless it is indicated 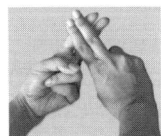 *Link anatomy with localization of signs* • Cranial nerves 9,10,11, and 12 are located in the medulla and have localizing value for lesions in this most caudal part of the brainstem
XI – Accessory nerve There are two parts, one is the cranial part linked closely to the vagus and a spinal part supplying the trapezius and the sternocleidomastoid muscles • This nerve has motor fibers that innervate the trapezius and sternocleidomastoid muscles • There is crossing and then recrossing of the corticobulbar tracts at the high cervical level. Hence, the cerebral hemisphere controls the sternocleidomastoid muscle on the same side 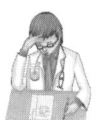 *"So if I want to use the left side of my body I would want to turn my head to the left so the right sternocleidomastoid must be actively used."*	Active shoulder and neck movements will examine both the trapezius and sternomastoid muscles. • Examine the trapezius for atrophy and asymmetry • This nerve is tested by shrugging of the shoulders. The examiner pushes the shoulders down against resistance. If normal, the examiner is unable to do this • In order to examine the nerve to the sternocleidomastoid muscle, ask the patient to turn his or her head to the opposite side against resistance and palpate the muscle. Wasting or weakness of the sternocleidomastoids are seen in conditions such as myopathies, motor neuron disease and myotonic dystrophy 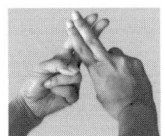 *Link anatomy with clinical test* The cerebral hemisphere controls the sternocleidomastoid muscle on the same side
XII – Hypoglossal nerve • Both hypoglossal nuclei innervate each genioglossus muscle • Bulbar palsy is lower motor neuron lesions involving CN IX, X, XI, XII. In upper motor neuron lesions involving the tracts, IX, X, XI, XII as well as V, VII are affected and is termed pseudobalbar palsy	The muscles of the tongue and its movements are supplied and controlled by the hypoglossal nerve. • Listen to the way the patient pronounces the words. Articulation can be affected by lesions of this nerve. • Unilateral lower motor neuron lesions cause wasting of the tongue on the affected side and deviation to that side when the tongue is protruded. Bilateral lower motor neuron lesions cause wasting of the tongue and fasciculations. Fasciculations are best seen when the tongue is in the mouth. Bilateral upper motor neuron lesions cause a spastic tongue with inability to move the tongue from side to side.

Developmental Assessment[24,25,32,34,36,39]

This is an area that can be tested with the neurological assessment. If developmental assessment is the focus of the examination, carry out this assessment before the physical examination in order to obtain maximum cooperation from the child. The four broad areas that are assessed include:

a. Movement and posture—the development and progress of locomotion (Gross motor).
b. Vision and manipulation—the advancement and maturity of eye-hand control (Fine motor).
c. Hearing and speech—the development and maturation of language skills (Hearing and Speech).
d. Personal and social behavior—the union of acquired skills to reflect a general understanding of the environment (Social).

Observation[24,25,32,34,36,39]

Observe everything that the child performs spontaneously. Sharp observation can be most informative about this assessment. Obtain as much cooperation as possible from the child.

Utilize your own toys and cubes to complete the assessment. The developmental assessment in a sick child is not a true picture of the milestones achieved. Normal developmental milestones include the following:[24,25,32,34,36,39]

Normal developmental milestones[24,25,32,34,36,39]	
At 6 weeks	Has a social smile. On ventral suspension, the head is held up briefly level with body. Tracks past the midline
At 3 months	The child holds a rattle placed in the hand and turns head to sound level with ear When pulled to sit from supine, there is no head lag
At 4 months	• Lifts up on hands • Rolls from front to back • Reaches the object of interest • Laughs and squeals
At 6 months	He or she is able to transfer objects from one hand to the other and sits with hands forward for support
At 10 months	• He or she uses the index finger approach to point at objects • Able to oppose finger and thumb and waves bye • Able to pull himself or herself up to stand • Gets into sitting position
At 13 months	• He or she walks with support and can say single words • Puts a block in a cup
At 15 months	• Scribbles • Stacks 2 blocks • Uses spoon and fork • Says 3–6 words • Follows commands

Contd...

Contd...	
At 18 months	• Runs, kicks a ball • Stacks 4 blocks • He or she tells mother that he or she wants to go to the potty and joins 2 or 3 words together to make a sentence
At 2 years	• Walks up and down stairs • He or she is mainly dry by day and can build a tower of 6 or 7 cubes • Points to pictures and knows body parts
At 3 years	He or she is mainly dry by night, dresses and undresses himself or herself
At 4 years	• Balances on each foot • Hops on one foot • Copies a circle • Dresses without help • Names colors • Understands adjectives
At 5 years	Heel-to-toe walks. Copies a square. Counts. Understands opposites
At 6 years	• Balances on one foot for about 6 seconds. Copies a triangle. • Draws a person with 6 parts • Defines words • Begins to understand right from left

Simple bedside test for hearing[24,25,32,34,36,39]	
	Age 6–18 months

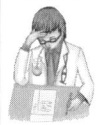
So the occupier should be sensitive to the child's needs and must be observant of the child's change in behavior to the sound stimulus and must decide whether the response was due to hearing, i.e. a response to the sound
	The distraction test[13]
	• The distraction test is best performed in a room that is of appropriate size and must be internally and externally quiet. All toys, pictures and bright, shiny objects should be covered or removed.
	• Both the testers must fulfill the following conditions:
	  – They must be appropriately trained
	  – They must be physically able to do the test
	  – They must be able to hear test stimuli
	  – They must not have a lisp or voice abnormality.
	• The occupier captures the child's attention by a fascinating toy or a bright object. The second tester, the distractor, makes a sound at a level horizontal with the baby's ear at a distance of one meter and at an angle of 45 degrees. The baby does not see it as it is outside the baby's field of vision.
	• The conditions of the test must be appropriate otherwise interpretation will not be meaningful. The baby must not be given olfactory, visual, or tactile clues. The sounds should have two high frequencies and one low frequency. A high frequency rattle and human voice are used as sound stimuli. The test is used for screening and for diagnosis.
	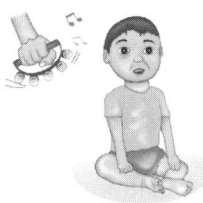
	The infant should sit by himself or on the mother's lap when performing the distraction test.

Pediatric Physical Examination

Reflections upon obtaining a positive distraction test[24,25,32,34,36,39]

- Ask yourself what a positive distraction test means.
- Ask yourself what you are testing and why the infant fails to respond. Were you doing it in a quiet room and was it conducted correctly? Think about the reliability of your technique
- Think about the history and the physical examination
- Think about all that you know about hearing problems in children.
- Ask yourself if there are any clues in the clinical history that you could link to the subsequent physical examination.
- Subsequently, conduct a focused physical examination to determine the anatomical site of the abnormality and the possible etiology.
- Then link the symptoms and facts (both positive and negative) in the history and the signs (both positive and negative) in the physical examination.

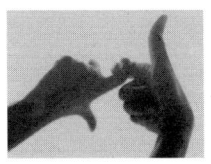 +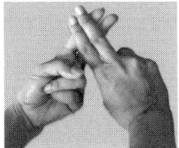

- Arrive at a differential diagnosis of the child's problem.

Suspected developmental delay: Physical links[24,25,32,34,36,39]

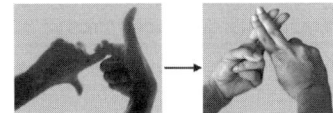

The history and its links lead you to a focused examination and the important links to seek in a case of developmental delay
- Physical examination signs (physical links) that you would search for in a child with possible developmental delay or signs that would alert you to a differential diagnosis of developmental delay.
- Measure and plot growth in gender and age appropriate charts. Some syndromes have their own charts too.

Growth[24,25,32,34,36]
Short stature is seen in:
- Williams syndrome
- Malnutrition

Obesity is seen in
- Prader–Willi syndrome
- Sotos syndrome
- Bardet Biedl syndrome
- Cohen syndrome
- Alström syndorme
- Carpenter syndrome
- Rubinstein-Taybi syndrome

Macrosomia

Congenital cardiac problems

Neonatal jaundice

Scoliosis

Renal anomalies

Macrodolichocephaly
Receding hairline
Apparent hypertelorism
Downward slanting eyes
Large ears, anteverted nostrils

Pointed chin
Large head and feet

Seizures

Hypotonia

Sotos syndrome: Large stature and developmental delay

Contd...

Contd...

Skin[24,25,32,34,36,39]
- Eczema
- Café au lait spots
- Hemangioma
- Telangiectasia
- Hypopigmented macules
- Adenoma sebaceum

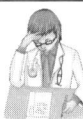

Can you link other skin manifestations that could be present in a child with developmental delay?

Hair[24,25,32,34,36,39]
- Hirsutism
- Confluence of both eyebrows (that meet in midline)

Extremities[24,25,32,34,36,39]
- Hands, feet
- Fingers— polydactyly, syndactyly, clinodactyly
- Simian crease
- Single transverse palmar crease more common in Down syndrome. When else can a single transverse crease be found?
- Sandal gap deformity between first and second toe, abnormal dermatoglyphics

Head and Face[24,25,32,34,36,39]
- Microcephaly and macrocephaly
- Abnormal shape of face or unusual facial shape
- Hypotelorism, hypertelorism, short palpebral fissures
- Coarse facies

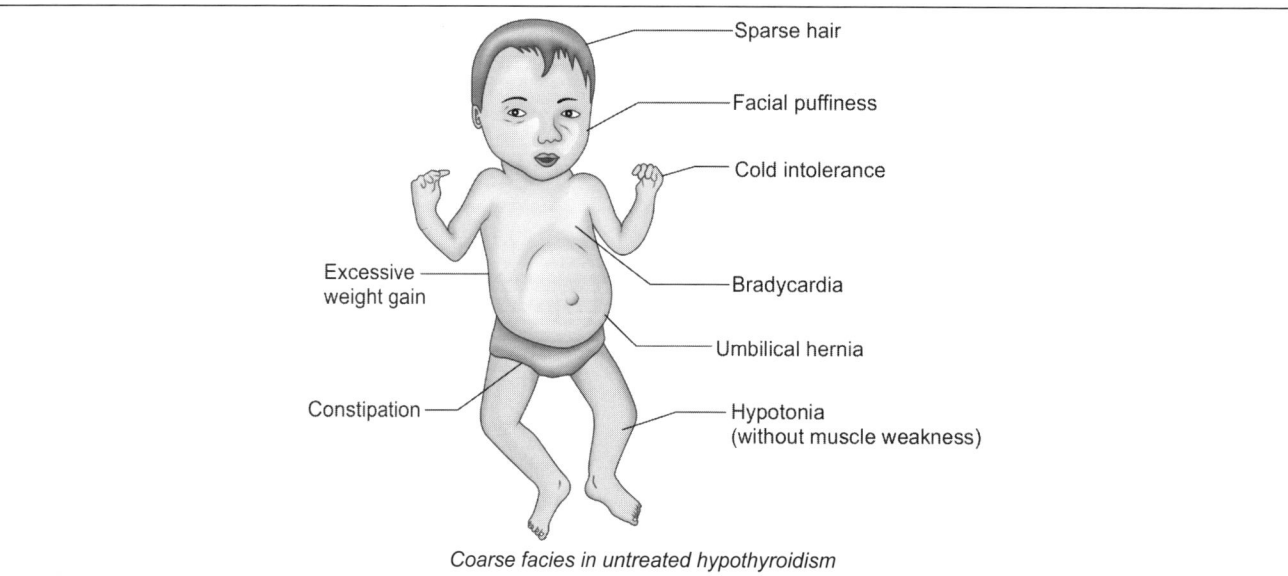

Coarse facies in untreated hypothyroidism

- Dysmorphism[24,25,32,34,36,39]

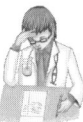

So the causes of developmental delay can be approached by looking for signs of dysmorphisms. Dysmorphisms can also be associated with developmental delay.

Contd...

Contd...

Eyes[24,25,32,34,36,39] • Cataracts • Cherry-red spots • Corneal cloudiness • Chorioretinitis • Blindness • Nystagmus
Ears[24,25,32,34,36,39] 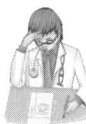 *What other systems are linked to anomalies of the ear?*
• Low set ears • Absence of pinnae • Malformed pinnae • Deafness
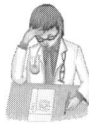 *Is deafness a cause or an effect of developmental delay? What are the causes? What are the effects of deafness to a young child? What other aspects of development will be affected? What are the historical and physical links?*
Heart[24,25,32,34,36,39] • Cyanosis • Structural problems murmurs and abnormal heart sounds • Hypertrophy
Liver[24,25,32,34,36,39] • Hepatomegaly
Genitalia[24,25,32,34,36,39] • Hypogenitalism • Macroorchidism
Neurologic[24,25,32,34,36,39] • Hypotonia 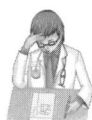 *What are the causes of hypotonia? How would you approach it in a patient? What are the links? The differentiation of central and peripheral hypotonia is clinically useful. Central causes have global developmental delay and dysmorphic features. A complete history is very important.* • Hypertonia • Asymmetry of strength • Asymmetry of tone • Ataxia.

> **POINTS TO REMEMBER**
> - Retention of primitive reflexes (*Primitive reflexes-described in Chapter 12*) beyond the normal age at which they are supposed to disappear is abnormal
> - Primitive reflexes represent spinal reflexes until the infant becomes older and higher cortical functions suppress them
> - Persistence beyond the expected normal age especially when involving more than one primitive reflex, failure to develop normal postural responses or asymmetry of the infantile reflexes are signs indicative of abnormal neuromuscular development
> - The special senses of hearing and vision, which are vital for development, must be examined first, as problems involving these senses will also result in associated developmental delay

MUSCULOSKELETAL SYSTEM[24,25,32,34,36,39]

General Observation must be done as mentioned earlier[24,25,32,34,36,39]

Specific Observation is Important[24,25,32,34,36,39]

This examination may be done together with the neurodevelopmental assessment. Human locomotion is a complex process. The attainment of normal gait in humans is complex, and involves physical maturation as well as conscious learning. It requires an intact musculoskeletal system as well as an intact neurological system. Assessment by inspection is of utmost importance. Correlate with the history, compare both limbs on examination, capture the diagnosis and confirm your findings with special examinations or necessary investigations.

Correlate, Compare, Capture and Confirm your findings CCCC[24,25,32,34,36,39]

Systemic features such as fever, rash and so on, that could link to musculoskeletal pathology must be looked for and could be relevant.

Inspection[24,25,32,34,36,39]

- Note the general appearance and whether there are any bandages, splints or tractions.
- Is there a Plaster of Paris (POP)? Any crutches or presence of a wheelchair?
- Any obvious deformities like kyphosis, scoliosis or contractures?
- Is there an obvious posture due to pain? A painful joint is often held in midflexion to minimize tension on the joint capsule
- Remember the existence of referred pain; hence, pain at distant sites may be relevant and could well link to the pathology at the joint.
- Pain in the knee may be referred from the hip joint and pain in the hip may be referred from the lower back.

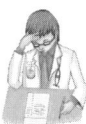

"I now remember that referred pain occurs in musculoskeletal diseases, ENT problems, gastrointestinal diseases and in some cardiovascular problems. Are there any other areas that I am missing? Why does it occur?"

- Look for deformity of a joint with associated wasting of the muscles due to disuse atrophy. Remember that growth and pubertal status are important to assess and if delayed it gives an indication of chronic disease. Systemic features like fever, salmon pink rash, psoriatic rash or vasculitic rashes must be looked for. Nail pitting, hepatosplenomegaly and lymphadenopathy must be checked. Uveitis, loss of vision and blindness are other signs that could be related to specific musculoskeletal diseases.

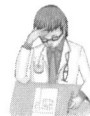

Remember to exclude simple causes of gait abnormalities like tight fitting shoes, paronychia or painful warts. These can be more quickly attended to and can get the patient back to normal activities of daily living

Limping Child[24,25,32,34,36,39]

A limp may be due to pain of the hip, knee or ankle. Toddlers will generally walk independently by 18 months; their **broad-based gait** does not have an associated arm swing. It takes several years for a mature gait pattern to evolve. Features of a mature gait pattern are a narrow base of support, smooth movements with minimal oscillations of the center of gravity and reciprocal arm swing.

Accurate description of the type of gait that a patient has, for clarity and useful clinical communication is essential. However, names of some specific gaits are well known. An **antalgic gait** is a gait caused by a limp due to pain. The Trendelenburg gait is due to weakness of the gluteus medius. It is characterized by the dropping of the pelvis on the unaffected side of the body at the moment of heel strike on the affected side. The pelvic drop lasts until heel strike on the unaffected side and is associated with an apparent lateral protrusion of the affected hip. There is shortening of the step on the unaffected side and a lateral deviation of the trunk associated with excessive swaying of the trunk.

The **waddling gait** refers to bilateral decrease in function of the gluteus muscle. Toe walking is a common complaint in early walkers. Any child who toe walks after the age of three years should be evaluated.

Muscular dystrophy is a differential diagnosis to exclude in an unusually clumsy 3- or 4-year-old boy particularly when hypertrophy of the calf muscles are seen.

In persistent toe walking beyond two years, you must exclude some conditions such as:
- Neuromuscular disorder
- Leg length discrepancy
- Achilles tendon contracture.

Normal developmental variations in the curvature of the child's legs[1,11,15,21,24,25,32,34,36,39]

Genu varum or bowlegs and medial tibial torsion are normal in newborn and infants. Maximal varus is present at 6 to 12 months of age. With normal growth, the lower limbs gradually straighten by 18 to 24 months of age when the infant begins to stand and walk.

Following this, knees gradually drift into valgus or knock knee position. This valgus deformity is maximal at around 3-4 years of age. Genu valgum spontaneously corrects by the age of 7 years to that of the adult alignment of the lower limbs. There is slightly greater valgus in the female than the male. The greater degree of valgus in females is due to their wider pelvis.

It must be understood that physiologic genu varum improves with growth, whereas pathologic genu varum increases with skeletal growth.

The indicators of a benign disorder of the bones are symmetrical bone deformities, the absence of symptoms of joint stiffness or systemic disorders or the association of syndromes. When deformities are asymmetrical and associated with pain, joint stiffness, systemic disorders or syndromes and more sinister underlying causes must be excluded.

Bowlegs after 2 years of age are considered abnormal. A pathologic condition or a growth disorder must be excluded by careful history and physical examination.

Genu valgum up to 7 years of age is physiologic. Above this age, it is pathological.

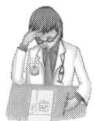

As often encountered in pediatrics, age related variations and physiological changes must be known and excluded first.

Compare both limbs. Children with asymmetrical genu valgum may have underlying diseases such as skeletal dysplasia or renal osteodystrophy.

Colors of the limbs	
Inflamed joints	Erythematous, painful, warm, swollen with limited range of movement
Vasculitis	Peripheral cyanosis with delayed capillary refill due to compromised circulation gives the limbs a dusky appearance and they are cold to touch

Disuse from pain may result in secondary stiffness, contractures, weakness and atrophy. Swelling of the joints due to effusion or synovial thickening is painful on movement. Examine the back from behind. The position of the pelvis must be assessed.

CCCC Gently expose both limbs. Compare both limbs first by meticulous inspection. Ascertain if pathology is unilateral or bilateral.

Compare both legs for difference in length. Measure both legs from similar points of measurement. Leg length difference produces pelvic obliquity resulting in compensatory scoliosis. When the pelvis is leveled, the spine is examined for symmetry and spinal curvature with the patient standing. In older children, ask them to stand straight, and then ask them to touch the toes. Inspect for asymmetry in the spine. The presence of a hump in this position is diagnostic of scoliosis. With the older child still bending forward, an angulation in the thoracolumbar area indicates a kyphotic deformity.

Palpation of the Limb[24,25,32,34,36,39]

Always enquire about pain before touching a limb. Do not begin examination at the point of pain.

Observe for any mass or abnormality; if present describe the mass or abnormal lesion. Compare the warmth over a painful joint and a normal one. Elicit tenderness, fluctuation, or effusion.

Movement[24,25,32,34,36,39]

Perform active movement before passive movement so as not to hurt the child. Inspect movements of the limb in older children.

Remember, benign nocturnal limb pains of childhood or growing pains is a benign musculoskeletal pain syndrome that occurs in some school aged children. It is diagnosed by a typical history and a normal physical examination.

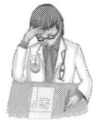

Benign nocturnal limb pain is a diagnosis of exclusion. A complete history and physical examination must be done first.

When moving the limbs, gently flex and extend at the joints. Joint hypermobility is suspected when the physical examination demonstrates exaggerated mobility at a joint. Here the range of motion may be exaggerated with excessive flexion or extension at the metacarpophalangeal joints, wrists, elbows or knees.

In a child with suspected juvenile arthritis, look for evidence of synovitis or arthritis. Exclude secondary causes for limb symptoms like infection, malignancy and reactive arthritis. You must also try to assess the subtype of arthritis, its severity and complications.

Decide whether the joint movement is limited by:
- Pain
- Contracture
- Neurological spasticity.

Examination of the spine.
Inspection (see section on inspection of the spine and back in this chapter and Chapter 12).

Scoliosis[24,25,32,34,36,39]

Stand behind the child if at an age where he or she can follow instructions, ask him or her to touch the toes.
A **postural scoliosis** will disappear on bending down to touch the toes.
A **structural scoliosis** will persist with a gibbus deformity, which is a hump due to increased convexity of the underlying ribs.

EAR, NOSE AND THROAT (ENT) EXAMINATION[24,25,32,34,36,39]

- General observation is done as already mentioned
- Specific observation is important and relevant

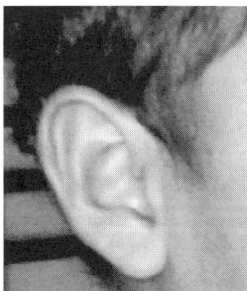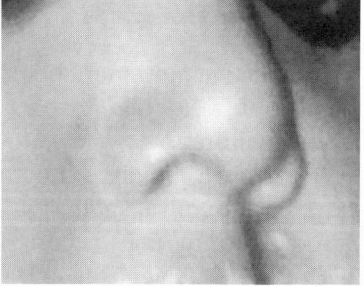

ENT examination is most unpleasant to the young child. Keep it to the last.

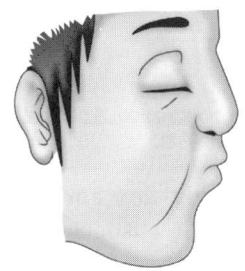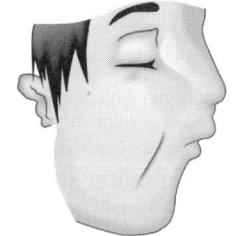

Normal pinna   Deformed abnormality of the pinna

Earlier on observation, you would have observed for abnormalities of the external ear.

- The ear, nose and throat are very commonly involved in childhood diseases, primarily, or as part of another disease.
- For a child, the most unpleasant examinations are those of the ear, nose and throat and these should be left until last.
- During examination of the nose, condensation on a surface like a mirror, under the nostrils, reflects patency of the nasal airways.
- The mucous membrane of the anterior nares can be inspected.
- Together with the suggestive history, pale, swollen inferior turbinates are characteristic of allergic rhinitis. Comment on the presence of nasal discharge; if present, note the color and nature.
- Inspect the pinna, then the mastoid area for swelling or redness. Then examine the external auditory meati and tympanic membranes. The differential diagnosis of obvious congenital anomalies here include microtia or small deformed pinna and complete atresia of the external canal, accessory auricles and preauricular sinuses.
- Discharge from the ear or otorrhea must be noted. Causes of ear discharge include otitis externa or otitis media.
- In otitis externa, there is local irritation, pain and tenderness on moving the pinna which usually has a bacterial etiology. It may be occasionally fungal. Remember that this could also be related to skin diseases, such as seborrheic dermatitis, contact eczema or psoriasis.

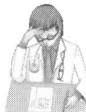

Observation of the ear discharge must not be forgotten. The color, the odor and the nature of the discharge are included in observation. Following that, a microscopic examination or a gram stain of the discharge clinches the exact etiology

- The nature of the discharge gives etiological clues. In acute suppurative otitis media, the otorrhea is mucoid or purulent. In chronic otitis media, the discharge has a foul odor.
- Furunculosis is very painful and may lead to cellulitis or pre or postauricular lymphadenitis. The red tender swelling can mimic mastoiditis which is associated with redness and pitting edema over the mastoid and marked tenderness on palpation.

Perichondritis is a very painful complication of local infection or trauma.

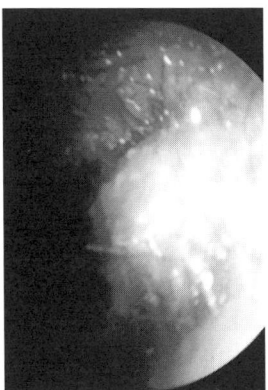

Furunculosis of the left ear (seen through an auroscope) (reprint with permission from Dr Raj Kumar, FRCS, MS)

Methods of Examination of the Ear in Resisting Children[24,25,32,34,36,39]

- Examination with an auroscope is an important part of the pediatric examination.
- The child will be put to ease if allowed to handle your instruments. To examine the ears of an infant, it is usually necessary to involve the mother who will gently restrain the child. Pull the auricle backward and downward; in the older child, the external ear is pulled backward and upward.
- Let the child sit on the mother's lap with the head resting on her chest facing to the side, and get her to hold the child firmly so that no sudden movement of the child occurs.

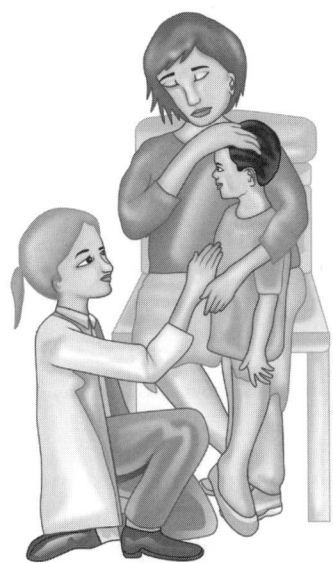

Mother stabilizes the child's ears by holding the head against her shoulder.

- Gently inspect the eardrums with the child held still.
- Remember in examining the ear, ask the mother to help with holding the child still and place one finger on the head to prevent injury resulting from sudden movement by the child. Use as large a speculum as possible. The speculum of the auroscope is inserted gently and not too deep, to avoid discomfort and to avoid pushing wax in front of the speculum so that it obscures the field. Foreign bodies inserted into the ear may be visualized, such as plasticine or beads.

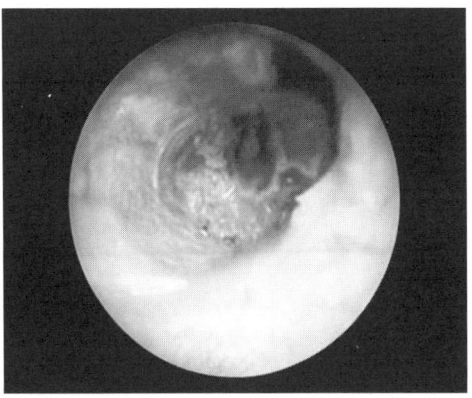

A view through the auroscope – plasticine in the ear of a child (reprint with kind permission of Dr Raj Kumar FRCS, MS)

Low-set Ears[24,25,32,34,36,39]

Definition

The ears are low-set if they are below a line drawn from the outer canthus of the eye to the external occipital protuberance. This condition is seen in a number of congenital syndromes, including several that are associated with mental retardation. Congenital anomalies of the urinary tract are frequently associated with abnormalities of the pinna.

Mouth and Throat[24,25,32,34,36,39]

Minimize the use of a spatula. Most children dread it. The uncooperative or very young child must be held by the mother as the child sits facing the examiner.

Buccal Mucosa[24,25,32,34,36,39]

The use of a spatula may sometimes be necessary and unavoidable to look at the throat. Place it as gently as possible between the teeth and onto the tongue, which is then depressed. Note the state of the teeth, the tongue, and the mucous membrane of the mouth. Look for Koplik spots which are seen in the catarrhal stage of measles and are small white spots with a red halo opposite the buccal mucosa adjacent to the lower first and second molar teeth. Detection of Koplik spots before the period of maximum infectivity is a useful control measure of the disease. Note the pharyngeal vesicles of varicella zoster. Note the milky white spots of oral thrush. Inspect the tonsils and pharynx for ulcers, erythema and vesicles. Accessory or aberrant salivary tissue can be seen in the mouth, the hard palate being the most common site. Petechiae on the palate are commonly seen in infectious mononucleosis in the older child, but can also be seen in any form of thrombocytopenia, in rubella and in streptococcal tonsillitis. Scrutinize the tonsils and the pharynx. Look for streaks of mucoid or purulent exudate on the posterior pharyngeal wall (post-nasal drip). This is sometimes clearly seen when the bigger child says 'ah'.

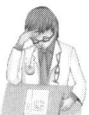

A post-nasal drip is a cause of nocturnal cough. What are the other causes? What are the historical and physical links in such a finding? Linkage and analysis are important in a focused clinical diagnosis.

Enlarged tonsils are covered with confluent white exudates in glandular fever with edema of the fauces and soft palate and erythema of the oropharynx. Adenotonsillar hypertrophy is associated with:
- Serous otitis media
- Open mouth position
- Feeding difficulties
- Failure to thrive
- An unusual nasal or hyponasal speech
- Daytime sleepiness
- Occasionally behavioral disturbances
- Sleep apnea.

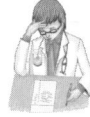

The general observation will reveal a very toxic child with high grade fever, chills and rigors in streptococcal pharyngitis, a peritonsillar abscess or, even more rarely, a retropharyngeal abscess. What important childhood conditions would need to be excluded in a child who presents with pallor and a retropharyngeal abscess?

In streptococcal pharyngitis, there are yellow punctate follicular exudates. White greenish colored membranous exudates are seen in diphtheria, now rare as diphtheria is an important disease prevented by immunization.

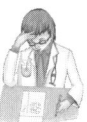

Can a nonimmunized child get diphtheria today? Has widespread immunization against this disease protected all children? What is herd immunity?

In varicella zoster, oral lesions appear prior to the rash. In herpangina due to coxsackie virus, vesicular or ulcerative lesions may be seen in the oropharynx, soft palate and uvula. Uncommonly, a peritonsillar abscess or quinsy may be seen. A retropharyngeal abscess forms a smooth, tense, tender swelling which is from the posterior wall of the oropharynx. Retract the cheek with a spatula and note the opening of the parotid duct which is a tiny swelling opposite the second molar tooth.

SKIN[24,25,32,34,36,39]

General observation is important and has been covered.[24,25,32,34,36,39]

Specific observation will give you more specific clues to the underlying condition.[24,25,32,34,36,39]

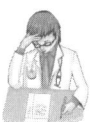

"In the specific observation I must observe the skin, the nails, the hair, the mouth and all mucous membranes, the palms and the soles."

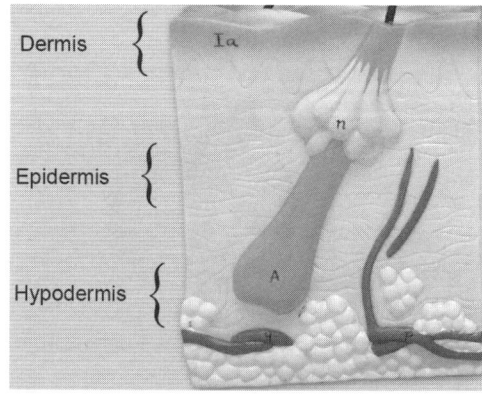

Skin model showing epidermis, dermis, and hypodermis

Examination of the skin must include inspection of the mucous membranes as well as the hair, nails and teeth. The description of a skin lesion must include the site, size, color, the shape and feel of the lesion. Stand a little away from the child and observe all these features. Most of all do not forget to note the distribution of the rash as an important diagnostic clue. The symmetry of a widely distributed rash is also important to observe.

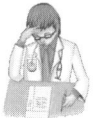

"In atopic eczema, lesions are distributed in infants on the cheeks, face and extensor surfaces of the limbs, knees and elbows. In older children flexural distribution predominates. In pityriasis rosea, a common condition in children the distribution of the rash is in a 'Christmas tree' pattern at the back of the body. In the pruritic rash of Sarcoptes scabiei, interdigital areas are involved in the older child. I realize that distribution is a vital observational link."

Remember that the skin also expresses manifestations of systemic diseases, the rashes of childhood infectious diseases and atopy. The skin therefore not only suffers from disease, but also tells the tale of internal disease.

Lesions on the skin[24,25,32,34,36,39]

Appreciate the following:
• A macule is flush with the skin
• A papule is raised above the surrounding skin
• A nodule is elevated to 1 cm
• A patch is a macule more than 1 cm
• An erythema is a patch of redness caused by capillary dilatation or hyperemia
• A plaque is a large solid elevated skin lesion
• A lichenified skin lesion is thickened
• An icthyotic lesion is dry and scaling
• Blisters, vesicles and bullae are fluid filled of different sizes
• Pigmentary changes—a hypopigmented lesion is lighter than the skin around it and a hyperpigmented lesion is darker than the surrounding skin
• Hemorrhagic skin lesions occur with anomalies of the vessel wall, thrombocytes and clotting factors. The skin may also manifest scratch marks of localized or generalized pruritus
• An ephemeral lesion with a raised center of pallor and redness in the periphery is a wheal that is typical of urticaria
• A scar is a patch of skin that has lost its normal surface anatomy
• Denudation of the epidermis results in atrophic changes
• A crust is a scab containing dried blood or transudation from the skin
• A scale is desquamation of keratin in the epidermis
• An erosion results from loss of top skin layers whereas an ulcer is discontinuity of skin or membrane
• A fissure is a groove or furrow on the skin

Morphology and pattern of rashes (Link to diagnosis)[24,25,32,34,36,39]
Annular—erythema marginatum, granuloma annulare or tinea corporis
Grouped lesions—vesicles of herpes simplex, dermatitis herpetiformis and herpes zoster
Linear—incontinent pigmenti or lichen striatus
Vesicular—varicella and herpes zoster
Dermatomal—herpes zoster (shingles) or epidermal nevus
Maculopapular—measles, rubella, toxic shock syndrome, roseola, parvovirus B19 infection and drug eruptions
Target lesions—erythema multiforme
Erythema marginatum—an area of redness surrounded by raised edges in rheumatic fever

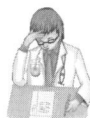

"Skin texture, moisture and turgor are what I will appreciate when I start palpation of the skin."

Palpation of the Skin[24,25,32,34,36,39]

Feel the texture of the skin and appreciate if it is rough, thin or thick.

Moisture[24,25,32,34,36,39]

Appreciate if it is dry or moist. If moist, see if it is generalized or localized.

Turgor[24,25,32,34,36,39]

- Healthy skin when pinched will immediately flatten but in dehydration it remains pinched or tented.
- One may also feel for pitting edema or the crepitus of subcutaneous emphysema.

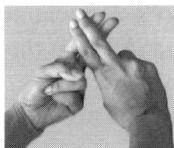

Visual Links to Abnormalities of the Nail[24,25,32,34,36,39]

- Separation of nails in onycholysis in fungal infections
- Beau's lines which is a transverse line tallying with arrested nail growth in severe illness
- Paronychia
- Pitted nails in psoriasis
- Koilonychias or spoon-shaped nails in chronic iron deficiency
- Leukonychia or diffusely white nails in hypoalbuminemia seen in nephrotic syndrome and liver diseases

- Deformed nails in epidermolysis bullosa
- Absent nails in ectodermal dysplasia
- Splinter hemorrhages in bacterial endocarditis.

Hair[24,25,32,34,36,39]

Ring worm infection of the scalp causes round bald areas covered with broken hair. Head lice or pediculosis capitis can be a cause of cervical and suboccipital lymphadenopathy.

Itchy Rashes[24,25,32,34,36,39]

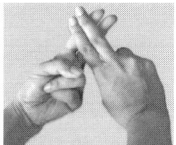

Visual links that tell you that a skin lesion is pruritic are the following:
- The presence of excoriation and lichenification
- Koebner phenomenon where lesions spread in a linear manner by autoinoculation by self-scratching
- When an older infant is still wearing mittens.

The **palms and soles** must be examined when examining the skin as certain lesions affect the palms and soles while others spare the palms and soles.

The palms and soles may be involved in the following:
- Vesicles in infections like hand-foot-mouth disease due to coxsackie A infections
- Erythema multiforme or Stevens Johnson syndrome
- Desquamation in the convalescent phase of Kawasaki disease
- Separation of the epidermis is Nikolsky's sign which is seen in Staphylococcal Scalded Skin (SSS) in the newborn due to staphylococcal exotoxin
- Eczema especially pompholyx where bullae are seen
- Pustular psoriasis
- Contact eczema.

Lesions that spare the palms and soles[24,25,32,34,36,39]

- Dermoid cysts
- Sebaceous cysts
- Benign nevus
- Lipomas.

Measles[24,25,32,34,36,39]

Look for the generalized erythematous maculopapules on the face, neck and upper trunk tending to be confluent and the staining and desquamation of the skin in the child with measles. Look for Koplik spots that are diagnostic but short lived. If vaccination has been given, the milder form is termed modified measles.

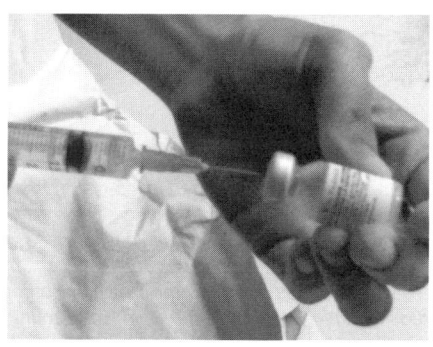

Measles is a dangerous disease in malnourished children. A vaccinated child is protected against measles. However vaccinated children may still sometimes get a milder form of measles and this form is termed as modified measles.

Scarlet Fever or Scarlatina[24,25,32,34,36,39]

Notice the red facial flush and circumoral pallor. The child may also have tiny punctate macules and papules on the limbs and trunk that start peeling after a week. Examine the tongue for its strawberry red color. Think also of other causes of similar appearances of the tongue.

Rubella[24,25,32,34,36,39]

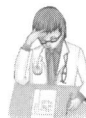

In clinical medicine, there are typical links that tie a specific rash to a related finding. This clinches the diagnosis. Suboccipital lymphadenopathy and rubella are examples of such a link.

Observe the discrete, pink maculopapules on the face, trunk and limbs in rubella. Check also for suboccipital lymphadenopathy and retroauricular lympadenopathy.

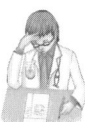

"I must not forget the sociodemographic impact of the influence of diseases. A febrile child who is also flushed, in the tropics, must make me link to all the other signs of dengue fever. The vital signs like the pulse rate and blood pressure are important".

Dengue Fever[24,25,32,34,36,39]

A febrile child may present with a flushed face and body. Look carefully for petechial hemorrhages.

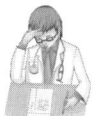

The lesions in chickenpox are polymorphous, some crust and dry while new vesicles emerge.

Varicella Zoster Rash[24,25,32,34,36,39]

Varicella zoster involves the trunk, limbs, scalp and mucous membranes. These vesicles appear in crops with different morphology and are pruritic.

Herpes Zoster[24,25,32,34,36,39]

In herpes zoster lesions occur as grouped vesicles along the lines of sensory nerves. They are painful and are described as a burning sensation over the area. The pain can precede the visible lesions.

Enteroviruses and Enteric Cytopathic Human Orphan (ECHO) Viruses[24,25,32,34,36,39]

Discrete, pink macules and papules that are nonpruritic are associated with these infections.

Hand-Foot-Mouth Disease[24,25,32,34,36,39]

These lesions have a predilection for the palms, soles, buttocks, nappy area and palate. The lesions in hand–foot–mouth disease and are painful. The palatal lesions, if significant, interfere with feeding due to pain.

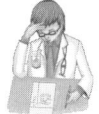

Where painful oral lesions occur, the feeding history is a factor in deciding on further management. This is especially so in a young infant with an infection such as hand-foot-mouth disease.

Molluscum Contagiosum[24,25,32,34,36,39]

These are umbilicated lesions on an erythematous base. They are painless, small, grayish-white tear drop lesions and are distributed, through autoinoculation, anywhere in the body.

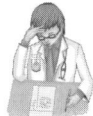

Autoinoculation can seed vital areas of the body with such infective lesions; hence, advise to the young child and parents is important. "Don't touch the lesions and scratch your eye with the same fingers" could be a useful practical advice.

Kawasaki Disease[24,25,32,34,36,39]

The skin manifestations in Kawasaki disease depends on the stage of presentation. The palms and soles become red and edematous, there are erythematous maculopapular eruptions on the trunk and limbs. Desquamation of the skin occurs later on in the disease.

Skin manifestations of childhood atopy include the following:[24,25,32,34,36,39]
• Atopic dermatitis or eczema
• Allergic contact dermatitis
• Urticaria
• Xerosis or dry skin
• Pruritus
• Hyperlinearity of the palms and soles
• White dermographism
• Pityriasis alba

As bronchial asthma is a disease with atopic etiology, one of the physical links outside the respiratory system is the skin.

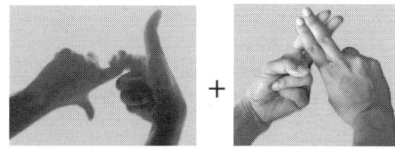

Use your knowledge of the historical links on skin manifestations of childhood atopy to look for all the mentioned physical signs in a child with bronchial asthma. The presence or absence of those signs must be mentioned as they are both significant. Remember the pertinent negatives in both the history and physical examination, they contribute in making the diagnosis.

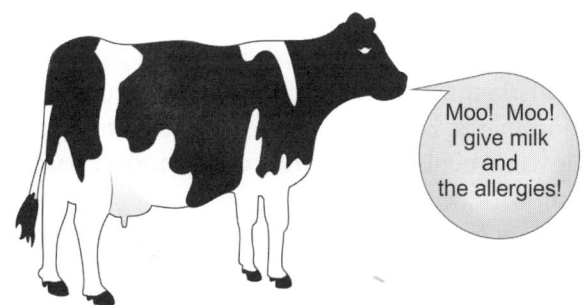

Skin manifestations of cow's milk protein allergy (CMPA)[17,19,24,25,32,34-39]	
IgE mediated cutaneous reaction	Immediate onset reactions which are acute urticaria, or angioedema potentially leading to anaphylaxis or contact urticaria
Late onset reactions	Atopic dermatitis
Non IgE mediated reactions (probably T-cell mediated)	Chronic, recurrent pruritic cutaneous inflammation
High levels of cow's milk - specific IgE	Early onset and greater severity of eczema

Skin manifestations of childhood inflammatory disorders[24,25,32,34,36,39]

In seborrheic dermatitis, you will notice soft, gray, yellow scales. Areas that are affected are the diaper area, the trunk, thighs and intertriginous areas of the groin and axilla, scalp (cradle cap), face, eyebrows, cheeks and back of ears. On the trunk, scaly lesions may be annular in shape.

The physical link helps in searching for other related signs.

Yellowish gray scales are seen in the scalp of an infant. You must examine other areas also known to be involved. Hence, do not leave the groin, neck, axilla and back of the ears unexamined. The area behind the ears can be missed if not meticulously examined. Excoriated skin can be a source of infection and must be attended appropriately.

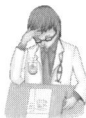

Age influences so many things in pediatrics. The pattern of distribution of the lesions in atopic eczema can also be influenced by age.

In atopic eczema, clinical features depend on the age of the child. It is a disease characterized by exacerbations and remissions. Morphologically, annular, red and scaly lesions occur in infants on the cheeks, face and extensor surfaces of the limbs, knees and elbows. It may involve the trunk but the napkin area is usually spared. A few infants may exhibit round patches in a discoid manner. In older children, flexural involvement predominates. Lesions may be excoriated and crusted, while wet, weeping lesions indicate secondary bacterial infection.

In toddlers with **xerosis leading to pruritus,** the areas commonly affected are the flexures. Areas involved are mainly the elbow, wrist, popliteal fossa, groin as well as the face especially the perioral and periorbital area and the neck.

Napkin dermatitis involves areas like the buttocks. The intertriginous areas are generally spared; this contrasts to the other disorders. Skin folds are spared in simple napkin dermatitis.

In **fungal infections,** look for the typical appearance and satellite lesions; confirm moniliasis by doing a fungal scrap.

Bacterial skin infections are common in children[24,25,32,34,36,39]

Below is a summary of the various types of bacterial skin infections:

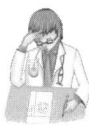

Description of skin lesions is an art that can be learnt. It gives clues to the diagnosis.

Disease[24,25,32,34,36,39]	Description[24,25,32,34,36,39]
Carbuncle	A few furuncles (abscesses from hair follicles) coalesce, linked by sinus tracts
Erysipelas	An angry red, painful infection of superficial skin with sharply demarcated borders
Impetigo	Large vesicles with crusted lesions. Link to the characteristics of the lesions: golden, brown, honey colored and crusted lesions are typical of impetigo
Cellulitis	Painful, erythematous infection of the deep skin with poorly defined edges
Folliculitis	Papular or pustular inflammation of the hair follicles
Furuncle	Painful, firm or fluctuant abscess from a hair follicle

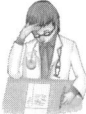

"In the neonate, vesicular and bullous lesions can be extensive, life-threatening and associated with other abnormalities (e.g. abnormalities of nails and teeth). Some lesions are acquired while others are inherited. Although it is difficult to memorize them all, I think that the antenatal history, the birth history for risk of infections, the neonatal history of illnesses and hospitalization, the social history of contact and the family history of skin diseases must be taken well… as these are links to the etiology and diagnosis."

Vesicular and bullous lesions in the neonate[24,25,32,34,36,39]

- Bullous impetigo due to staphylococcal skin infections and not the exotoxin as in Staphylococcal Scalded Skin Syndrome
- Herpes simplex

- Epidermolysis bullosa is autosomally inherited with nail changes
- In incontinentia pigmenti, look for hyperpigmented lesions and dental abnormalities.

Documentation of the physical findings[24,25,32,34,36,39]

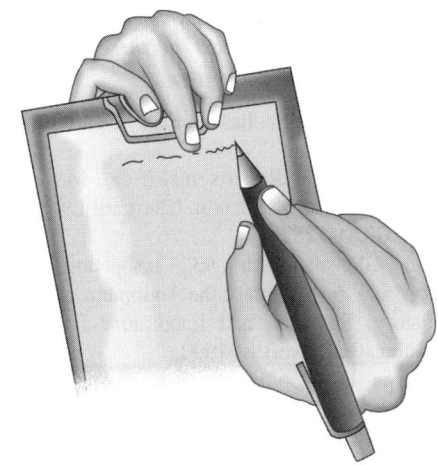

Documentation of the date, time, and the physical findings are important.

The importance of accurate and clear documentation of the physical examination must be inculcated from the beginning of your career. It is important for many reasons. Patients' records are vital to keep when you practice clinical medicine. These records are completely private and confidential. Clearly and legibly document the physical findings. Document the date and time of the examination. Document all aspects of the examination under the specific systems. Include all temporal details of the examination in your notes. Document your clinical impression of the problem(s) based on the history and physical examination. After completion of the history and physical examination, your differential diagnosis now becomes more certain. This is the provisional diagnosis and may be your definitive diagnosis if investigations are not required. A good history and physical examination can do away with unnecessary investigation.

REFERENCES

1. Arazi M, Oğün TC, Memik R. Normal development of the tibiofemoral angle in children: a clinical study of 590 normal subjects from 3 to 17 years of age. J Pediatr Orthop. 2001;21:264-7.
2. Adkins III, David W. Hannon, Murmurs in Pediatric Patients: When Do You Refer? Am Fam Physician. 1999; 60(2):558-64.
3. Baujat G, Cormier-Daire V. Sotos syndrome. Orphanet J Rare Dis. 2007;2:36.
4. Brillman J, Kahan S. In: A Page Neurology. Blackwell Publishing.2005.
5. Cranial nerve: Anatomy and function. University of Georgia's Interactive Cranial Nerve Anatomy and Function website. Available at http://vmerc.uga.edu/CranialNerves/index.html. Accessed in December 2013.
6. Douglas G, Nicol F, Robertson C (Eds). Macleod's Clinical Examination Graham (13th Ed.) Churchill Livingstone, 2013. ISBN 9780702047282
7. Devlin A. Pediatric neurological examination. Advances in Psychiatric Treatment. 2003;9:125-34.
8. D'Alessandro DM, D'Alessandro MP (Curators). What causes different types of cries? A Pediatric Digital Library and Learning Collaboratory. Available at http://www.pediatriceducation.org. Accessed in January 2015.
9. Difference between Kwashiorkor and Marasmus. Available at http://www.difference between.net/science/health/difference-between-kwashiorkor-and-marasmus. Accessed in Jan 2015.
10. Behrman RE (comps), Kliegman RM, Nelson WE, Vaughan VC III (Eds). Nelson's Textbook of Pediatrics, 14th edn. Philadelphia: WB Saunders, 1992.
11. Espandar R, Mortazavi SMJ, Baghdadi T. Angular Deformities of the Lower Limb in Children. Asian J Sports Med. 2010 Mar;1(1):46-53.
12. Ferguson CM. Chapter 93: Inspection, Auscultation, Palpation, and Percussion of the Abdomen. Clinical Methods: The History, Physical, and Laboratory Examinations (3rd ed.). Boston: Butterworths; 1990.
13. Glasgow M. Distraction test. Available at http://www.batod.org.uk/content/resources/audiology/refreshers/testing/T3-distraction.pdf. Accessed in February 2015.
14. Goldenberg D, Goldstein BJ. Section 6: Pediatric Otolaryngology. Handbook of Otolaryngology: Head and Neck Surgery. Thieme Medical Publishers, Inc 2011.
15. Gray CS. Children & Chiropractic Care. Why do children need Chiropractic care? Available at http://www.grayfamilychiropractic.com. Accessed in December 2013.
16. Growth & Development: WHO working group on Infant Growth. Available at http://www.breastfeedingbasics.org/cgi-bin/deliver.cgi/content/Growth/gro05_research_who_workgroup.html. Accessed in April 2013
17. Guidelines for the management of cow's milk protein allergy in children 2012 (CMPA in children). Available at http://www.allergymsai.org/file_dir/6296706325048109343baa.pdf. Accessed in April 2015.
18. Hills W. Pediatric and Infant Neurologic Examination. Available at http://www.ohsu.edu/xd/health/services/doern-becher/research-education/education/med-education/upload/ped-neuro-exam-edit-05-8-13.
19. Koletzko S, Niggemann B, Arato A, et al. Diagnostic approach and management of cow's milk protein allergy in infants and children: ESPGHAN GI Committee practical guidelines. J Pediatr Gastroenterol Nutr. 2012;55(2):221-9.
20. KV Krishna Das, Thomas M (Eds). New Delhi: Clinical Medicine (A textbook of Clinical Methods and Laboratory Investigations). Jaypee Brothers Medical Publishers (P) Ltd; 2007.

21. Keen M. Early Development and Attainment of Normal Mature Gait. Available at http://www.oandp.org/jpo/library/1993_02_035.asp. Accessed in Jan 2015.
22. L Tewfik TL, Yoskovitch A. Congenital malformations of the Neck. Available at http://emedicine.medscape.com. Accessed in December 2013.
23. MJ Robinson, Lee EL. Pediatric problems in tropical countries. Pelanduk Publications (M) Sdn Bhd.1994.
24. Mason S, Swash M. Hutchinson's Clinical Methods (17th ed). Cassell Ltd. 1980.
25. Marcdante K, Kliegman RM, Jenson HB, Behrman RE (eds). Nelson's Essentials of Pediatrics (6th ed). Saunders Elsevier, 2010.
26. Nervous: Cranial Nerves Exam. Available at http://www.clinicalexam.com/pda/n_cranial_nerves_exam.htm
27. Neurological examination. Available at library.med.utah.edu/neurologicexam/html/cranialnerve_anatomy.html. Accessed February 2015.
28. Normal growth of young children. Available at http://pediatrics.about.com. Accessed in April 2013.
29. Normal breath sounds. Available at http://www.rnceus.com/resp/respnorm.html. Accessed in Jan 2015.
30. Neurological examination. Available at http://library.med.utah.edu/neurologicexam/html/coordination_anatomy.html. Accessed February 2015.
31. Pediatric Clerkship. The University of Chicago. Diaper rash. Available at https://pedclerk.bsd.uchicago.edu/page/diaper-rash. Accessed in Jan 2015.
32. Talley NJ, O'Connor S. Clinical examination: A systematic guide to physical diagnosis. India: Reed Elsevier India (P) Ltd. 2010.
33. Sasidharan P. An approach to diagnosis and management of cyanosis and tachypnea in term infants. Pediatr Clin North Am. 2004;Aug:51(4):999-1021, ix.
34. Stephenson T, Wallace H. Clinical Pediatrics for postgraduate examinations; ELSEVIER Churchill Livingstone. 1991.
35. Spergel JM. Nonimmunoglobulin: E–Mediated Immune Reactions to Foods. Allergy, Asthma & Clinical Immunology. 2006;2:78-85
36. Snell RS. Clinical Anatomy: An illustrated review with questions and explanations. Wolters Kluwer Health. Lippincott Williams & Wilkins. 2008.
37. Walker HK. Chapter 65 Cranial Nerve XII: The Hypoglossal Nerve. Clinical Methods: The History, Physical, and Laboratory Examinations. (3rd ed). Boston: Butterworths; 1990.
38. World Health Organization charts for Weight-for-age charts and Length-for-age charts (- z-scores: girls for Birth to 6 months, - z-scores: boys for Birth to 6 months, - z-scores: girls for Birth to 6 months and - z-scores: boys for Birth to 6 months). Available at http://www.who.int/childgrowth/standards/cht.
39. Milner AD, Hull D. Hospital Pediatrics. 3rd edn. ELBS with Churchill Livingstone. 1998.
40. Habib Ur Rehman, Methemoglobinemia. West J Med. 2001 Sep; 175(3):193-196.
41. Weighing a child using a taring scale. Available at http://www.who.int/childgrowth/training/jobaid_weighing_measuring.pdf. Accessed in Dec 2014.

The essence of the relevant chapters in the following books have also been numbered as references in this chapter. We recommend for further reading, the rich text in these books for greater integration and deeper understanding.

1. Brillman J, Kahan S. In: A Page Neurology. Blackwell Publishing. 2005.
2. Douglas G, Nicol F, Robertson C (Eds). Macleod's Clinical Examination Graham, 13th edn. Churchill Livingstone, 2013. ISBN 9780702047282
3. Ferguson CM. Chapter 93, Inspection, Auscultation, Palpation, and Percussion of the Abdomen. Clinical Methods: The History, Physical, and Laboratory Examinations, 3rd edn. Boston: Butterworths. 1990.
4. Goldenberg D, Goldstein BJ. Section 6: Pediatric Otolaryngology. Handbook of Otolaryngology: Head and Neck Surgery. Thieme Medical Publishers, Inc. 2011.
5. KV Krishna Das, Thomas M (Eds). New Delhi: Clinical Medicine (A textbook of Clinical Methods and Laboratory Investigations). Jaypee Brothers Medical Publishers (P) Ltd. 2007.
6. Marcdante K, Kliegman RM, Jenson HB, Behrman RE (eds). Nelson's Essentials of Pediatrics, 6th edn. Saunders Elsevier. 2010.
7. Mason S, Swash M. Hutchinson's Clinical Methods, 17th edn. Cassell Ltd. 1980.
8. Milner AD, Hull D. Hospital Pediatrics. 3rd edn. ELBS with Churchill Livingstone. 1998.
9. Robinson MJ, Lee EL. Pediatric problems in tropical countries. Pelanduk Publications (M) Sdn Bhd. 1994.
10. Behrman RE (comps), Kliegman RM, Nelson WE, Vaughan VC III (Eds). Nelson's Textbook of Pediatrics, 14th edn. Philadelphia: WB Saunders; 1992.
11. Snell RS. Clinical Anatomy: An illustrated review with questions and explanations. Wolters Kluwer Health. Lippincott Williams & Wilkins. 2008.
12. Stephenson T, Wallace H. Clinical Pediatrics for postgraduate examinations; ELSEVIER Churchill Livingstone. 1991.
13. Talley NJ, O'Connor S. Clinical examination: A systematic guide to physical diagnosis. India: Reed Elsevier India (P) Ltd. 2010.
14. Walker HK. Chapter 65, Cranial Nerve XII: The Hypoglossal Nerve. Clinical Methods: The History, Physical, and Laboratory Examinations, 3rd edn. Boston: Butterworths. 1990.

Chapter 11

Layout of a Complete Pediatric Physical Examination

Gather all the positive and negative physical findings and present them in a systematic manner. Remember that the pediatric physical examination must adapt and accommodate to the level of cooperation, mood and the general will of the pediatric patient. Various methods have been mentioned in this book as examination techniques that we may use in the young patient. The important factor throughout the physical examination is to keep the child at ease and as comfortable as possible.

Having done all that we can do to keep our young patient happy, the findings both positive and negative must be analyzed. The analysis is made easier by the clinical links already mentioned.

No matter how we adapt ourselves to the examination technique and accommodate our examination to keep the young patient comfortable, the presentation of the physical examination must be systematic and complete just like in the adult physical examination. This must be borne in mind at all times.

A young child will hardly cooperate and so it is best to let them be on their own while you observe from afar.

Ensure that the child is comfortable, be it on the parent's lap or the examination couch.

You may not be able to undress the child and examine in a sequential manner as in the adult physical examination. Therefore, it is always advisable to complete the examination in whichever manner that is comfortable to the child.

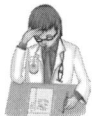

"In the physical examination, I must systematically analyze the positive and negative signs. The history and physical examination will help make a reasonable provisional diagnosis and then, a definitive diagnosis."

General observation
• **At this point you formulate a few (2–3 differential diagnoses) based on the history and the general observation**
• You are thinking of the general condition of the child, obtaining clues from the surrounding and trying to make an impression about the anatomical site of the disease
Specific observation
• At this point you sharpen your thinking by observation and reinforce your impression of the anatomical site and start to formulate the pathophysiology of the disease
Specific examination
• You examine the most likely system involved first
• **You become certain of the system involved and are fairly sure of the pathology**
• You consider the positive and negative signs in the system directly involved in the disease
• **You strengthen your impression of the system involved and are certain of the pathology**
• You use physical links and examine other relevant systems affected by the disease
• **You now think of etiology and become more focused on pathophysiology**
• Positive and negative signs are reflected upon
• **You strengthen the system involved and are certain of the pathology and are thinking about etiology**
• Positive and negative signs are reflected upon and more possible signs are looked for
• **You strengthen the system involved and are more certain of the pathology and etiology and will eliminate uncertainties**
• Examine all systems thoroughly
• **Analyze**
• Arrive at a provisional diagnosis
• **Analyze**
• Arrive at a definitive diagnosis
• **Analyze**
• Discussion with team
• Decision on important investigations to arrive at the diagnosis or to support the diagnosis
• If clinical history-taking and examination cannot arrive at the definitive diagnosis, investigations are needed
• Investigations may also be required to diagnose and monitor complications of the disease, if any
• Detect and monitor comorbidities, if any

212 *The Link*: Pediatric History-Taking and Physical Examination

The following layout of the pediatric physical examination will help you achieve this objective. Deduce and analyze from your history and continue to think and analyze in the physical examination.

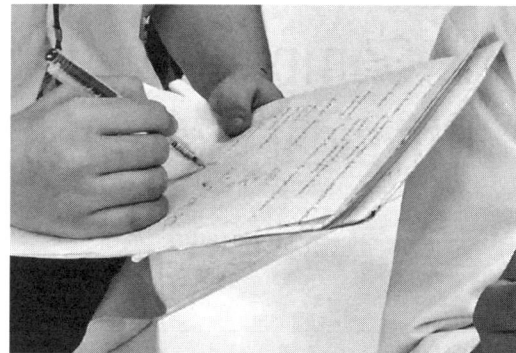

The layout of a complete pediatric physical examination is as follows:

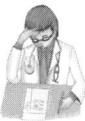

"Now it is time I use my analytical mind."

As the physical examination is done immediately after history-taking:
- Date and time of clerking as written in the layout of the history
- Patient's particulars, i.e. name, gender, address, date of birth and race as written in the layout of the history.

PHYSICAL EXAMINATION[1-8]

General examination

Vital signs

Blood pressure (done at the end of physical examination using appropriate size cuff):

Standing ▢ mmHg; Sitting ▢ mmHg; Lying ▢ mmHg.

Pulse rate (radial pulses e.g. bradycardia) [describe the rhythm, volume and character (e.g. bounding pulses, anacrotic, bisferiens, pulsus paradoxus)]:

Respiration rate: ▢ (with/without recession) If with recession: Subcostal/intercostal/substernal/suprasternal

Temperature: ▢ °C/°F   (Continuous/intermittent/remittent/tertian/quartan/quotidian/others)

Measurements

Height/length (plot growth chart): ▢ m/cm
Weight (may use tared weighing method; plot growth chart): ▢ kg
BMI (plot growth chart): ▢ kg/m^2
Head circumference using occipitofrontal circumference (if below 2 years and plot growth chart): ▢ Note the shape of the head where relevant (brachycephaly, microcephaly)

Arm span (helps diagnose Marfan's/Klinefelter's syndrome):
Mid-arm circumference (measures nutritional status):
Torso ratios (helps check nutritional status):
Chest circumference (level of nipples in mid inspiration):

Layout of a Complete Pediatric Physical Examination

Remember to use the Cardinal Ten (Physical)
1. Alertness (Looking around the room or at the observer, shiny and bright eyes, happily follows instructions).
2. Appearance (looks happy, squealing with excitement, laughing aloud).
3. Appreciation (by sense of smell, sense of hearing and sense of touch).
4. Activity of patient (sitting and moving arms and legs, playing with toys, stacking up building blocks).
5. Adjunct or surroundings.
6. Asymmetry.
7. Color.
8. Posture.
9. Swelling.

If an abnormality is found, define it by using these parameters:
- Site
- Size
- Shape
- Edge
- Tenderness
- Surface
- Contour
- Consistency
- Mobility
- Ability to get above the swelling
- Pulsatility (pulsatile or not)
- Maneuvers to define exact location and nature, e.g. intra- or extra-abdominal, transilluminability
- Comparison with other masses, if present, e.g. on other limb
- Percussion note over the swelling (done over nontender masses to differentiate cystic from solid
- Auscultation
- Observation (Observe parental-child interaction).

Note: General observation: Observation of surroundings/nasal oxygen/nebulizer/IVD/perfusion pump/urine container/stool in container/crutches/wheelchairs

General (circle all the appropriate)
- Well looking (looks happy, squealing with excitement, laughing aloud)/ill-looking/very ill-looking
- Well-nourished/thin/emaciated
- Alertness (looking around the room or at the observer, shiny and bright eyes, happily follows instructions)
- Active/playful/sitting and moving arms and legs/playing with toy/stacking up building blocks/uninterested/quiet
- Lethargic/irritable/dull/difficult to awaken/poor response/delirious/comatose
- Comfortable/uncomfortable
- Slow/not responding to surrounding atmosphere
- In older child: Oriented to place, time and person
- Stature: Appropriate/inappropriate for age (short and fat, thin and tall boy or girl)
- Color of skin/lips/nails
- Odor (If present, describe)
- Photophobic

I/O chart
- Input (oral/parental) ☐
- Output (urine/stool/vomitus) ☐

Facies
- Dysmorphism (If present, describe, e.g. Down, Turner or William syndrome facies)
- Drooling of saliva   Yes/No
- Expression

Mucous membranes
- Lip color: Pink/dusky/pale/striking pallor
- Conjuctiva: Pink/hyperemic/pale/striking pallor
- Under tongue: Cyanosis present/absent
- Other abnormalities:

Skin
- Rashes: Present/absent (If yes, describe):
- Mottling: Present/absent
- Subcutaneous bleeding
- Pitting edema
- Other abnormalities (ichthyosis, bruises, pyoderma, erythema nodosum)

Posture
- Sitting (describe), e.g. head and chin forward
- Standing (describe)
- Other abnormalities

Movements
- Floppy/jerky/stiffness
- Other abnormalities

Cry
- Normal/weak/shrill/husky/stridorous/muted
- Other types

Hydration (circle the appropriate one)
- Alert — Yes/No
- Sunken eyes — Present/Absent
- Tears — Present/Absent
- Dry mouth — Yes/No
- Dry tongue — Yes/No
- Dyspneic — Yes/No
- Skin turgor — Normal/Abnormal
- Excessive thirst — Yes/No
- Respiratory rate — Normal/Increased/Reduced
- Heart rate — Normal/Increased/Reduced
- Restlessness — Yes/No
- Irritability — Yes/No
- Oliguria — Yes/No
- Capillary refill time — Normal/Prolonged
- Anterior fontanel — Normal/Bulging/Sunken
- Coated tongue — Yes/No

Nutrition
Features
- Marasmus — Present/Absent
- Kwashiorkor — Present/Absent
- Vitamin deficiency — Present/Absent
  - Vitamin A deficiency — Night blindness, bitot spots, dry scaly skin
  - Vitamin B complex — Seborrheic dermatitis, cheilosis, glossitis, apathy, drowsiness
  - Vitamin C deficiency — Petechial hemorrhages, sicca syndrome.
  - Vitamin D deficiency — Harrison's grove, bow legs, knock knees.
  - Vitamin K deficiency — Hemorrhages
- Other abnormalities

Head (describe the following)
- Skull (secondaries, histiocytosis)
- Shape (scaphocephaly, oxycephaly)
- Fontanel (closed/open anterior and posterior, depressed or tensed)
- Scalp (swelling: caput, cephalhematoma)
- Other abnormalities

Hair (describe the following)
- Texture (thin, sparse, coarse)
- Pattern (posterior balding, generalized alopecia)
- Hair line
- Other abnormalities and bulging, pulsatile)

Facial appearance (describe where applicable)
- Abnormal facies: Yes/No. If yes, describe (widened facies, Down syndrome facies, cretin, rounded face).
- Eyes (upward slant, epicanthal folds, hypertelorism)
- Ears (low set)
- Nose (depressed nasal bridge)
- Skin (coarse, dry, rough)
- Nails (pale, pigmented, constant nail biting, splinter hemorrhages, koilonychia)
- Mouth (false macroglossia, small mouth)
- Other abnormalities

Oral Cavity and Lips (describe where applicable)
Tongue
- Color (cyanoses/pale/erythematous/yellow discoloration)
- Size (macroglossia, microglossia)
- Moisture
- Papillae
- Fury/Thrush/Ulcers/Coated/Geographical/Forchheimer spots
- Cysts
- Other abnormalities.

Buccal mucosa—normal/abnormal.
Gums—normal/abnormal (Note for any gingivitis, malignat infiltrations).
Teeth—Dental caries in cardiac case.
- Specific anomalies: Trauma/Discoloration/Enamel hypoplasia

Palate, tonsils, fauces and pharynx
- Ulcers
- Erythema
- Vessels
- Rashes
- Pigmentation
- Other abnormalities.

Neck (describe where applicable)
- Position (torticollis, opisthotonos, inability to support head)
- Webbing
- Fistula
- Sinuses
- Cysts (cystic hygroma, ranula, sublingual dermoid cyst, thyroglossal cyst, lipomas)
- Lymph nodes
- Swellings
- Skin laxity
- Thyroid gland (size, contour, briot, nodules, tenderness)
- Tracheal location
- Other abnormalities (hemangioma, vascular/lymphatic malformation, vascular tumors).

Arms (describe where applicable)
- Scars (vaccination scars)
- Muscle wasting
- Edema
- Deformities
- Axillae
- Other abnormalities.

Hands (describe where applicable)
- Capillary refill
- Palms
- Fingertips
- Finger clubbing
- Peripheral perfusion/capillary refill/cyanosis
- Nail changes
- Other abnormalities.

Legs and feet (describe where applicable)
- Edema (ankle edema)
- Foot deformities (see body posture)
- Muscle wasting
- Talipes equinovarus, rocker bottom feet, pes cavus
- Other abnormalities.

Spine and back (describe where applicable)
- Deformities
- Edema
- Other abnormalities.

Genitalia (describe where applicable)
- Confirm gender

Boys
- Testes: Retractability/Undescended/Hydrocele/Labia
- Penis size
- Scrotum
- Other abnormalities

Girls
- Vulva
- Discharge
- Other abnormalities

Anal orifice (describe where applicable)
- Patency
- Fissures
- Sinuses
- Anal tags
- Polyps
- Visible hemorrhoids
- Prolapse
- Other abnormalities

SYSTEMIC EXAMINATION

Compare, Contrast, Capture and Consolidate (CCCC)

A. Thorax

Inspection
- Respiratory rate (tachypnea)
- Chest expansion/recession
- Nasal flaring
- Recessions of chest wall/hyperinflated chest wall
- Wheezing/stridor
- Cough (brasy, dry, whoop)
- Shape (pectus excavatum, pectus carinatum)
- Other abnormalities (How is the child lying down? Harison's sulcus, spinal deformities)

Auscultation
- Breath sounds (reduced/absent/prolonged)
- Adventitious sounds (rhonchi, crackles)
- Added breath sounds
- Other abnormalities

Palpation
- Chest expansion
- Trachea centrality
- Cardiac impulses
- Palpable rhonchi
- Vocal fremitus
- Tactile fremitus
- Other abnormalities

Percussion
(Done above 2 years)
- Appreciate percussion note
- Resonant
- Dull
- Stony dull

B. Abdomen

Inspection
- Movements of all abdominal regions
- Mass/swelling
- Any peristaltic movements
- Umbilicus: Shape/inverted/everted
- Hernia orifices
- Dilated veins

Palpation
- Liver (measure span and note level of upper border
- Kidney: Ballotable/not ballotable
- Spleen

Percussion
- Liver

- Operation scars: Site and size
- Rashes
- Muscle wasting (gluteal region)
- Any pampers around (note the stools)
- Perianal region: Redness/excoriation/fistulae/fissures/prolapse

Auscultation
- Bowel sounds
- Bruits
- Other abnormalities

- Bladder
- Spleen
- Other masses: Solid or cystic

C. Genital Region

Male Inspection

Penis
- Circumcision
- Meatal opening
- Hypospadias/epispadias
- Phimosis
- Adherent foreskin
- Other abnormalities (nappy rash)

Testes

Scrotum
- Hydrocele/translumination test
- Swelling/Hernia

Palpation
- Cremesteric reflex

Female Inspection
- Imperforate hymen
- Discharge
- Adhesion
- Hypertrophy of clitoris
- Other abnormalities

Pubertal changes in genitalia
- Pigmentation of skin/areola/nipples/skin creases/genitalia
- Hair growth over pubic area and axillae
- Other abnormalities

Tanner staging of puberty

Boys—development of external genitalia
Stage 1: Prepubertal stage.
Stage 2: Scrotum and testes enlarge; scrotal skin becomes reddened and rugae are seen.
Stage 3: Penis enlarges in length; testes grows further.
Stage 4: Penis increases in length and breadth; glans develops; testes and scrotum enlarge and scrotal skin darkens.
Stage 5: Genitalia is adult size.

Girls—breast development
Stage 1: Prepubertal stage.
Stage 2: Breast bud seen; papilla elevate areola and areola enlarges.
Stage 3: Breast and areola continue to enlarge; no distinction between both.
Stage 4: A distinction between the areola and breast is seen.
Stage 5: Papilla projections on the areola seen.

Boys and girls—pubic hair
Stage 1: Velus hair seen.
Stage 2: Sparse pigmented curly or straight hair seen at the base of penis or along labia.

Stage 3: Hair become dark and curly and spread over mons pubis.
Stage 4: Adult type hair seen over the mons pubis.
Stage 5: Adult type hair seen with spread over the medial aspects of the thighs.

Rectal examination
- Inspection
- Perianal rash
- Stool
- Perianal skin tags.

D. CARDIOVASCULAR SYSTEM
- Inspection
- Apex beat
- Pulsations over precordium
- Neck pulsations: JVP/Other pulsations
- Scars
- Other abnormalities (xanthomata, child's growth, activity and color, chest recessions)

Palpation
- Apex beat
- Palpable thrills

Auscultation

	Area heard	Grade	Radiation	Maneuvers done
• Murmurs (describe)				
• Added sounds				
• Rhythm of the heart sounds		S1	S2	
• Other abnormalities				

E. CENTRAL NERVOUS SYSTEM

Head
- Fontanels (bulging, sunken)
- Rashes
- Head circumference
- Other abnormalities

Nose
- Rhinorrhea
- Other nasal discharge
- Transverse nasal crease
- Other abnormalities.

Eye
- Epicanthal fold
- Hypertelorism
- Palpable fissure
- Ptosis
- Corneal opacity
- Blue sclerae
- Iris colobomata
- Other abnormalities.

Ear
- Discharge
- Otitis
- Tenderness
- Preauricular sinuses and pits
- Other abnormalities.

Limbs
- Abnormal posture
- Muscle bulk
- Deformities
- Abnormal movements
- Tremors involuntary movements
- Other abnormalities.

Jaw
- Macrognathia/micrognathia
- Other abnormalities.

Gait
- Standing
- Walking
- Jumping
- Other abnormalities.

Muscle tone (hypotonia/hypertonia/ cogwheel rigidity/lead pipe rigidity)

Tongue
- Macroglossia/microglossia
- Other abnormalities.

Muscle power (use standard grading).

Head
- Posture: Torticollis/strabismus/hemianopia
- Neck: Retraction with ached back (tetanus)/nuchal rigidity.

Trunk
- Posture: Scoliosis/kyphosis/lordosis/spinal hemangiocele/spinal bifida
- Others

Limb posture
- Frog leg posture
- Other abnormalities.

Scalp
- Dilated veins
- Other abnormalities.

Eyes
- Down turning eyes/sunset sign
- Cataracts/scleral discoloration/keratitis
- Other abnormalities.

Musculoskeletal system
- Foot deformities
- Spinal deformities
- Gait
- Joint abnormalities
- Other abnormalities.

Skin
- Neurocutaneous stigmata
- Café-au-lait spots
- Neurofibromas
- Adenoma sebaceum
- Facial hemangiomata
- Pigmented macules
- Other abnormalities.

Developmental assessment
Inspection
- Movements and postures
- Vision and manipulation
- Learning and speech
- Personal and social behavior
- Activities of daily living.

F. ENT
Ear
- Pinna
- Mastoid area
- External auditory meatus discharge
- Tympanic membrane.

Reflexes (grade)
- Normal/Abnormal reflexes (brisk, very brisk)
- Presence/absence of clonus.

Cerebellar signs
- Ataxia
- Coordination
- Position sense
- Other abnormalities

Cranial nerves
- Examine cranial nerves 1-12.

Mouth
- Buccal mucosa
- Teeth
- Gums
- Throat/tonsils.

- Other abnormalities.

- Palate
- Fauces
- Pharynx
- Other abnormalities.

Nose
- Deformities
- Discharge
- Septum
- Abnormal growths
- Skin on nose
- Mucous membranes of the anterior nares
- Other abnormalities.

Summary:
- Summarize the physical examination.
- This must be brief and succinct and should contain the main positive findings of the physical examination.
- Important negative signs that are absent and that contribute to the diagnosis must also be mentioned.

Note:
Thank the patient and parents. After completion of the physical examination, summarize your findings, then review the history and physical examination, obtain all the information and deduce a number of differential diagnosis and then make your provisional diagnosis. When this is confirmed by deduction and analysis, make up your mind on the definitive diagnosis.

REFERENCES

1. Goel KM, Gupta DK. Hutchinson's Pediatrics, 1st edn. India: Jaypee Brothers Medical Publishers (P) Ltd. 2009
2. Krishna Das KV, Thomas M (Eds): Clinical Medicine: A Textbook of Clinical Methods and Laboratory Investigations). Jaypee Brothers Medical Publishers (P) Ltd. 2005.
3. Marcdante K, Kliegman RM, Jenson HB, Behrman RE (Eds). Nelson's Essentials of Pediatrics. 6th edn. Saunders Elsevier, 2010.
4. Mason S, Swash M (Eds). Hutchinson's Clinical Methods (17th edn). A Bailllere Tindall book published by Cassell Ltd; 1980.
5. Milner AD, Hull D. Hospital Pediatrics. 3rd edn. ELBS with Churchill Livingstone. 1998.
6. Behrman RE (comps). Kliegman RM, Nelson WE, Vaughan III VC (Eds). Nelson's Textbook of Pediatrics (14th ed). Philadelphia: WB Saunders; 1992.
7. Stephenson T, Wallace H (Eds). Clinical Pediatrics for Postgraduate Examinations. UK: Churchill Livingstone; 1991.
8. Douglas G, Nicol F, Robertson (Eds). Macleod's Clinical Examination Graham (13th ed). Churchill Livingstone 2013.

The essence of the relevant chapters in the following books have also been numbered as references in this chapter. We recommend for further reading, the rich text in these books for greater integration and deeper understanding.

1. Douglas G, Nicol F, Robertson (Eds). Macleod's clinical examination Graham, 13th edn. Churchill Livingstone 2013.
2. Goel KM, Gupta DK. Hutchinson's Pediatrics, 1st edn. Jaypee Brothers Medical Publishers (P) Ltd, India. 2009.
3. Krishna Das KV (Eds), Thomas M. Clinical Medicine: A Textbook of Clinical Methods and Laboratory Investigations). Jaypee Brothers Medical Publishers (P) Ltd 2005.
4. Marcdante K, Kliegman RM, Jenson HB, Behrman RE (Eds). Nelson's Essentials of Pediatrics. 6th edn. Saunders Elsevier, 2010.
5. Mason S, Swash M (Eds). Hutchinson's Clinical Methods, 17th edn. A Baillere Tindall book published by Cassell Ltd. 1980.
6. Milner AD, Hull D. Hospital Pediatrics, 3rd edn. ELBS with Churchill Livingstone. 1998.
7. Behrman RE (comps), Kliegman RM, Nelson WE, Vaughan VC III (Eds). Nelson's Textbook of Pediatrics, 14th edn. Philadelphia: WB Saunders. 1992.
8. Robinson MJ, Lam LE. Paediatric Problems in Tropical Countries. Pelanduk Publications (M) Sdn Bhd 1994.
9. Stephenson T, Wallace H (Eds). Clinical Pediatrics for Post-graduate Examinations. UK: Churchill Livingstone. 1991.

SECTION 3

NEWBORN: HISTORICAL AND PHYSICAL LINKS

- Newborn

Chapter 12

Newborn

TERMS AND DEFINITIONS[1-27]

Gestational Age

Period of gestation is measured from the first day of the last menstrual period up to the time the pregnant mother reviews with her obstetrician or family physician.

The gestational age of the neonate is obtained from the following:
- The last menstrual period (LMP)
- Fetal ultrasound
- Neonatal methods
- Dubowitz score
- The Ballard score.

The gestational age is expressed either in completed days or completed weeks.

Fetal growth measurements are expressed according to a specific week of gestational age. For example, X cm at 12 weeks.

The mean birth weight at 40 weeks is the birth weight that is obtained at 280–286 days of gestation.

> **Note:** The Dubowitz and the Ballard score measure gestational age by the assessment of many physical criteria and neuromuscular characteristics.

The physical and neurological criteria are used in scoring infants because recognized physical and neurologic features mature with advancing gestational age:

These physical criteria are:[15,18,23]
• Decreasing opacity of skin
• Increasing firmness of the pinna of the ear
• Increasing size of breast tissue
• Decreasing fine immature lanugo hair over back
• Plantar creases with increased indentations on palm with increasing age
• Genitalia with descent of testes into scrotum and maturing features of scrotum, such as rugae in the male and in the female the labia majora enlarges with small labia minora

These neurological criteria are:[15,18,23]
• Increased flexion of hips, arms and legs
• Increased tone of the muscles for flexion of the neck
• Decreased joint laxity
• Arm recoil, popliteal angle, square window, scarf sign and heel to ear are used to assess limb flexibility

Definitions[15,23,27]

Term
• 37 completed weeks to less than 42 completed weeks
Preterm
• Less than 37 completed weeks (from the first day of the last menstrual period)
Post-term
• 42 completed weeks or more
Low birth weight (LBW)*
• Less than 2,500 g
Very low birth weight (VLBW)
• Less than 1,500 g
Extremely low birth weight (ELBW)
• Less than 1,000 g
Small for gestational age or SGA
• Birth weight less than 10th percentile for estimated gestational age
Appropriate for gestational age or AGA
• Birth weight between 10th and 90th percentile for estimated gestational age
Large for gestational age or LGA
• Birth weight more than 90th percentile for estimated gestational age

* Note:
Low birth weight infants (LBW)
A low birth weight may be simply due to prematurity or intrauterine growth restriction (IUGR) or both.
Prematurity is the most common cause in developed countries.
Intrauterine growth restriction (IUGR) is the most common cause in some developing countries.

NORMAL FULL-TERM NEONATE

Newborn: A Full-term Infant[15,18-23]

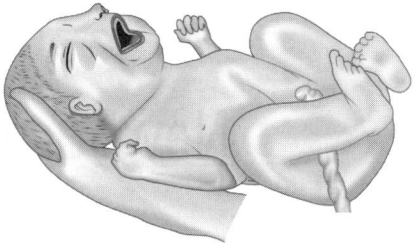

A healthy full-term newborn infant has a flexed posture and a lusty cry.

Characteristic features of a full-term infant[15,18-23]	
General appearance on observation	• Average weight of 2.7 to 3.8 kg and in the initial week after birth, the healthy term neonate loses about 5% to 7% of his or her body weight due to fluid resorption • Approximately 50 cm in length • The skin may be cracking with pale areas and rare veins. Vernix caseosa may be seen on the skin • There are bald lanugo areas. Creases are present on the anterior two thirds of the plantar surface of the feet. The areola of the breast is raised with a 3–4 mm bud; the ears have well curved pinnas which are soft but with instant recoil. In the male, the testes are bilaterally descended with good rugae. In the female, the labia majora is big and the labia minora is smaller
Head	The head appears large for the body. Moulding, which occurs in labor and delivery, can cause the head to be irregular on palpation. 'Caput' usually disappears in 1–2 days. The head circumference is 33–35 cm
Fontanel	Two areas on the head where bone formation is incomplete at birth. The larger one is diamond shaped, anteriorly situated and closes by 18 months. The smaller one is triangular, posteriorly situated and usually closes by 2 months
Heart	The heart rate is 120–140 beats per minute
Respiratory rate	The respiratory rate averages 30–40 breaths/minute. Breathing may stop up to an average of about 10 seconds but less than 20 seconds known as periodic breathing, a common finding in the normal newborn
Color	Peripheral cyanosis is commonly seen at birth. It is not significant. 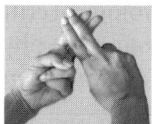 Hypothermia is one reason for peripheral cyanosis in the newborn. Link pathophysiology with other causes of peripheral cyanosis

Contd...

Activity	Vigorous spontaneous activity and extremities are in a flexed position
Reflexes	Reflexes: Primitive reflexes develop at different times during gestation. Some newborn reflexes seem essential for survival and to nurture the newborn's physical and emotional needs. The Moro reflex and the palmar grasp are such reflexes. Term infants are born with a rooting reflex using which they seek the nipple and a sucking reflex enabling them to effectively obtain nutrition from the lactating mammary gland.

PREMATURE NEONATE

Newborn: A Preterm Infant[15,18,22,23]

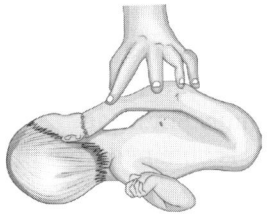

A preterm infant. The hips are flexed completely towards the abdomen and the heel to the ear.

Characteristic features of a preterm infant[15,18,23]
General appearance: This depends on the age of gestation, hence a premature neonate has different characteristics from a full-term neonate but as gestational age increases the characteristics become less noticeable. The premature infant is small, usually weighing less than 2.5 kg. Lanugo is sparse, or abundant, plantar surfaces may have only faint red marks or none at all depending on gestational age. The breasts may be barely perceptible or with a flat areola without a breast bud. The eyelids may be fused or open and the pinna may be flat which stays folded or with slow recoil depending on the gestational period
Skin and cartilage: The skin is thin, shiny, pink and transparent. There is little subcutaneous fat and little external ear cartilage compared to the term infant, in the preterm. These features explain the transparency of the skin and slow recoil of the external ear. The skin may be covered by vernix caseosa which is a creamy white layer covering the skin *Can you understand that the lack of subcutaneous fat contributes to problems with temperature control in a premature infant? Link the covering vernix with temperature control in the preterm. Could it have a role to play in the early maintenance of body temperature?*
Activity: Spontaneous activity and tone are reduced compared to the full term newborn. In preterm infants the extremities are not in a flexed position. Increased flexibility is evident. The preterm infant is able to bring the heel to ear and extend the arms right across the shoulders

Contd...

Newborn

Contd...

Genitalia: The premature male neonate has less rugae on the scrotum and the testis may be undescended. Depending on gestation, the scrotum may be empty and the testis may be in the upper canal. In premature female infants, the clitoris may be prominent and the labia minora are small. 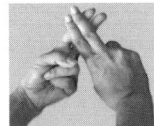 *When do the testes fully descend? Link to embryology. What is an undescended testis? How does that differ from an ectopic testis?*	
In a premature female, the labia majora do not yet cover the labia minora and look equally prominent	

Prematurity: Risk Factors[15,18,22,23]

Maternal risk factors predisposing to prematurity[15,18,23]
• A previous premature birth
• Multiple pregnancy
• Less than six months between one pregnancy and another
• Anatomical and functional problems with the placenta, uterus and/or the cervix
• Smoking cigarettes, drinking alcohol or using illicit drugs
• Malnutrition
• Maternal infections involving the lower genital; chorioamnionitis
• Certain chronic medical conditions, such as high blood pressure and diabetes mellitus
• Mother who is significantly underweight or overweight before pregnancy
• Extreme psychological stresses during pregnancy such as the sudden death of a loved one or domestic violence
• Many miscarriages or abortions
• Physical injury or trauma during pregnancy

Fetal risk factors in the preterm infant[15,18,23]
• Respiratory distress syndrome due to hyaline membrane disease
• Hypothermia
• Necrotizing enterocolitis
• Apnea of prematurity
• Hyperbilirubinemia
• Retinopathy of prematurity (retrolental fibroplasia)

POSTMATURE NEONATE

Newborn: Post-term Infant[15,18-23]

Some characteristic features of a post-term infant[15,18-23]	
General appearance	• Wizened "old" appearance with long nails and shrivelled skin
	• Bright and alert eyes
	• Parchment-like skin. The lanugo will be mostly bald. There will be creases over the entire sole. The areola is full with a breast bud of 5–10 mm. The ears are well formed with instant recoil or the ears may be stiff

Contd...

Contd...

	due to thick cartilage. The testes which are bilaterally descended, are pendulous and the scrotum has deep rugae. The labia majora is large and labia minora is small or the labia majora may cover the clitoris and the labia minora
Skin	• Dry desquamation with cracking around the creases of the ankles, wrist and neck
	• Wrinkled and loose skin
	• Reduced or absent vernix caseosa
Nails	• Long and brittle nails
Limbs	• Thin arms and legs
Hair	• More scalp hair and less lanugo hair
Meconium	• May stain skin yellowish green
	• Increased risk of meconium aspiration (MAS)

Post-maturity: Causes and Effects[15,18-23]

Causes and effects of post-maturity

Causes[15,18,23]
Error in dates
Factors associated with decreased fetal estrogen production
• Placental sulfatase deficiency
• Anencephaly
• Fetal adrenal hypoplasia
Effects[15,18,23]
Maternal effects[15,18,23]
Increased Cesarean section rates
Postpartum hemorrhage
Traumatic delivery, e.g. shoulder dystocia
Fetal effects[15,18,23]
Increased perinatal mortality
Fetal distress
Meconium aspiration syndrome (MAS)
Fetal trauma, e.g. brachial plexus injuries, clavicle fracture
Dysmaturity syndrome is linked to prolonged gestation and placental insufficiency with reduced amount of subcutaneous fat, wrinkling and meconium staining of the skin and long nails.

Small for Gestational Age[15,17,18,22,23]

Risk Factors for SGA (IUGR)

Maternal risk factors
Genetics
- Short stature
- Low weight

Ethnicities
- Certain ethnicities have higher incidence

Maternal medical history
- Chronic hypertension
- Kidney disease

- Severe diabetes mellitus
- Connective tissue diseases.

Maternal infections
- Urinary tract infection
- Malaria
- Intrauterine infections.

Risk factors developing in pregnancy
- Per vaginal hemorrhage in early pregnancy
- Pre eclampsia
- Abruptio placentae
- Gestational hypertension
- Placental and uterine abnormalities
- Poor nutrition (cause or effect).

Maternal medication
- Antimetabolites
- Heavy metals
- Hydantoin
- Steroids
- Warfarin
- Substance abuse and illicit drug use
- Cocaine
- Cigarette smoking.

Problems linked to SGA (IUGR)[15,18,23]

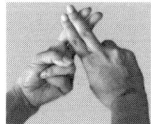

Fetal risk factors in SGA[15,17,18,23]

Intrauterine fetal death
Temperature instability
Prenatal asphyxia
Hypoglycemia
Polycythemia
Hypothermia
Pulmonary hemorrhage
Dysmorphism
Chromosomal anomalies
Nonchromosomal syndromes
Congenital infections
Insulin resistance due to reduced production of insulin or insulin-like growth factor 1

Large for gestational age[3,15,18, 20,22,23]

Risk factors for LGA

Maternal risk factors
Diabetes mellitus
Infant risk factors

Contd...

Contd...

Birth injury due to macrosomia resulting in clavicular fracture, injury to the brachial plexus and shoulder dystocia.
Facial nerve injury, cephalhematoma, asphyxia, increased perinatal and neonatal mortality
Increased incidence of Cesarean section
All risk factors associated with infant of diabetic mother (IDM) (see below)

* Note
An IDM can also be an SGA. Can you think of the cause? Think of the effects of diabetes mellitus on the blood vessels in the body and on the placental vasculature.

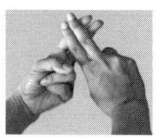

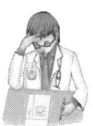

The IDM is a clear example of how maternal disease can adversely affect the newborn. This delicate equilibrium is reflected by the numerous morbidities linked to neonatal hypo- and hyperglycemia

The common problems in the infant of diabetic mothers (IDM)[3,20]

Immediate problems of IDM
• Congenital anomalies
• Large size for dates
• Respiratory distress
• Hypoglycemia
• Birth trauma
• Birth asphyxia

Neonatal complications of IDM[3,20]

Metabolic Derangement

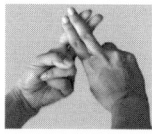

Link pathophysiology to explain neonatal hypoglycemia: The newborn IDM abruptly faces an interruption in the delivery of glucose in the postpartum period, which when linked to high circulating insulin levels results in hypoglycemia.
Hypomagnesemia—occurs within the first 72 hours of birth
Hypocalcemia—occurs within the first 72 hours of birth

Contd...

Contd...

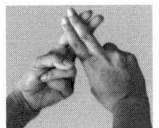

Why does an IDM look "puffy and red"? Polycythemia. How would that affect the IDM?

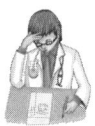

The IDM manifests many of the symptoms and signs of a premature infant. Additionally many problems associated with the IDM have been listed. Others include organomegaly, short- and long-term neurological instability, renal vein thrombosis, small left colon syndrome and transient hematuria.

Polycythemia
Increased erythrocyte mass
Ineffective erythropoiesis
Relative immaturity of hepatic bilirubin conjugation and excretion
Hyperbilirubinemia
Respiratory distress
Surfactant deficiency
Transient tachypnea of the newborn
Cardiac abnormality
Truncus arteriosus
Intraventricular septal hypertrophy
Hypertrophic obstructive cardiomyopathy
Double outlet right ventricle
Increased incidence of patent ductus arteriosus (PDA) and other cardiac lesions
Central nervous system changes
Perinatal asphyxia
Caudal regression
Glucose and electrolyte abnormalities affecting brain physiology
Birth trauma affecting the CNS
Seizures
Lethargy
Jitteriness
Changes in tone
Abnormal movements

APGAR Score[23]

A 5-point scoring system in the delivery room that reflects fetal well-being and adaptation (2 marks for each point on a 5 point scale; minimum score 0, maximum score 10).

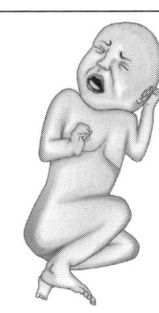

The **APGAR** score rates:
Appearance (skin color of body and extremities)
Pulse/Heart rate
Grimace (Reflexes/Irritability)
Activity (Muscle tone)
Respiration

Dr Virginia Apgar, (June 7, 1909,—August 7, 1974) was an American Obstetric Anesthesiologist. She was a pioneer in the fields of anesthesiology and teratology, and introduced parameters of obstetrical importance to the established field of neonatology.

Interpretation of score at 1 minute:	Tolerance of the newborn to the process of delivery
Interpretation of score at 5 minutes:	Adaptation to extrauterine environment

Normal Newborn[15,18,23,25,27]

Recognition of features in the normal newborn

Rationale

- There are differences in the thickness and nature of the skin of the newborn from that of the older child and adult. The thickness of newborn skin is about 50% less than that of adult skin. Dermatologically, the newborn skin has intercellular attachments which are weaker and there is less production of sweat.
- Several physical features that are seen in the normal newborn must be known and it must be appreciated that neonatal skin changes show a wide geographic and ethnic variation.
- The range of 'normal' occurrences in the newborn needs accurate identification so as to avoid unnecessary treatment to the newborn.
- Some other features that have been described occur frequently during the newborn period and may not be entirely normal. Some such lesions require urgent treatment or urgent referral for specialist opinion. Yet others may only require close observation and follow-up.

IMPORTANT PHYSICAL FEATURES OF THE NEWBORN[15,18,19-27]

Various types of skin rashes in a newborn are summarized below:

Descriptive types of physiological skin rashes and other clinical manifestations in the newborn that require no specific treatment

Skin rashes[6]	Description[6]
Milia	• Milia are epithelial cysts plugged with keratin • Fine white spots on the nose and cheeks or chin • These must be differentiated from septic spots • Disappear spontaneously
Miliaria neonatorum	• As a result of heat therapy • Vesicular sweat retention cysts as a result of plugging of the immature eccrine ducts • Common on the forehead and face especially the bridge of the nose
Sebacious gland hyperplasia	• These are common lesions seen in the newborn • Different from milia, more pronounced papules on the nose may be due to sebaceous gland hyperplasia. Compared to milia, the lesions are more yellow in color and occur due to maternal androgen exposure in utero. Parents can be reassured that these lesions will resolve with time.
Cutis marmorata *Since temperature control is very important in the newborn, the newborn infant is placed in a "thermoneutral environment". This is the environmental temperature at which oxygen consumption and metabolism are minimal while the newborn maintains a normal body temperature.*	• As a result of cold. Due to dilation of capillaries and venules and disappears on warming. • Mottled, lacy discoloration of skin • They are also seen in conditions associated with poor perfusion, CNS disturbances and hypothyroidism
Erythema toxicum *This is important to know as a normal occurrence and unnecessary treatment must be avoided.*	• These consist of vesicles with eosinophils and are thus also known as eosinophil rash. • They are very common and appear within the first 24 hours of life • Widespread fluctuating erythematous maculopapular rash beginning after birth • Individual lesions consist of white central papules surrounded by erythematous flare or halo • May be mistaken for septic spots and disappear spontaneously • They appear on the face, trunk and upper extremities
Suckling blister	• Probably a consequence of vigorous sucking of the baby *in utero* or soon after birth • Presents in the accessible areas such as the hand and forearm • To be differentiated from neonatal herpes and bullous impetigo
Acne neonatorum	• Seen on the cheeks due to sebaceous gland stimulation by androgens. They are sometimes referred to as "the puberty of the newborn", and are present due the exposure to maternal hormones • They tend to appear in the first 2–4 weeks of life • Most undergo resolution without treatment

Contd...

Contd...

Vernix caseosa	• Describes an oily substance on the skin of some newborns at birth over the face, neck, ears and groin. The vernix may also have thermoregulatory, antioxidant, wound healing, moisturizing and anti-infective properties[6,10] • It dries and flakes off a few hours after birth. In a series by Farhana TTSH and Arun C. I (2014)[6] vernix caseosa was seen in 92.8% full-term, 5.9% preterm and 1.5% post-term neonates
Lanugo	• Soft and fine hair on the body of the newborn. Although this is present to a much greater degree in premature infants, term babies also have variable amounts of lanugo present at birth
Harlequin color change	• Immaturity of the central control of the tone of peripheral vasculature • Upon lying on one side, the upper or lower part of the body reddens while the other blanches
Seborrheic dermatitis	• Erythematous scaly lesions on the scalp, referred to as the cradle cap • In addition to cradle cap, a non pruritic mild rash appears on the eyebrows, on the skin next to the nose, in skin creases around the neck, behind the ears or in the axilla. It can also cause a nappy rash in the groin creases. The condition most frequently is observed in the first six weeks of life • Secondary infection with bacteria and fungi can commonly occur • Usually self-limiting, it may need emollients and scalp oil
Capillary nevi	• These are frequently seen on the forehead and upper eyelids where they are referred to as salmon patch • If such nevi appear at the posterior aspect of the neck they are called stork mark or stork bite nevi • They disappear in a few months
Port wine stains or nevus flammeus	• Also known as venous hemangioma; they are flat, purplish marks found commonly on the face or neck. Commonly unilaterally distributed • In some cases, a port wine stain may affect a large surface area and specific underlying conditions must be excluded such as if it occurs on the spine, it is important to check for occult spinal dysraphism • When present in the forehead it may be linked to Sturge–Weber syndrome and those on the extremities may be seen in Klippel-Trenaunay-Weber syndrome, linked to overgrowth of an extremity • Some become lighter but they rarely disappear
Strawberry nevus *Although these lesions will disappear gradually, lesions in the diaper area or near vital structures such as the eye must be observed for infection or bleeding and may require treatment when they grow and become raised*	• These are crimson-red raised vascular papules, a consequence of abnormal collections of venous capillaries of the skin • They appear a few days to few weeks of birth, in any part of the body and enlarge over the next 6 months • Even large hemangiomas potentially regress spontaneously over a period of time. Involution is thus the natural history of these lesions
Mongolian blue spots *Differentiation from multiple ecchymosis in nonaccidental injury (NAI) is sometimes required*	• They are large, flat black or blue-black areas, commonly present over the lower back and buttocks. They have no pathologic significance • They are commonly present in Asians and less common in some other races and are due to dermal arrest of neural crest cells • These disappear spontaneously by the second year. In cases where it persists, there is no risk of malignancy
Café-au-lait spots	• These usually number less than three, occurring in about 20% of normal children • The presence of six or more café-au-lait spots, exceeding 0.5 cm in diameter is considered to be a major clue to the diagnosis of neurofibromatosis
Linea nigra	• The appearance of a line between the umbilicus and the pubis in some newborns especially if darker skinned • Benign condition may be related to maternal hormonal levels

Mouth[19-27]

Various types of abnormalities found in the mouth of a newborn

Abnormalities[19-27]	Description[19-27]
Epithelial pearl	• They are also known as milk spots or epidermal cysts • They occur as clusters of white spots in the mouth at the junction of the soft and hard palate in the midline and sometimes are seen over the gingiva • Not to be mistaken for oral thrush, they disappear spontaneously
Natal teeth *"I remember an infant who was brought for hematemesis by the mother. When examined it was found that the mother had cracked nipples due to the natal teeth of the infant ! The "hematemesis" was due to swallowed blood as a result of that.... This indicates the importance of examining both mother and infant."*	• These are uncommon and sometimes a family history is present • It may be loosely attached and often found in the area of the lower incisors • Remove early to prevent aspiration
Mucus retention cysts	• These cysts are also known as ranulae or superficial cysts and are situated in the anterior part of the floor of the mouth under the tongue • They disappear spontaneously and need no intervention unless they interfere with feeding • Larger cysts need surgical intervention

Eyes[19-27]

In general, babies begin to focus on objects from the 6th week onwards. The infant responds to the mother or the most familiar face at this age with a "social smile."

The various types of abnormalities of the eyes of a newborn[19-27]

Abnormalities[19-27]	Description[19-27]
Squints	• A term newborn should fix, follow and turn to light but may have a nonparalytic strabismus. Mild squints are commonly seen, many correcting themselves by 3–4 months. Temporary dysconjugate eye movements especially when the infant is falling asleep are common *In pediatrics, some 'apparent' abnormalities are linked to age. Mild dysconjugate eye movements in the first 2 months is an example* • However, if the dysconjugate eye movements are fixed, an ophthalmological opinion must be sought • Any persistent squint should be referred to the ophthalmologist
Retinal hemorrhages[26]	• These are usually observed in a small percentage of normal newborns. Birth-related retinal hemorrhages in infants are more common after instrumental deliveries. Frequently bilateral, they resolve quickly.
Epiphora	• This is a result of partial patency of the nasolacrimal duct in early infancy; the duct usually opens spontaneously by one year of age
Eyelid edema	• Seen in many infants after birth; resolves in a few days
Subconjunctival hemorrhage	• Occurs due to the rupture of small vessels during delivery. Does not affect vision. Clears spontaneously

Contd...

Contd...

Gonococcal conjunctivitis	• A pediatric emergency, it is associated with copious eye discharge in the first few early days of life. There is marked edema of the eyelids: With slight pressure on the lids, purulent material oozes out. Aggressive therapy, monitoring and intravenous antibiotics are urgently required. *Severe eyelid edema and purulent eye discharge are physical links indicating urgent eye management; gonococcal ophthalmia is an important reason for urgent intervention. Do you know of other bacterial causes?* *The prepregnancy history, the history of birth and delivery and the neonatal history are important to determine the source and etiology of the conjunctivitis. Chlamydial ophthalmia, gonococcal ophthalmia as well as ophthalmia due to other bacteria and herpetic keratoconjunctivitis are important to detect and treat early. The clinical presentation and when they present after birth may help you differentiate their etiology. Systemic, topical, or combined antimicrobial therapy are used.*
Dacrocystoceles	*A doctor explains the position of the nasolacrimal duct* • It is caused by obstructions at both ends of the nasolacrimal duct. An ENT referral is required.(for internal nasal evaluation)
Dacryostenosis	• Nasolacrimal duct obstruction can cause persistent tearing and ocular discharge in infants. In this condition, eye discharge occurs with the sclera remaining clear. It resolves in weeks to months.
Congenital cataracts	• They are seen alone or with other defects: there is absence of the red reflex. They could be inherited, due to intrauterine infection like congenital rubella, Lowe's syndrome, galactosemia (not present at birth but may appear by second week) *Any one congenital anomaly can be associated with another. Sometimes specific anomalies occur in clusters. In congenital cataracts, search for other abnormalities in the newborn. Examine all systems using a head-to-toe approach*
Congenital glaucoma	• There is a hazy and broad corneal appearance. Buphthalmos is extreme enlargement of the eyeball in the later stages. It may be inherited or due to congenital rubella *Examine all other systems carefully using a head-to-toe approach*
Coloboma	• It is a defect or hole in a component of the eye. It may be associated with other eye abnormalities or linked to other disorders: **C**HARGE association **C**oloboma **H**eart disease **A**tresia choanae **R**etarded growth **G**enital abnormality **E**ar anomalies

Ear Anomalies[12,19-27]

Abnormalities	Description
Normal ear	• Great variations of normality exist. In the normal ear the helix, antihelix, tragus, antitragus, scaphoid or triangular fossa and external auditory canal are all present and well formed.
Ear pits	• If isolated maybe a normal finding; however, it is important to look for associated renal abnormalities if there is a family history of hearing defects, maternal gestational diabetes or other auricular malformations
Ear tags	• May be a familial trait. If isolated may be a normal finding; However it is important to look for associated renal abnormalities if there is a family history of hearing defects, maternal gestational diabetes and other auricular malformations *Deformed and abnormal pinna Normal shaped pinna* • Here, exclusion of other related abnormalities are important. External ear anomalies are linked to renal tract anomalies. Pulmonary hypoplasia is linked to some renal anomalies.
Microtia	• The pinna is smaller than the normal ear and is not properly formed. Hearing assessment is mandatory. Renal tract anomalies must be excluded. Look for other congenital anomalies. Look for features of known syndromes
Low set ears	• If an imaginary line is drawn from the outer canthus of the eye to the occiput a low set ear will fall completely below the line. Normally set ears will cross or touch the same line. In association with some syndromes like trisomy 18, trisomy13, CHARGE syndrome, Turner syndrome and Noonan syndrome
Normal umbilical cord	• In the newborn, it is bluish white and then may become pale yellowish in color. A normal cord has two arteries and one vein • A single umbilical artery is linked to other congenital anomalies including chromosomal and renal anomalies • The umbilical cord gradually separates in about ten days of life • Delayed separation is linked to disorders of granulocyte function *Thick walled artery* *Thin walled vein* *Fresh umbilical cord of a newborn. Cross sectional diagram of umbilicus*
	One umbilical artery is associated with renal anomalies

Contd...

Contd...

Other conditions in the umbilical area	• Umbilical hernias, omphalitis (an important condition to treat immediately), Wharton's jelly cyst and umbilical hemangiomas
Meconium[21] *Delayed or non-passage of the meconium may denote conditions such as anorectal malformations, intestinal atresia, meconium ileus, neonatal sepsis, Hirschsprung's disease, neonatal asphyxia and hypothyroidism. The passage of the first stool, therefore, is a pivotal observation in the newborn.*	• Meconium is an accumulation of desquamated gut epithelium, residues from swallowed amniotic fluid, lanugo hair, mucus, and bile in the fetal gut • It is sticky, tarry greenish black stool passed within 24-48 hours of life • The passage of meconium in the first 24 to 48 hours is an important sign of fetal well being • It may be passed in utero if there is fetal distress • Inhalation can cause pneumonitis with severe respiratory distress
Meconium staining of the cord[21]	• This gives it a greenish color. Meconium stained liquor is a sign of fetal distress and infants must be observed for respiratory distress and sepsis. Meconium stained airways are vigorously suctioned to minimize the risk of meconium aspiration *Meconium-stained liquor is due to fetal distress as hypoxia relaxes the anal sphincter and allows for the passage of meconium into the amniotic fluid. The neonate must be observed for respiratory distress*

Breast and Genitalia[19-27]

This table summarizes the various types of abnormalities of the breast and genitalia.

Various types of abnormalities of the breast and genitalia

Abnormalities[19-27]	Description[19-27]
Breast engorgement	• It is present in many full-term babies of both sexes. The breasts must not be squeezed as this can cause an infection or lead to an abscess • The effect of maternal hormones may also cause some fluid to leak or milk to be secreted from the infant's nipples. This is sometimes called "witch's milk".
Mucous vaginal discharge leukorrhea and vaginal bleeding	• This is common around the end of the first week of life and are temporarily observed in the newborn girl. • Caused by withdrawal of maternal estrogenic hormones
Vulval tags	• Tags of mucous membrane are common in the posterior vulval region; are often long and pedunculated • They shrink and disappear within a few days
Hypospadias is the incomplete development of the anterior urethra and corpus spongiosum.	• Diagnosed during newborn screening (Refer to Chapter 10)

234 *The Link*: Pediatric History-Taking and Physical Examination

Hands and Feet[15,18,23,25]

- Count the number of digits in the hands and feet
- Examine the palmar creases for a single simian crease
- Look for conditions like
- Polydacytyly or extra digits
- Clinodactyly or incurving of the little finger
- Syndactyly or fusion of the fingers
- Brachydactyly or short fingers

- Note if the thumbs or the toes are unusually broad
- Note if the distance between the first toe and second toe is unusually wide. Do you know in which syndrome it is seen?

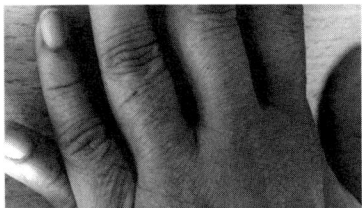
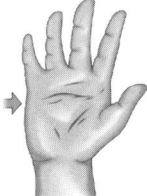
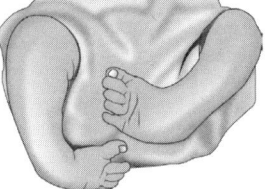

Polydactyly   *Simian crease*   *Talipes equinovalgus*

Back and Hips[1,19-27]

Abnormalities of the back and hips

Abnormalities[1,19-27]	Description[1,19-27]
Sacral pits and dimples (also known as sacrococcygeal or coccygeal dimples or pits)	• Generally harmless, they are common and often seen over the sacrum and they occur at the lower sacral region close to or within the natal cleft • Fistulae at the sacrum (blind ending) need to be excluded • May be associated with hairy nevus tuft of hair, skin tag, lipoma or skin discoloration • No intervention required once other conditions are excluded

Hips[1] 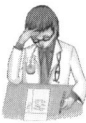
 	
Embryologically, the head of the femur and acetabulum has its origin in closely related mesenchymal cells. A division separates these mesenchymal cells at around 8 weeks of intrauterine life. By the 11th week of gestation, the hip joint has fully developed. In the newborn, the acetabulum which continues to develop postnatally and the femoral head are mainly cartilaginous. The embryological formation of the hip makes it possible that hip dysplasia may occur in utero, anytime perinatally, in infancy or in early childhood. A dislocation at 11 weeks is termed teratologic.
	• The hips are screened soon after birth as the early diagnosis of developmental dysplasia of the hip (DDH), includes observation and examination. It was previously called congenital dislocation of the hip (CDH) and is an important early screening examination. It is known that girls, due to the sensitivity to the maternal hormone relaxin, partly causing laxity of the ligaments are at a higher risk of instability of the hip. There is an observed slightly greater involvement of the right hip.
	• Dislocation of an unstable hip is Barlow's sign.
	• Reduction of the dislocated hip is Ortalani's sign.
	• The observational diagnosis is important although not pathognomonic. Asymmetrical thigh or gluteal folds is more easily observed when the child is prone. Apparent limb length difference and reduced motion, mainly abduction, are significant signs:
	  – Dislocation of an unstable hip is Barlow's sign.
	  – Reduction of the dislocated hip is Ortalani's sign.
	• The Ortolani is a test that makes the examiner feel the dislocated hip reducing, and the Barlow is a clinical test that uncovers the unstable hip dislocating from the acetabulum. The Ortolani is done with the newborn lying supine and the index and middle finger of the examiner at the greater trochanter. The examiner's thumb is held along the thigh. The hip is flexed hip at 90 degrees while the leg is held in neutral position. Gentle abduction of the hip while anteriorly lifting the leg will make the dislocated head of the femur reduce into the acetabula fossa which indicates that the test is positive.[1,19-27]
	• The Barlow provocative test is done with the newborn lying supine and the hips flexed to 90°. The leg is then gently adducted while posteriorly directed pressure is placed on the knee. A positive test is when a clunk is felt.[1,19-27]

Contd...

Contd...

At 18 weeks of intrauterine life, various problems involving nerves and muscles such as arthrogryposis and myelodysplasia contribute to this anomaly. During the last 4 weeks of pregnancy, oligohydramnios or breech position predispose to DDH. Postnatally, the manner in which an infant is positioned for routinely or for prolonged periods such as swaddling, contribute to DDH.	• The Ortolani and Barlow maneuvers are performed 1 hip at a time and these tests must be done with minimum force. Caution must be taken to avoid excessive pressure and the examination must be conducted in a gentle manner as injury can occur to the seal between the head of the femur and labrum.

Primitive Reflexes[15,18,23,25]

Newborn reflexes, infantile reflexes, or primitive reflexes.

The following are the important characteristics of the newborn reflexes:
• Newborn reflexes are reflexes that are unique in the neonatal period and in infancy. These reflexes continue for some months and disappear with maturation of the nervous system. They start at different times and are fully developed at different ages. These reflexes disappear or are inhibited by the frontal lobes as a child progresses through normal development • It may be hypothesized that some of these reflexes in response to different stimuli may be essential for survival, nurturing the fetus and the young infant • A primitive reflex in infants is linked to abnormality when it is absent or inadequate, when it ought to be actively elicitable • An heightened reflex can be abnormal • Any condition that results in pain, bony fractures or injury involving the muscles or peripheral nervous system can also result in asymmetry of these reflexes
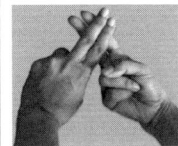 *Abnormal persistence of newborn reflexes are linked to anomalies of the brain.*

Palmar Grasp

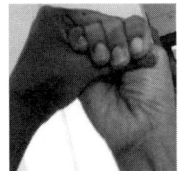

The teacher demonstrates a palmar grasp.

Infantile Reflexes[15,18,23,25]

Reflex	Infant's response
Sucking reflex	The infant sucks in response to nipple stimulation or a finger in or around the mouth
Rooting reflex	This reflex occurs when the infant's cheek is stroked. The positive response is when the infant turns to the side that is stroked and starts to make sucking movements
Palmar grasp reflex	When a finger is inserted into the palm of the infant from the ulnar aspect and exerts gentle pressure to the palm, with the infant awake and lying on a flat surface, symmetrically and supine. Flexion of all fingers around the examiner's finger is the response seen
Plantar grasp	The plantar grasp reflex is a reflex that is elicited by pressure against the sole of the foot behind the toes where flexion of the toes are seen.

Contd...

Contd...

Moro or startle reflex[4] 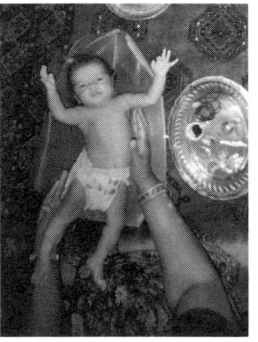	• The Moro reflex was first described by Ernst Moro in 1918. It occurs when the infant is held on back with head supported and the head is suddenly allowed to drop slightly • Arms and fingers will spread and then flex back to body. • Occurs when the infant's head is turned to one side. If the Moro reflex is absent at birth or if it persists for more than six months of age it is abnormal. • Its absence during the neonatal period and early infancy is linked to disorders such as severe birth asphyxia, infections, and malformations of the central nervous system. An exaggerated response is seen in neonatal withdrawal from maternal drug abuse including drugs such as heroin and opioids. • An unequal or asymmetric response is due to an injury to the cervical cord, peripheral nerve or a clavicular fracture which may inhibit the reflex on the side which is affected. • Persistence of the reflex is linked to conditions such as cerebral palsy, sometimes seen in Down syndrome and severe brain malformation.
The Moro reflex is characterized by:[4,8] The first phase of the reflex is when the head moves backwards, arms are held up and abducted with hands spread and the second phase is when the infant curls forwards, pulls legs up, adducts arms and folds arms across the chest. The infant then breathes out as in a cry for help.	
Tonic neck reflex	• As in the fencer's position, this reflex is observed when the head of an infant who is relaxed and lying supine is moved to the side. The arm on the same side where the head is facing stretches away from the body with the hand partially open. The arm on the side away from the face is held flexed and the fist is clenched.
Parachute reflex	• Here in the older infant, hold the infant upright and quickly rotate the body to face forward as if falling. The infant extends arms forward as if to protect from a fall • This reflex is a prerequisite to walking.

Newborn reflexes: appearance and full manifestation[8]
• Palmar grasp starts at 28 weeks and is fully developed at 32 weeks • Rooting reflex starts at 32 weeks and is fully mature at 36 weeks • Moro reflex starts at 30 weeks and is fully developed by 37 weeks • Tonic neck reflex commences at 35 weeks and is fully mature at 1 month • Parachute reflex has its onset at 7-8 months and is fully developed at 10–11 months.

REFERENCES

1. American Academy of Pediatrics. Committee on Quality Improvement, Subcommittee on Developmental Dysplasia of the Hip. Clinical Practice Guideline: Early Detection of Developmental Dysplasia of the Hip. PEDIATRICS Vol. 105 No. 4 April 1, 2000. pp. 896-905.
2. Brillman J, Kahan S. In: A Page Neurology. Lippincott Williams & Wilkins. ISBN 978-1-4051-0432-6. Accessed in April 2013.
3. Cowett RM. The Infant of the Diabetic Mother. NeoReviews. 2002;3:173.
4. Moro E, "Das erste Trimenon," Münchener Medizinische Wochenschrift. 1918;65:1147-50.
5. Elizabeth KE. Clinical Pediatrics for Undergraduates. India: Jaypee Brothers Medical Publishers (P) Ltd. 2009.
6. Haveri FT and Inamadar AC. A Cross-sectional Prospective Study of Cutaneous Lesions in Newborn. Dermatol. 2014;360590. Also available at http://dx.doi.org/10.1155/2014/360590.
7. Fletcher MA. Physical Diagnosis in Neonatology. (1st ed). Philadelphia Lippincott-Raven. 1998.
8. Futagi Y, Toribe Y, Suzuki Y. The Grasp Reflex and Moro Reflex in Infants: Hierarchy of Primitive Reflex Responses. International Journal of Pediatrics. Volume-2012; Article ID 191562. Also available at http://dx.doi.org/10.1155/2012/191562.
9. Goel KM, Gupta DK. Hutchinson's Pediatrics, 1st edn. India: Jaypee Brothers Medical Publishers (P) Ltd; 2009
10. Gurcharan Singh, G Archana. Unraveling the mystery of vernix caseosa. Indian J Dermatol. 2008;53(2):54-60.

11. Information on child growth from WHO. Available at http://www.who.int/childgrowth. Accessed in April 2013.
12. Information on ear deformities. Available at http://newborns.stanford.edu.
13. Krishna Das KV, Thomas M (Eds). Clinical Medicine: A Textbook of Clinical Methods and Laboratory Investigations. Jaypee Brothers Medical Publishers (P) Ltd. 2005.
14. Levene MI, Tudehope DI, Thearle MJ. Essentials of Neonatal Medicine. 3rd edition. Blackwell Science. 2000.
15. Marcdante K, Kliegman RM, Jenson HB, Behrman RE (Eds). Nelson's Essentials of Pediatrics. 6th edn. Saunders Elsevier, 2010.
16. Mason S, Swash M (Eds). Hutchinson's Clinical Methods (17th edn). A Bailllere Tindall book published by Cassell Ltd; 1980.
17. McCowan L, Horgan RP. Risk factors for small for gestational age infants. Best Pract Res Clin Obstet Gynaecol. 2009;23(6):779-93.
18. Milner AD, Hull D. Hospital Pediatrics. 3rd edn. ELBS with Churchill Livingstone. 1998.
19. Newborn examination. Available in newborns.stanford.edu. Accessed in February 2015.
20. Nold JL, Georgieff MK. Infants of diabetic mothers. Pediatr Clin North Am. 2004;51:619-37.
21. Okoro PE, Enyindah CE. Time of passage of First Stool in Newborns in a Tertiary Health Facility in Southern Nigeria. Niger J Surg. 2013 Jan-Jun;19(1):20-2.
22. Problems in the newborn. Stacy Gray & Alisha Davis 4908 Professional Court, Raleigh, NC. Available at http://www.grayfamilychiropractic.com/info/children-and-infants.
23. Behrman RE (comps), Kliegman RM, Nelson WE, Vaughan VC III (Eds). Nelson's Textbook of Pediatrics, 14th edn. Philadelphia: WB Saunders. 1992.
24. Robinson MJ, Lam LE. Paediatric Problems in Tropical Countries. Pelanduk Publications (M) Sdn Bhd. 1994.
25. Stephenson T, Wallace H. Clinical Paediatrics for Postgraduate Examinations UK: Churchill Livingstone; 1991.
26. Watts P, Maguire S, Kwok T, Talabani B, Mann M, Wiener J, et al. Newborn retinal hemorrhages: a systematic review. J AAPOS. 2013 Feb;17(1):70-8. doi: 10.1016/j.jaapos.2012.07.012. Epub 2013 Jan 28.
27. Kassim Z. Consice Neonatology. International Islamic University Malaysia Press. 2003.

The essence of the relevant chapters in the following books have also been numbered as references in this chapter. We recommend for further reading, the rich text in these books for greater integration and deeper understanding.

1. Elizabeth KE. Clinical Pediatrics for Undergraduates. Jaypee Brothers Medical Publishers (P) Ltd, India 2009.
2. Goel KM, Gupta DK. Hutchinson's Pediatrics, 1st edn. Jaypee Brothers Medical Publishers (P) Ltd, India 2009.
3. Kassim Z. Consice Neonatology. International Islamic University Malaysia Press. 2003.
4. Krishna Das KV, Thomas M (Eds). Clinical Medicine: A Textbook of Clinical Methods and Laboratory Investigations. Jaypee Brothers Medical Publishers (P) Ltd. 2005.
5. Marcdante K, Kliegman RM, Jenson HB, Behrman RE (Eds). Nelson's Essentials of Pediatrics, 6th Edn. Saunders Elsevier. 2010.
6. Mason S, Swash M (Eds). Hutchinson's Clinical Methods, 17th edn. A Bailllere Tindall book published by Cassell Ltd. 1980.
7. Milner AD, Hull D. Hospital Pediatrics. 3rd edn. ELBS with Churchill Livingstone. 1998.
8. Behrman RE (comps), Kliegman RM, Nelson WE, Vaughan VC III. (Eds). Nelson's Textbook of Pediatrics, 14th edn. Philadelphia: WB Saunders. 1992.
9. Robinson MJ, Lam LE. Paediatric Problems in tropical countries. Pelanduk Publications (M) Sdn Bhd. 1994.
10. Stephenson T, Wallace H (Eds). Clinical Pediatrics for postgraduate examinations. UK: Churchill Livingstone; 1991.

SECTION 4

DIFFERENTIAL DIAGNOSIS AND PROVISIONAL DIAGNOSIS WITH SELECTED CASE STUDIES

- Formulation of Differential Diagnosis and Provisional Diagnosis

Chapter 13

Formulation of Differential Diagnosis and Provisional Diagnosis

PROCESS OF FORMULATION OF THE PROVISIONAL DIAGNOSIS

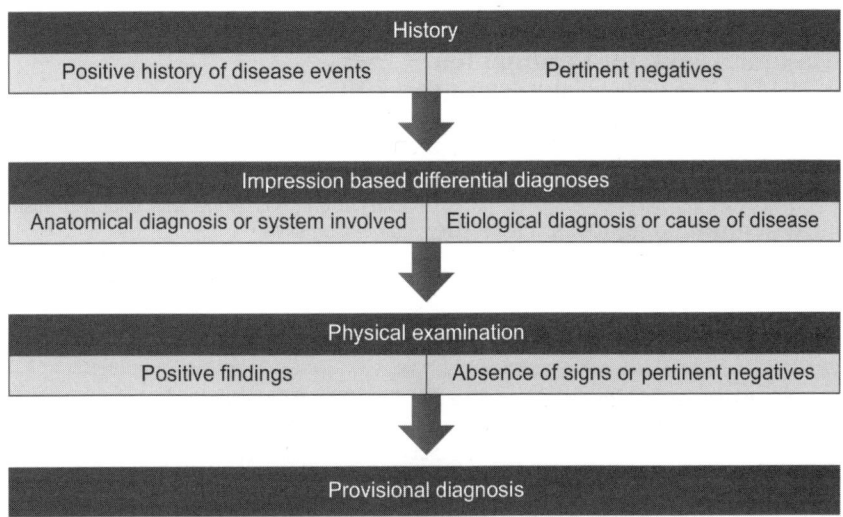

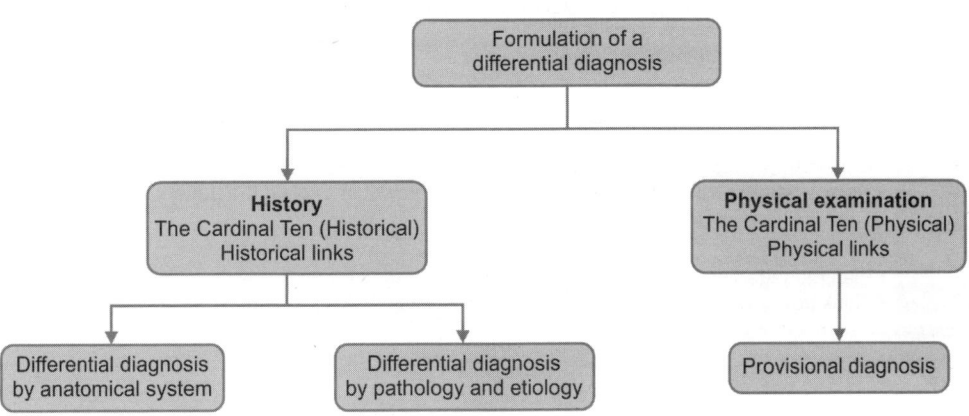

The aim of a good pediatric history is to reach a reasonable differential diagnoses. In doing so, you must analyze the history of the presenting illness (HOPI) in terms of the system involved in the disease of the presenting illness, think of common conditions that affect the age group, the gender, and the socioenvironment. After the HOPI, your 5 differential diagnoses is re-evaluated in all other parts of the history where you listen to the patient, then ask open-ended questions and directed questions. Once the differential diagnoses are considered, put in priority; the most likely is to be mentioned first.

A complete examination of the patient as a whole is always desirable. However, the history will then help you focus on your physical examination. The focused physical examination will help you narrow your differential diagnosis. Narrow the possibilities based on your knowledge of the pathophysiology of the disease which you have accurately elicited by **The Cardinal Ten (Historical)**, the historical links, **The Cardinal Ten (Physical)** which are tested by the physical links and confirmed by inspection, palpation, percussion and auscultation.

Based on your history and physical examination, you critically analyze your differential diagnoses. Here the analysis is based on the positive and negative responses and the historical links that emerge from your history taking. Weigh the pros and cons of each symptom (the presence or the absence of related symptoms).

All this is given value by the physical findings, both the positive and negative ones. The narrowed list of differential diagnoses will now form your provisional diagnosis. The provisional diagnosis may require investigations or interventions for confirmation and to arrive at the definitive diagnosis.

Where you are unable to make a definitive diagnosis on clinical grounds alone, do only necessary investigations that may be needed to confirm or to exclude the possible differential diagnosis.

These investigations may include blood tests, imaging studies and any other special tests you deem fit in order to arrive at the definitive diagnosis.

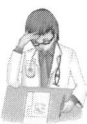

Remember, a definitive diagnosis may sometimes also be made on clinical grounds alone with excellent history-taking and physical examination skills.

Differential diagnoses
- History using historical links and **The Cardinal Ten (Historical)**
- Physical examination using the physical links and **The Cardinal Ten (Physical)**

Analyze
- Analyze the history in the light of the positive and negative information
- Analyze the physical examination in the light of the positive and negative findings

Provisional diagnoses
- Weigh the pros and cons of the history and physical examination
- Use your knowledge, your understanding and reasoning to decide on the most likely diagnosis or diagnoses
- Formulate your provisional diagnosis

Analyze
- Plan investigations if necessary
- Use noninvasive investigations where possible
- Consider radiation hazards
- Think what you would tell the family and how you would explain the patient's problems to them

Definitive diagnosis
- Plan management strategies
- Think how you will approach the patient and family

ANALYTIC THINKING DURING THE PROCESS OF FORMULATION OF THE DIAGNOSIS

1. Analysis during the process of information gathering from the patient[1-25]

Explore established clinical patterns of diseases:

- When a history is elicited think of all diseases that could present in that manner and work out a differential diagnosis and enlist these diagnoses in order of priority
- Explore the history with relevant questions by the historical link
- Look for possibilities of these differential diagnoses when asking questions in the history using **The Cardinal Ten (Historical)** and the historical link
- It is for these purposes that you must always bear the differential diagnoses in mind as you progress in the history-taking and the subsequent examination of the patient
- Astutely observe the clear clinical signs and search for other possible clinical findings to strengthen or eliminate the possible diagnosis
- Use **The Cardinal Ten (Physical)** and all relevant tools to help you compare and confirm your findings.

2. Analysis of the information gathered from the patient and the signs on physical examination[1-25]

- Analyze the clinical symptoms and signs during history-taking and physical examination
- Consider the anatomical site of the problem
- Consider similar symptoms and signs that may be present in all diseases thinking of the common diseases first
- Understand that sometimes "clustering" of similar symptoms help you broadly categorize diseases. Such clustering of related symptoms and signs make you ask for historical links and look for physical links that should be sought in a certain disease or disease group that may share anatomical site, pathophysiological processes, or etiology.
- Consider pathophysiological processes that result in symptomatology in the diseases that you think of
- Consider the underlying pathophysiological processes of the signs of the diseases that you think of.

3. Analysis of the differential diagnoses, provisional diagnosis, and definitive diagnosis[1-25]

Consider demographical and historical clues:
- Such as age of patient and gender, thinking of the common diseases first
- Where diseases with clinical patterns that need urgent intervention or counseling are important to exclude[1]
- Where environment and socioeconomic status influences are well-known[2]
- Where vaccination history would make certain diseases more likely
- When the birth history provides evidence for events that have a bearing on diagnosis
- When the family history is suggestive, especially in inherited, genetic or familial diseases.

4. Analysis on decision of diagnostic tools or investigations to clinch the definitive diagnosis[1-25]

- These are used as adjuncts to the history and physical examination where necessary and as such it is important not to be completely reliant on these tools
- When considering investigations, think of a plan to minimize investigations and maximize yield
- Think of simple laboratory investigations that will help confirm the diagnosis
- Think of noninvasive investigations first before invasive ones
- Give priority to minimize radiation hazards although you may sometimes need to use some radiological investigations to confirm your clinical diagnosis
- Consider more complex investigations if the diagnosis remains uncertain; here again, think which investigation(s) will give the maximum yield in confirming your diagnosis.

The synthesis of facts, observations and links in the formulation of the differential diagnosis and provisional diagnosis is necessary.

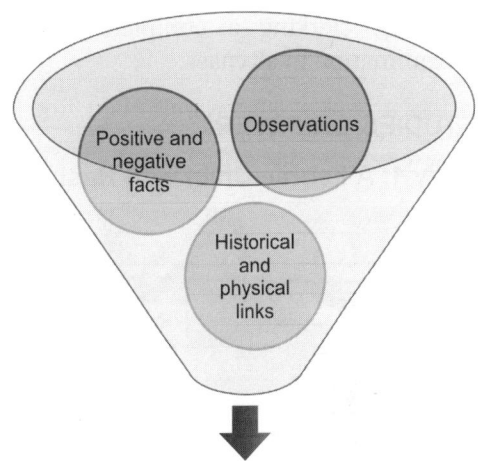

Clinical impressions or differential diagnoses and provisional diagnosis.

The tools you will need to be able to reach a diagnosis

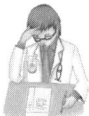

To come to a diagnosis, I must think of the history and the physical examination considering each one separately, then, linking them to everything I have learnt in the case study of my patient.

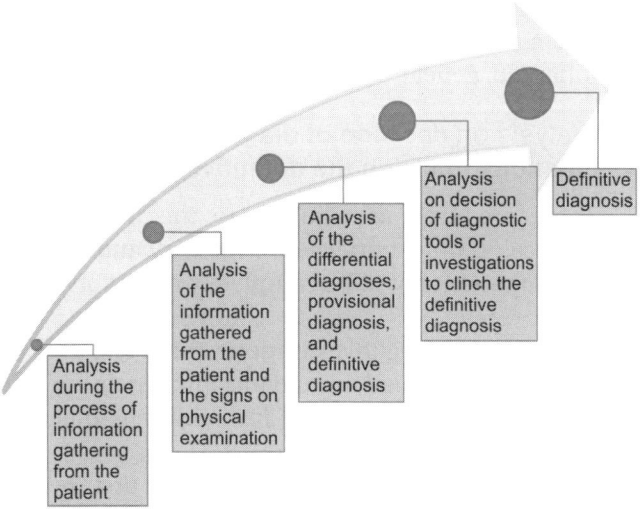

- Analysis during the process of information gathering from the patient
- Analysis of the information gathered from the patient and the signs on physical examination
- Analysis of the differential diagnoses, provisional diagnosis, and definitive diagnosis
- Analysis on decision of diagnostic tools or investigations to clinch the definitive diagnosis
- Definitive diagnosis

CASE STUDIES[1-25]

In this section, some simple summaries of clinical case studies will be discussed. These case studies consist of cases based on real life encountered clinical scenarios. The names used are fictitious. In these examples, due to the nature and focus of the book, only aspects of the history and physical examination that are relevant to the discussion of the case and the subsequent teaching points including patient approach are highlighted. The student is advised on always, consistently and conscientiously, clerking a complete history, and physical examination in all cases.

CASE STUDIES ON FEVER[1-5]

Case Study 1: A Febrile Child with Rash[8,14,17,20,23]

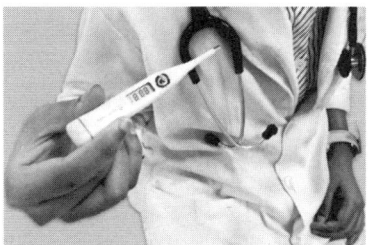

The height of the temperature, the duration of fever, the time of onset of rash and the activity of the child are important diagnostic clues.

An infant of 8 months is brought by his parents looking miserable and unwell. The infant has a mild cough and coryza. The infant has been having fever for the past 4 days not responding to the antibiotics prescribed by the general practitioner. He is taken care in the daycare center. There is a history of a few other children who recently recovered from fever in the daycare center. On examination, the child looks toxic. His height and weight are above the 25th percentile for age. The temperature is 38.5°C. The throat and conjunctivae are injected. There is a fine red maculopapular rash behind both ears and on the face, spreading down to involve the entire body. There were also small raised 'bumps' on top of the red macules. The spots were noted to become confluent as they moved from the head to the rest of the body. The mother says the rash began as flat red spots on the face and at the hairline and has spread downward now to the neck, trunk, arms, legs, and feet. The doctor looked for Koplik spots or little white lesions like grains of salt surrounded by a reddish area on the mucous membranes opposite the 2nd molars, but could not appreciate them. All systems were examined. The ears were normal and the chest was clear. Examination of the nervous system was unremarkable.

Relevant history: Age of infant, duration of fever, contact with other children with fever.

Relevant examination: Toxic appearance of child, nature of rash.

Points to note: At 8 months of age, there is little to no protection from transplacental maternal antibodies, hence the child is susceptible to many infections. The infant who attends a daycare center where other children are febrile, may have contracted an infection there. The differential diagnosis of viral exanthems is considered. Aerosol droplets and respiratory secretions make some viral exanthems easily communicable. Of the viral exanthems, the history of the rash appearing on the fourth day of the fever, the presence of cough, coryza, and injection of the conjunctivae associated with a centripetal rash starting behind the ears, makes the diagnosis of measles likely.[10] The MMR is given at 12 months in some countries and at others at 15 months; hence, this child has little protection against measles after maternal antibodies wane from 6 months up to the time of vaccination at 12–15 months. The doctor actively looks for Koplik spots. In measles, the transmission is via droplets. It is easily communicable. The incubation period is 7–14 days. Koplik spots occur in the pre-eruptive stage and disappear as the rash becomes evident; hence, although pathognomonic, is often not present on examination. Complications due to measles can occur particularly in children who are malnourished. The complications to exclude are secondary bacterial infections like otitis media, secondary bacterial pneumonias, and bronchitis.[6] Post-infectious encephalitis is uncommon. Hepatitis, myocarditis, and blindness as a result of measles keratitis are also recognized. Also remember that if the child contracted measles from the daycare center, it is of public health importance that it should be reported to appropriate health authorities to ensure adequate preventive measures of a measles outbreak.

Case Study 2: Simple Febrile Seizures[8,14,17,20,23]

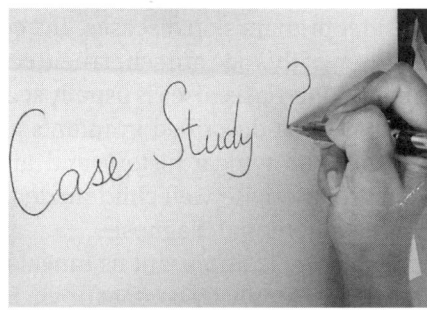

Documentation of the history and physical examination is important.

A previously well one-year-old child is admitted with high fever. During his hospital stay, he develops a generalized convulsion on the first day of fever as the temperature reaches 39°C. On examination, there is eye redness, irritability and runny nose. After the convulsion, he is tired but alert and well hydrated. The CNS examination is normal. The throat is mildly injected. The anterior fontanel is normotensive. There is no neck stiffness.

The child is observed in the ward. The fever lasts for 4 days. Despite the fever, the child, though tired-looking is alert and does not appear ill. When the fever subsides, the child develops a rash which appears on the middle of the body with tiny red bumps then spreads to the arms, legs, neck, and face. Re-examination reveals that the rashes are pink in color. They are slightly raised. The rash lasts 2 days then fades. They do not itch.

The child has been previously healthy and developmentally normal. The birth history and the history of the neonatal period are uneventful. The family history is noncontributory as there is no known member with seizures, epilepsy or mental retardation. The parents are nonconsanguineous.

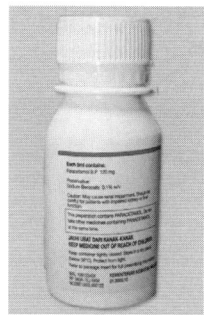

Tepid sponging, antipyretics and reassurance are all that may be needed in managing simple febrile seizures.

Relevant history: High fever, fits, appearance of rash as fever is about to subside, nature of rash. Past history, birth history and developmental history are normal.

Relevant examination: Normotensive anterior fontanel, normal CNS examination.

Points to note: Note that the convulsions occur with steep rises in temperature. The child who seems well on admission develops a seizure on the first day of fever when the temperature rises very quickly. The child is active and has no neurological signs after the seizure. Taking the age of the patient, the clinical history and the normal neurological findings, the likely diagnosis is a febrile seizure.

Simple febrile seizures last 15 minutes or less, have no focal features, and do not occur more than once in 24 hours. There is a typical rash suggestive of a viral exanthem. A common viral exanthem that is considered is roseola infantum, also known as exanthem subitum or sixth disease. It is due to human herpes virus 6 (HHV-6). It is associated with febrile seizures in a third of affected children. The description of the rash is fairly typical.

Complex febrile seizures are prolonged, last more than 15 minutes and there are more than one seizure within 24 hours. They are associated with focal seizures and sometimes with Todd's paralysis. Intracranial causes of seizures are unlikely in this case as a thorough physical examination shows no abnormal neurological signs. Additionally, the history reveals that the child remains alert and active although tired. Most children with febrile seizures 'outgrow' or will not have such seizures at an older age. Their growth and development are normal. A small subgroup with complex febrile seizures who have additional predisposing factors will be at a slightly increased risk of epilepsy.

Case Study 3: An Active Child with Skin Lesions[3,8,14,17,20,23]

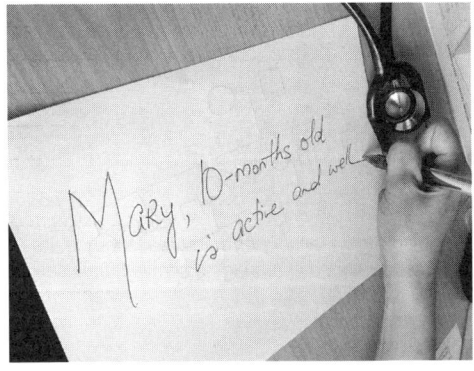

Mary's general activity and the morphology, pattern and distribution of her skin lesions helped the doctor come to a diagnosis.

Mary, a 10-month-old infant is otherwise active and well except for the presenting skin lesions. She is brought by her mother who says that Mary has been having a "red spotty rash on the body."

The mother says that these rashes have been present for almost a month now although she did not seem to be worried about it initially. While history-taking, the doctor glanced at the rash. Based on what he saw by first impression, the doctor enquired about the appearance of a specific type of rash... the mother remembers a "fungal" lesion which she describes as an oval, scaling lesion on the right thigh about 2 weeks prior to the other lesions. The mother felt that Mary was uncomfortable due to the new rash and that it might have been itchy as Mary often wriggled her body when asleep. The family history is negative for allergic skin rashes or any current illnesses. The child was born full-term with an APGAR score of 10 at 5 minutes, and was a product of a spontaneous vaginal delivery. The child was exclusively breastfed and had no recognized food allergies now or when complementary feeding was introduced.

On examination, the child is active and afebrile. A head-to-toe inspection of the child's skin revealed multiple discreet oval lesions, pinkish to brownish in color, less than 1 cm in diameter and slightly raised. Many lesions are covered by fine scales. The lesions are noted to clear centrally producing a collarette of scales attached only at the periphery. They are distributed on the trunk and arms. Further inspection reveals that these macules are arranged parallel to the skin tension lines, where the length of the lesions are typically arranged along the creases of the skin. There are no rashes on the palms and soles. Examination of the scalp, genitalia and fingernails were normal. The oral mucosa and conjunctivae were normal. All systems examination was entirely normal.

Relevant history: Well child, previous rash, distribution of rash.

Relevant examination: Nature of rashes described, symmetrical distribution of rash, mainly on trunk.

Points to note: Skin diseases in children may be primary dermatological problems affecting the skin or dermatological manifestations of systemic diseases. The presence or absence of fever and the child's general activity are important factors that will help decide the nature and origin of the rash. In rashes associated with fever, consider acute viral exanthems and other systemic diseases that involve or manifest on the skin. In a well, afebrile child where examination of all systems are normal, consider primary skin diseases. The commoner rashes in children of this age are seborrheic eczema and atopic dermatitis. Pityriasis rosea is usually seen in older children but has been described in infants and young children.[3] Hence the typical history and appearance of the rash in an otherwise well child made the doctor think of it in the differential diagnosis.

The family history is important as fungal infections can spread within a family by contact or via fomites. In this case, the doctor's knowledge, the appearance of the rash, its site and distribution prompted enquiry of the herald patch (which the mother thought was a fungal lesion). This is an example where the historical link is made use of.

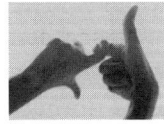

A maculopapular rash with the preceding herald patch in a well-child is suggestive of the diagnosis of pityriasis rosea. In the dermatological examination, inspection from head to toe must be done for a thorough approach to examination of an infant. It is reemphasized that examination of the scalp by parting the hair of the head to inspect the scalp and examination of the nails are important parts of the skin examination.

Case Study 4: Infantile Seborrheic Dermatitis[8,12,14,17,20,23]

A male infant of 2 months who appears comfortable has rashes in the napkin area and develops one or two areas of intertrigo. The lesions consist of sharply demarcated red patches with yellowish waxy exudates. The child also has thick whitish scaly lesions on the scalp.

The lesions have appeared for the past few months. There are no constitutional symptoms. The typical appearance of this common rash in a child who is

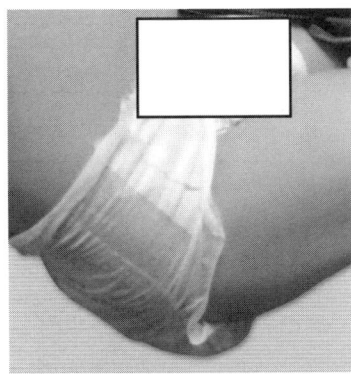

The nappy area is important to examine for both skin conditions and as an initial site for specific systemic infections.

well, allowed the doctor to make a diagnosis and in addition to topical creams, advices that the diapers be changed frequently and as soon as possible after the passage of stool. He advises that the skin be gently but thoroughly cleansed with warm water after each diaper change and then gently patted dry with a soft, smooth, cotton cloth. He explains that keeping the diaper area clean, dry, and exposed to air promotes resolution of the inflammation. He advises that the infant be left without a diaper for about half an hour several times a day, as this practice promotes rapid healing.

Relevant history: Age of child, duration of rashes.

Relevant examination: No constitutional symptoms, nature of rash.

Points to note: The gradual onset and the yellowish waxy nature of the nappy rash must prompt examination of the scalp. Cradle cap refers to thick whitish scaly lesions in the scalp usually seen with the findings in the nappy area. The physical examination of the skin must be looked for thoroughly by conducting a head to toe inspection. The scalp, the teeth and nails are part of the integumentary system. The mucosae are continuous to this system; hence, the conjunctivae, the oral and genital mucosae must also be included in the examination of the skin. By examining the mucosae, important positive or negative findings can be useful in discerning the differential diagnosis. Remember that seborrheic dermatitis involves the genitocrural flexures, the scalp and other flexures.[12] In atopic eczema, the infant is usually older.[12] The cheeks, forehead, forearms, cubital and popliteal fossae are involved and there is associated pruritis which may manifest itself as a "wriggly infant". In this case, in an infant not perturbed by his skin lesions, examining the scalp after checking the nappy area is a simple physical link which makes the diagnosis.[12]

Case Study 5: The Child with "an Irritating Habit of not Responding to His Mother's Call"[8,14,17,20,23]

Osmond, a 4-year-old child develops sneezing, cough, watery eyes, and complains of a pain in the throat. The parents smoke at home. The father volunteers the information that he smokes a packet of unfiltered cigarettes a day. The mother says she smokes much less. The child was never breastfed and the parents say that he is quite well although the mother says that young Osmond often has the "irritating habit of not responding to her call". Osmond's temperature is 37.8°C. Examination reveals diffuse inflammation of the oropharynx. Although the child did not complain of symptoms in the ear, examination revealed bilateral serous otits media. Developmental testing is done. Osmond is very shy. He can make 3-word sentences but on initial testing, does not have a vocabulary of more than 10 words.

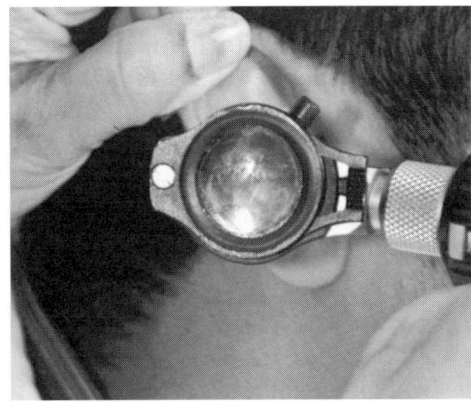

Otoscopic examination of the ear

Relevant history: Sneezing, cough, watery eyes. Exposure to smoke at home. No breastfeeding.

Relevant examination: Findings in the pharynx and ears.

Points to note: The clinical diagnosis of his symptoms suggest pharyngitis. There are symptoms of allergy,

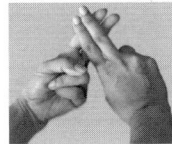

The appearance of a rash makes you examine associated areas in the body.

such as sneezing, cough, watery eyes, and runny nose. There is a low-grade fever, suggestive of a secondary infective viral etiology. The throat is examined and the doctor proceeds to a complete ear and nose examination. Note how important it is to examine the ears in this case. A positive finding in the throat must prompt you to search for all other relevant pathology. Without knowledge of the physical link, one would miss the ear findings.

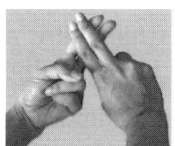

In allergic manifestations, the physical links are the eyes, ears, throat and nose. What other system(s) would you include in your examination of such conditions?

Unlike adults, children do not always complain of all symptoms. Clinically, it seems that they are 'asymptomatic' but often they do not know better and hence remain silent about important symptomatology. *This should reiterate the importance of a thorough physical examination in the pediatric age group.* Moreover, serous otitis media is more commonly underdiagnosed because of its lack of acute or obvious symptoms (compared to acute otitis media (AOM)). Hearing difficulties, loss of balance and delayed speech development can occur with recurrent acute otitis media (AOM). Structural changes to the tympanic membrane can occur. Problems with speech and language development with permanent hearing loss can result if undiagnosed. Like Osmond, the problems with decreased hearing secondary to fluid in the middle ear can "irritate" an adult who is not aware that the child is genuinely unable to hear. Various forms of nonaccidental injury as a result of undetected hearing impairment can potentially occur.

CCCC

Correlate (with other clinical signs), *Compare* (with the other ear), *Capture* (the abnormality) and *Confirm* (the diagnosis).

Case Study 6: Persistent Rhinorrhea and Sneezing in a Cat Lover[6,8,14,17,20,23]

A polite 6-year-old primary school Indian boy gives a history of persistent nasal airway obstruction associated with clear rhinorrhea, which at times

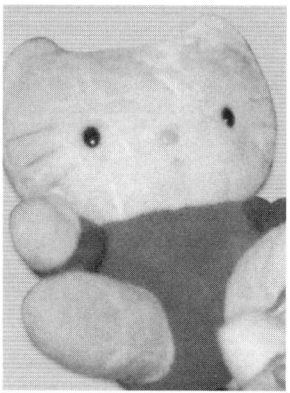

Contact with unclean furry toys, furry pets and pigeon droppings can cause persistent rhinorrhea in a child.

becomes purulent. He constantly sneezes, especially in the morning. He often has watery itchy eyes. He also tells the doctor that even his throat and ears itch as the doctor takes the history from both the mother and the young boy. The doctor asks him if he sometimes feels a tickle in his throat and he says 'yes, sir', especially when he goes to sleep. He has been to a number of clinics and has been treated with repeated courses of antibiotics. He frequently misses his activities at his school due to feeling somewhat unwell. The social history reveals that the apartment where they live is near an active construction site and that there are eight kittens at home. 'Some stray kittens are brought home for shelter', he says. Further enquiry also reveals that a pigeon is reared in the neighbor's unit. The mother who did a cyber-search asks the doctor if her not giving breast milk to the boy could explain his symptoms. There is a positive family history of bronchial asthma in his mother when she was young. His older sister has atopic eczema.

Observation of the child reveals that the child is sniffing due to a stuffy nose. The child is mouth breathing. He often rubs his nose. He has a crease over his nasal bridge and the doctor writes in his notes "allergic salute". Examination of the nasal mucosa shows pale congested mucosae especially over the turbinates, and the presence of clear mucous in the nostrils. Dark circles are visible around his eyes.

Relevant history: Persistent rhinorrhea, sneezes especially in the mornings. Watery itchy eyes. Throat and ears itch, a tickle in the throat, eight kittens, a pigeon. Positive family history of allergic disorders.[6,10]

Relevant examination: Pale nasal mucosae, allergic salute, dark circles under his eyes or allergic shiners.[6,10]

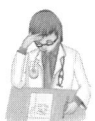

Common complications of a disease are important to ask for in the history and to exclude in the physical examination.

Points to note: Persistent nasal obstruction, clear rhinorrhea, constant morning sneezes, watery itchy eyes, throat and ears and a tickle in the throat are suggestive of an allergic condition including a differential diagnosis of allergic rhinitis. Note the recurrence of symptoms due to the persistent precipitating factors in the history that refer to allergies in various forms. Note the important social history and how his illness has impacted his life by missing school. Cat fur and pigeon droppings are contributory factors. Complications associated with this condition include sinusitis and mucopurulent nasal discharge as a result of secondary bacterial infection. Nasal obstruction, headache and facial pain are symptoms of sinusitis and ear pain is a symptom of otitis media.[6,10] Such complications are historical and physical links if rhinitis is considered as a differential diagnosis. Hence ask about them and look for the relevant signs. Although in clinical practice one must avoid hurting the feelings of patients (especially where self-blame is not a good thing in a mother who feels guilty for not breastfeeding), a gentle reminder that breastfeeding is associated with some protection even in the long-term, against this problem is truthful and may encourage her to breastfeed her future children.

Case Study 7: Nasal Beans, Beads or Ball frame?[8,14,17,20,23]

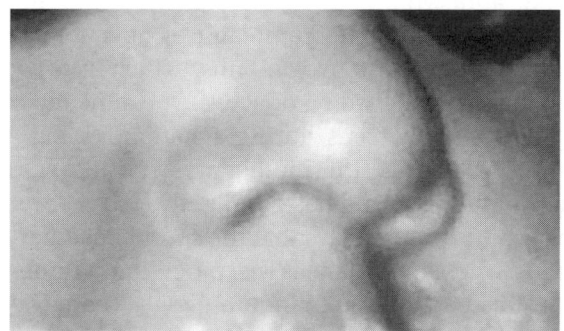

As examination of the nose in a child requires cooperation, take a good history and gather the historical links before the examination.

A mother brings her 4-year-old son who has a purulent unilateral nasal discharge, which is offensive and occasionally blood stained from the left nose of five days duration. Although the boy did not tell his parents anything about putting a bead into his nose, he tells the doctor that he had inserted a small ball frame bead into his left nose a week ago. The boy says that there is some pain in the left nose but experiences no other difficulty. The general practitioner examines the nose and sees part of a red colored object deep in the left nasal cavity. He then refers the case to the ENT for removal of the foreign body as he is cautious not to push a foreign body down the back of the boy's throat where it may be aspirated into the trachea. He also feels that in order to remove the foreign body from the nose he would have to use a topical anesthetic and vasoconstrictor and prefers to refer the case to the ENT for a second opinion and for expert removal.

Relevant history: Purulent unilateral rhinorrhea, occasionally blood stained, inserted a small ball frame bead into nose.

Relevant examination: Observation of part of a red colored object deep in the nasal cavity.

Points to note: Remember never to ignore a unilateral nasal discharge in a child. It must be assumed to be secondary to a foreign body until proven otherwise. The young boy volunteers the history of the ballframe to the doctor. The typical history must lead to a detailed examination of the nose. These foreign bodies usually lodge on the floor of the anterior or middle third of the nasal cavity. A referral to the ENT may be required to remove the bead. The examination of the nose must be done by speculum and a good light. Small toys or erasers too can be hidden in the nose. Beans or other foodstuff, beads, pebbles and paper wads have also been reported.[6,10]

Case Study 8: The Importance of Examination of the Ear in a Febrile Child[6,8,10,14,17,20,23]

A 3-year-old girl is brought to the office by her mother because she has a fever and suddenly complained that her ear hurts. The mother says that she was crying during the night and had little sleep. She has no significant medical history except for cough and a runny nose 3 days ago. It was not easy to examine the distressed young girl. Her temperature was 37.8°C (100°C), respiratory rate was 28 breaths/minute and pulse 110 beats/minute with regular rhythm and good volume. There was no neck stiffness and the reflexes were normal. The plantars were downgoing. The abdominal examination revealed no tenderness including in the suprapubic area and the kidneys were not ballotable. There was no perianal redness or tender swelling in the perianal area.

250 *The Link*: Pediatric History-Taking and Physical Examination

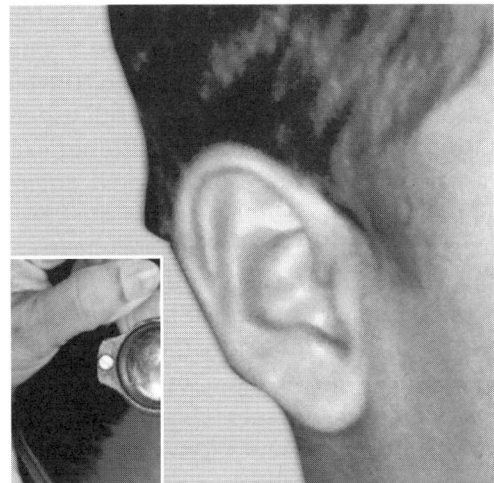

Ear examination is kept to the last in children.

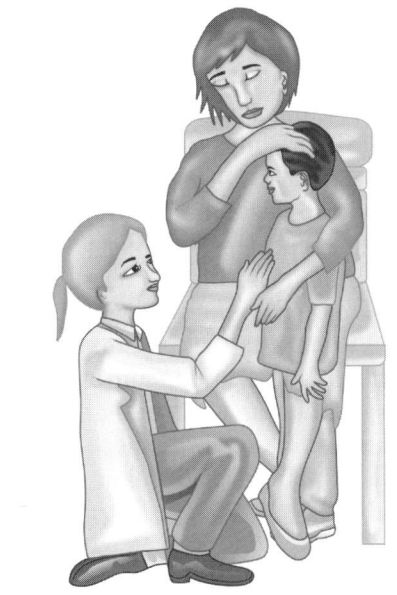

Ear examination is done as the mother gently restrains the child and holds the child's head towards her.

The rest of the physical examination done was normal except for some redness of the throat and thick green mucus in the nose. The child was seated on the mother's lap with her hands and head held. The mother repeated her favorite nursery rhyme to keep her very still. She then cooperated and allowed her ear to be examined with an otoscope. The doctor looked carefully at the tympanic membrane; there was erythema different from the normal tympanic membrane which is pearl gray. The tympanic membrane was bulging. The light reflex was distorted. He looked for a hole in the membrane which would confirm perforation but could see none.

Relevant history: Fever, ear pain.

Relevant examination: There is redness, bulging of the ear drum.

Points to note: Symptoms of middle-ear infection as indicated by either otalgia or discomfort referable to the ears resulting in interference with normal activity or sleep are important. A history of recent upper respiratory illness may be obtained in many children. In such cases, remember that examination of the ears is important to make the diagnosis and should be a part of the examination of a child with fever. In this child, the signs and symptoms are of *acute onset* and examination reveals *middle ear infection* as evidenced by redness of the tympanic membrane; the history and physical examination support a diagnosis of acute otitis media. In younger children with fever and irritability, and who may not complain of pain, remember the middle ear, the meninges, the urinary tract and the perianal area as possible "occult" sources of infection, fever and irritability. The negative examination of the systems attempt to exclude these causes of fever in this 3-year-old girl.

CCCC

Correlate (with other clinical signs), *Compare* (with the other ear), *Capture* (the abnormality) and *Confirm* (the diagnosis).

Case Study 9: Lucy's Mother and Aunt are Reassured[8,14,17,20,23]

Lucy, a 3-month-old infant is brought by her mother and her aunt who takes care of her when the mother is at work, with a chief complaint of noisy breathing noticed for the past two months, which gets worse when the infant is feeding or active. The aunt adds that the noise also worsens during agitation, crying, and supine positioning. The mother was not too worried initially, but the sound has got slightly louder recently. However, the mother says that the sound becomes less obvious when the infant is sleeping. The stridor was first noticed at about one month of age. There was no antenatal history of decreased fetal movements and the pregnancy was uneventful. The birth history was unremarkable with an Apgar score of 7 and 9. Lucy is exclusively breastfed. She takes expressed breast milk when mum is at work. The mother does not think that the sound interferes with the baby's feeding although the aunt says that occasionally when she is spoon fed

Formulation of Differential Diagnosis and Provisional Diagnosis

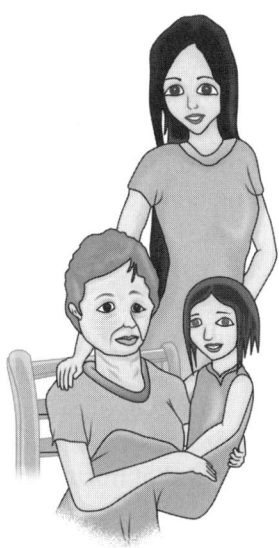

Listening to the members of the family who take care of the child is important.

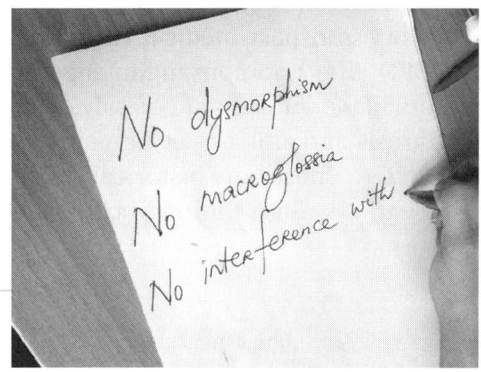

What diagnoses are the negative observations attempting to exclude?

expressed breast milk, she does cough and vomit a little. The aunt also remembers one episode where the baby's noisy breathing had got worse when she suffered from a blocked nose. Lucy was taken to a GP then who told her mother to continue vigorous breastfeeding and to come back for a review if she got any worse. She had recovered in a week's time.

On examination, the child was alert and active. There was no dysmorphism. There was no micrognathia or macroglossia. The facies were not coarse. There was no umbilical hernia. The skin showed no hemangiomata. Her growth parameters of weight, length and circumference of head (COH) were between the 25th and 50th percentile. She was afebrile. There was inspiratory stridor. The chest was clear. All other systems examination was normal.

Relevant history: Age, worsening factors associated with the noisy breathing.

Relevant examination: Normal growth and chest examination, inspiratory stridor.

Points to note: Laryngomalacia is a differential diagnosis in a well child with stridor that has been persistent. It is the most common cause of chronic stridor in infants. The history and age of presentation is fairly typical. However, it is important to differentiate this condition from other causes of noisy breathing (Refer to Chapters 3 and 10).

The pertinent negatives mentioned in the physical examination attempt to exclude other causes of stridor.

Also to note is that children with laryngomalacia cope poorly with upper respiratory illness or croup. Thus, in children with laryngomalacia, a mild respiratory infection can result in respiratory compromise and the advice and close observation (by calling back for review) done by the GP in the past history was indeed required of Lucy's condition. Lucy had luckily recovered uneventfully.

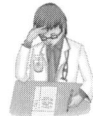

The negatives in the history and physical examination help in the diagnosis and dictate conservative management for Lucy.

The absence of respiratory distress and the normal growth of the child help make a clinical diagnosis. A "wait" and "watch" attitude can be adopted and the infant followed up to ensure that growth is normal and that the stridor gradually improves. Although it is generally a benign condition and both the mother and the aunt can be reassured, sometimes other associated symptoms that may be observed in this condition such as regurgitation, vomiting, cough, choking, and slow feeding due to difficulty in coordinating sucking, swallowing and breathing as a result of the upper airway obstruction are potential complications.

Case Study 10: The Most Common Viral Respiratory Illness in Children under 2 years of Age[8,14,17,20,23]

A male infant of 6 months has a short history of coryzal symptoms. This was followed by a history of coughing, wheezing, and breathlessness. Many members of the family have just recovered from an upper respiratory tract infection.

There is no previous history of wheezing episodes and the child has been well prior to the illness. The child was born full-term and had an uneventful neonatal

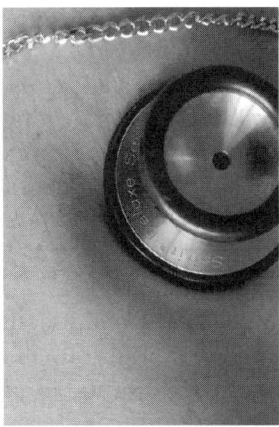
In an infant, auscultation of the chest is performed soon after observation

period. There is no previous history to suggest feeding difficulties, scalp sweating during feeds or poor weight gain.

There is no family history of asthma. The parents are non-consanguineous. There is no known family history of inherited respiratory disorders. No one smokes at home.

The child whose growth percentiles are on the 50th centile has tachypnea with a respiratory rate of 50 per minute and difficulty with taking his usual feeds due to the high respiratory rate. The temperature is 37.8°C. Although the infant is distressed, he is not irritable. On examination of the chest, gross hyperinflation of the chest is evident. normal. There are chest retractions. On auscultation, there are generalized fine crackles and diffuse wheezing. The liver is palpated 2 cm below the right costal margin, although the liver span is normal.

Relevant history: Age, coryzal symptoms, family history of coryza.

Relevant examination: The chest findings on inspection and auscultation.

Points to note: While many differential diagnosis are excluded in the history, it is fair to consider bronchiolitis as one of the most likely differential diagnosis in this case. This is based on the age and the clinical presentation. Other family members with a respiratory tract infection is an important event to elicit in the history-taking of children with respiratory diseases. Based on the history and physical findings, another possible differential diagnosis in this case is viral pneumonitis. In viral pneumonitis, fever, nonproductive cough, upper respiratory illness and systemic symptoms like myalgia and headaches may occur making the young child miserable and irritable.

Although most congenital lesions present early in life and the history in this case is acute in nature, it is good practice to exclude congenital problems in all infants. Excluding conditions such as prematurity and underlying chronic lung diseases is useful as such children are at higher risk of complications in an acute respiratory illness. Remember also that you must ask questions that will differentiate it from other causes of wheezing. The absence of recurrent wheezing episodes and the absence of a family history of asthma are important negative points. The history of being well previously and of normal growth are asked to attempt to differentiate congenital lung diseases that cause wheezing, for example, congenital cystic adenomatoid malformation of the lung or a vascular ring, congenital lobar emphysema, and cardiac causes of wheezing, such as heart failure. The normal neonatal history and past medical history attempts to exclude BPD. The non-consanguineous marriage of the parents make autosomal recessive conditions like cystic fibrosis and alpha-1-antitrypsin deficiency (ATD) less likely. These are historical links in the family history to ask, for a thorough clinical clerking of the case.

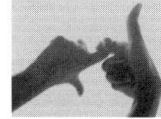
Historical links add weight to the provisional diagnosis.

In acute bronchiolitis, a condition common under two years of age, bronchiolar inflammation causes narrowing of the airways and air trapping. Air trapping produces hyperinflation of the lungs and pushes the liver downwards. Although most normal children will recover, high risk groups include bronchiolitis in the very young infant, bronchiolitis with underlying heart disease, chronic lung diseases or immunodeficiencies syndromes. Treatment is supportive aiming at maintaining fluid intake. Remember that a tachypneic infant must be helped by nasogastric tube feeding both to conserve the energy utilization during feeding as well as to prevent aspiration. Intravenous fluids may also be used. Hypoxia must be prevented and pulse oximetry is useful in monitoring these infants. Hypoxia is indicated by a oxygen saturation below 93%.

Formulation of Differential Diagnosis and Provisional Diagnosis

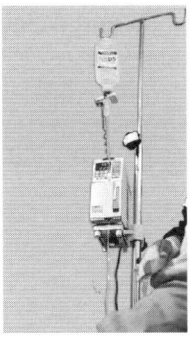

Intravenous fluids may be used in a tachypneic child for many important reasons. What are they?

Case Study 11: History of Recurrence of Illness, Reactivation by Trigger Factors and Response—Bronchial Asthma[8,14,17,20,23]

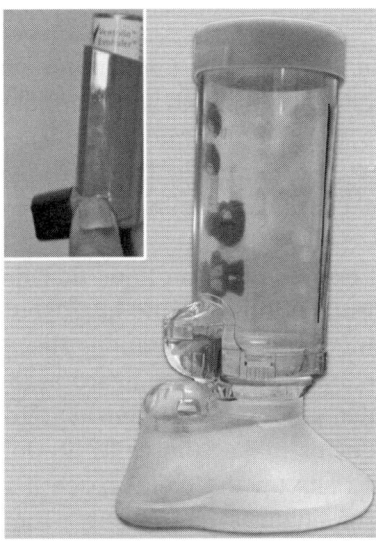

The AeroChamber with mask is a spacer device which can be used along with some metered-dose inhalers to treat bronchial asthma in children.

Abdullah, a 4-year-old Malay boy is brought for an acute attack of wheezing and cough, associated with upper respiratory infections for the past two days. There is a history of nocturnal cough in the past one month. Smoke and strong odors precipitate the symptoms.

The past medical history indicates that the child gets episodes of coughing and wheezing about once in 6 months and these are relieved by nebulizers that he takes regularly at a nearby clinic. He also has suffered from dry skin and eczema as an infant. Both his parents smoke at home and Abdullah loves his pet hamster which he rears in a cage in his room. There is a family history of eczema and asthma in the siblings.

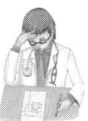

"The general examination, including observation on growth and nutritional deficiencies are important in a growing child with a chronic disease. Observation of deformities of the chest tells me something about the trend and duration of the illness and, the severity and the control of bronchial asthma. Atopic manifestations like flexural eczema and xerosis can give me an indication of etiology. Observation is very important in pediatrics!"

On examination, the child's height and weight are on the 10th centile. His parents are well built and of medium height. The child is not pale and there are no signs of nutritional deficiencies. Observation of the chest indicates hyperinflation, recession and the use of accessory muscles and a Harrison's sulcus deformity. There are dry lichenified areas noted at the flexures of the elbows and knees. There is pityriasis alba and xerosis noted on the skin of the face and body.

The child looks tired and has a cough. There is tachypnea and tachycardia. There are intercostal retractions. There is no cyanosis.

Auscultation of the chest reveals a prolonged expiratory phase. There is generalized wheezing.

There are no crackles. The CVS examination is normal. All other systems are unremarkable.

History: *Recurrence* of attacks, *reactivation* of symptoms by flu, and *response* to bronchodilators.

Examination: Atopic eczema, pityriasis alba and xerosis as signs of atopy. Prolonged expiratory phase with wheezing.

Points to note: Recurrence of symptoms, reactivation of symptoms by identifiable precipitating factors and good response to bronchodilators make the most likely diagnosis in Abdullah be bronchial asthma. The relief of symptoms by bronchodilators is highly suggestive of reversible airway disease. The history should elicit the frequency of attacks, the severity of the attacks indicating the nature of the asthma and exacerbating and relieving factors. Physical examination must assess the severity of the present attack. All related signs of atopy and chronicity must be sought. The height and weight are important to assess. A comparison with parents is made as genetics influence growth in height. In Abdullah, weight and height are unsatisfactory. Various factors like frequent viral infections and persistent nasal allergies can interfere with a child's appetite. Daily symptoms of nocturnal cough and exacerbations of asthma increase energy utilization in the growing child. Nocturnal cough causes vomiting and, if it occurs regularly, can contribute to the poor weight gain. Exacerbations of attacks of asthma itself are associated with increased energy expenditure in the form of tachypnea, tachycardia, and usage of accessory muscles of respiration. Growth, both height and weight, must be monitored in all asthmatic patients both as a reflection of severity of asthma as well as an indicator of control. Remember also to dwell on the attacks and the impact of the disease on Abdullah's daily activities. It is clear that besides objective measurements of the severity of asthma like peak flow monitoring in a child who can cooperate, the control and severity of asthma can be well assessed by both a good history and a thorough physical examination; one complementing the other.

SYSTEM: CARDIOVASCULAR[1]

Case Study 12: An Asymptomatic Child with a Heart Murmur[1,8,14,17,20,22,23]

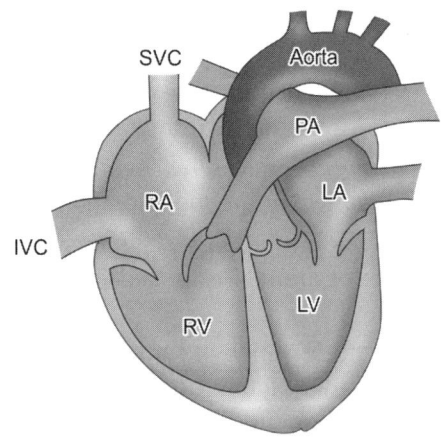

Functional murmurs may be heard in normal hearts in childhood. What are the features of such a murmur?

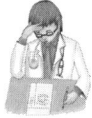

"Although the child is growing well, the heart sounds on auscultation are not normal and there is a murmur that does not fulfill the criteria of a physiological murmur. I think that such a cardiac lesion in this well thriving child who is asymptomatic is not causing hemodynamic problems... What could it be?"

An 18-month-old infant is brought for routine vaccination. The doctor who auscultates the child and plots growth percentiles before vaccination of all children finds that there is a fixed splitting of the second heart sound. The height and weight are just under the 50th centile for age.

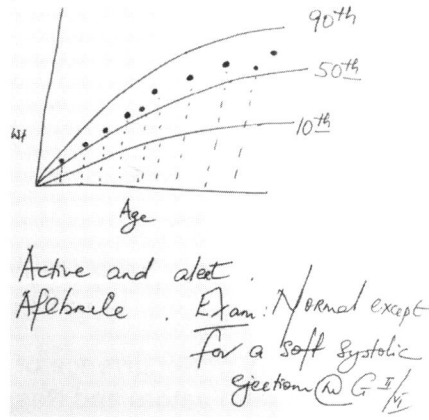

Growth is an important consideration in suspected heart diseases.

The child was not pale, temperature was 37°C, the pulse rate was 110 beats/min with normal rate, rhythm and volume and the respiratory rate was 30 breaths/min. His BP was 90/55 mmHg. There is no dysmorphism. There is no chest cage deformity or obvious spinal deformity.

On CVS examination, he finds that the first heart sound is normal but the second heart sound is split in both expiration and in inspiration. He appreciates a systolic ejection murmur best heard at the left upper sternal border, grade 2/6 in intensity, radiating to the back. The doctor makes the child lie down with his legs up, then sits up the child to see if the murmur disappears or changes in intensity. The absence of tachycardia, or fever, the nature of the murmur, and the fact that it does not disappear with changing of the child's position makes him think that it is caused by an underlying cardiac pathology. The fixed splitting of the second heart sound, instead of the physiological split confirms underlying cardiac abnormality. He then puts his findings together to make the most likely diagnosis.

Relevant history: Routine vaccination.

Relevant examination: No chest cage deformity or obvious spinal deformity, first heart sound is normal but the second heart sound is split in both expiration and in inspiration, systolic ejection murmur best heard at the left upper sternal border and radiating to the back.

Points to note: The doctor does a detailed cardiovascular examination. He noticed that the infant was not pale or febrile. Pallor and fever can cause a child to have a functional murmur. A fixed split of the second heart sound is diagnostic of an atrial septal defect (ASD). In ASD, patients may have a systolic ejection murmur best heard at the left upper sternal border; this murmur is caused by the excess volume of blood crossing the pulmonary valve. With moderate or larger defects, an additional mid-diastolic murmur may be appreciated along the lower sternal border due to the volume of blood crossing the tricuspid valve. Children are commonly asymptomatic with this heart condition. Hence, the differentiation from an innocent murmur is important.[1] He re-examined the murmur and noted that it did not change in intensity upon change of posture.

The diagnostic points here are the second heart sound which has a fixed split and the features of the murmur. Fixed splitting of the second heart sound is characteristic of an ASD.[22] To remind you, a split S2 is caused physiologically during inspiration as the increase in venous return overloads the right ventricle and delays the closure of the pulmonary valve. With an atrial septal defect, the right ventricle is 'overloaded' because of the left to right shunt, producing a widely split S2. Because the atria are linked via the defect, there is no net pressure change between the atria in inspiration, and inspiration does not influence the splitting of S2.[22] Therefore, S2 is split to the same extent during inspiration and expiration, and is termed as "fixed".[22] The differentiation of a physiological murmur from a pathological murmur in an asymptomatic child is based on the abnormal second heart sound, the murmur not changing in intensity when the child sits up or lies down with legs lifted (this happens in a venous hum), and the radiation of the murmur to the back which does not occur in a physiological murmur. A physiological murmur occurs in a normal heart where heart sounds are normal, it changes with position and does not radiate (remember the 10 links beginning with 'S'[23]—*refer to Chapter 10*). In children, physiological murmurs include Still's murmurs, low-pitched murmurs heard at the lower left sternal area; pulmonary flow murmurs, high-pitched, harsher murmurs heard at the upper left sternal border; systemic flow murmurs, caused by normal blood flow into the aorta and the vessels of the head and neck are heard higher up in the chest and above the clavicles.[1,16] Venous hums are physiological murmurs that are low-pitched continuous murmurs produced by blood returning from the great veins to the heart.[1,16]

Case Study 13: A 5-month-old with a VSD[1,8,14,17,20,22,23]

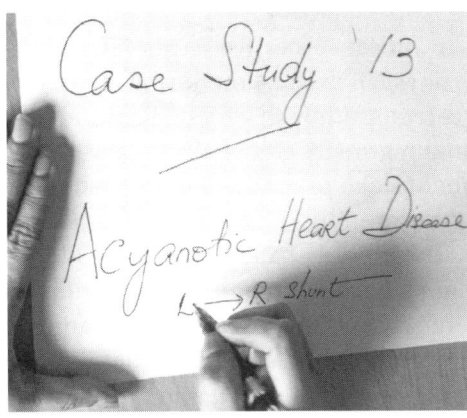

A ventricular septal defect is the most common acyanotic heart disease in children. Tachypnea, tachycardia, cardiomegaly, hepatomegaly, fine basal crackles, and failure to thrive are the cardinal signs of heart failure in infancy.

Siva, a 5-month old Indian male infant is brought by his mother with excessive scalp sweating. The sweating is especially notable during feeds. The mother also says that he looks very tired during feeds and most of the bottle feeds go unfinished though he sucks vigorously. The child is noticed to be small for his age. The mother is concerned that the child is not putting on weight like his other siblings. His past history indicates hospitalization at three and a half months for pneumonia. The infant is a product of a spontaneous vaginal delivery (SVD) born at term at 2.5 kg. The history of pregnancy and delivery are normal and he is the third child in the family. His two other older siblings are well.

Examination: An alert looking infant. Crying off and on. Not cyanosed. Slightly pale. Growth in weight and length are below the third percentile. Mild subcostal chest recessions are seen. Temperature is 37°C, heart rate 181 beats/min, respiratory rate 60 breaths/minute, CVS examination: S1 and S2 are normal. The apex beat is located on the 5th intercostal space at the midclavicular line. A pansystolic mumur grade 3/6 is heard, loudest at the lower left sternal edge. A mid-diastolic murmur is heard at apex. There are fine crackles in the lung bases. The liver is just palpable.

Relevant history: Sweating during feeding, tired during feeds, hospitalization at three and a half months for pneumonia.

Relevant examination: Tachycardia and tachypnea. Apex beat is located on the 5th intercostal space. A pansystolic mumur is heard at the lower left sternal edge. The fine crackles at bases of lungs. The liver is just palpable 2 cm below the costal margin.

Points to note: Excessive scalp sweating during feeding, physical exhaustion during feeds, inability to complete feeds although very hungry and an inability to maintain growth either secondary to decreased nutritional intake or an increased catabolic state are important symptoms of significant cardiac disease in infancy. The child is failing to thrive as indicated by the mother's observation and the growth percentiles on examination. The excessive sweating is as a consequence of increased sympathetic tone seen in children who are in heart failure. The auscultatory signs are indicative of a VSD. The mid-diastolic murmur indicates that the flow caused by the VSD is significant and in this case, as can be seen from the history and physical examination, has caused heart failure in this infant. In this infant, the VSD has resulted in problems of growth, although a more detailed nutritional history is warranted. Additionally, it is important to look for nutritional deficiencies in the physical examination of this infant. Pallor is one important sign that has been obtained. Other positive or negative signs pertaining to nutritional assessment must be mentioned.

The child is tachycardic and tachypneic for age. The apex beat is on the 5th intercostal space at the mid clavicular line; hence, there is cardiomegaly on examination. The liver is just palpable and the lung bases have fine crackles which indicate heart failure.

Tachypnea, tachycardia, cardiomegaly, fine crackles in the lung bases, hepatomegaly, scalp sweating, and failure to thrive are cardinal signs and symptoms of cardiac failure in infancy. The size of the VSD determines much of the clinical manifestations. The location of the defect at the interventricular septum, such as if at the muscular part of the interventricular septum, membranous, inlet or oulet VSD also bears influence on whether or not the VSD will spontaneously close. While a small VSD may be asymptomatic, moderate to large shunts cause pulmonary congestion with signs and symptoms of heart failure. Siva's growth must be closely monitored and he must be immediately started on antifailure medication. He must also be urgently referred for further assessment including a chest X-ray, ECG and echocardiography and for surgical management of the VSD.

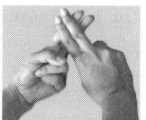

Link and search for respiratory infections in a child with acyanotic cardiac disease with a left to right shunt like a VSD.

Respiratory infections are a result of increased pulmonary blood flow leading to pulmonary vascular congestion. Symptoms of a VSD, may be clearly apparent by the age of 2–3 months when pulmonary vascular resistance decreases (pulmonary pressures decrease).

Case Study 14: An Infant with Colic[2,4,7,8,11,13,14,17,20,21,23]

A tense lady, who is a teacher and a mother of a two and a half month old baby boy, reports to you that her baby has been crying much more often than the baby had, before in the past three weeks. She says that the crying in the evening is inconsolable and can last for 2–3 hours and describes the cry as "a piercing, high-pitched scream." The baby is well in between episodes of crying. The baby is fully breastfed and the mother says that her own diet has not changed in the past three weeks except that she admits to have been eating a lot of chocolates, brought by her sister from Switzerland, for the past few weeks. The mother has not been on excessive cow's milk products. The young infant passes loose seedy greenish yellow stool once to twice every day. The mother is happy with the weight of the child and feels that he is putting on weight adequately. The mother who is keen on her child's weekly weight gain, says the child puts on about 200 g/week.

The child is afebrile and is held comfortably in the mother's arms at the time of examination. The baby coos at the red ball in front of him, smiles and babbles in response to his mother's overtures. On physical examination, the baby's weight, length and circumference of head are on the 50th centile and no abnormalities were detected. The baby has a lusty cry. The fontanel is normotensive. The abdomen is not distended. On palpation, it is soft. There are no abnormal masses felt. The hernial orifices are normal. Both testes are descended into the scrotal sac and are normal. Sometimes borborygmi can be heard and the baby passes flatus with some relief.[4] There is no perianal fissure, mass, redness or excoriation. The ears are carefully examined and are normal. A developmental assessment indicates that all aspects of his development

Formulation of Differential Diagnosis and Provisional Diagnosis

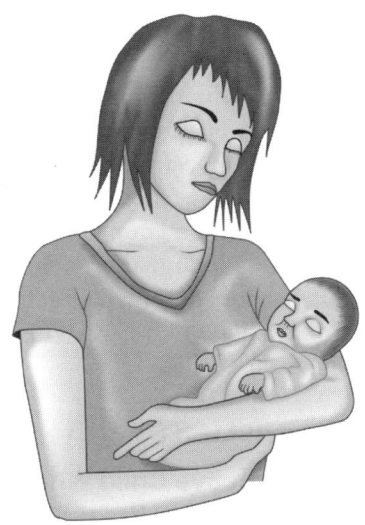

Infantile colic is a diagnosis of exclusion.

are normal for age. The doctor elicits the Moro reflex: when the infant is held on his back with head supported, and head suddenly allowed to drop slightly, the arms spread and then flex back to body bilaterally. This is interpreted to be normal.

Relevant history: Crying at same time every day, well in between episodes, loose seedy stools.

Relevant examination: Weight, height and circumference of head are on the 50th percentiles, normal baby, normal examination.

Points to note: The baby is growing well. The stools are typical of normal breastfed infant stools. The normal growth parameters including the COH and normotensive fontanel are important as CNS abnormalities and subdural hematomas can cause excessive crying in infants. Gastrointestinal causes such as constipation, cow's milk protein intolerance, gastroesophageal reflux, lactose intolerance and rectal fissures are vital to exclude in the physical examination of such an infant as well.[4] Infective causes such as middle ear infection and urinary tract infections must always be looked for. It is important to exclude otitis media, and meningitis, urinary tract infection and any other focus of sepsis. The lusty cry of an active child and the completely normal physical examination, including abdominal examination for masses, and the examination of the genitalia and hernial orifices are done to exclude all other conditions that can cause the infant pain and result in unconsolable crying episodes. Infantile colic is a diagnosis of exclusion.

The mother not taking excessive cow's milk is an important historical point as cow's milk protein, when excessive in the mother's diet, can enter human milk and trigger symptoms of cow's milk protein allergy (CMPA). Mothers who breastfeed must not stop breastfeeding if the infant has colic as this does not relieve symptoms and deprives the baby numerous benefits of breastfeeding. A systematic review of randomized controlled trials found a possible therapeutic benefit from eliminating milk products, eggs, wheat, and nuts from the diet of breastfeeding mothers.[7] Could the chocolates containing cow's milk have contributed to the symptoms? Crying at a particular time each day without vomiting or alteration in bowel habit suggests that the differential diagnosis to consider is infantile colic. This is a diagnosis of exclusion after a complete and detailed examination of the abdomen, the ears and the anterior fontanels are done. In infantile colic, maternal anxiety must be allayed as anxiety potentially aggravates the situation. If colic is confirmed, the mother should be told that these symptoms will reduce after 3 months or so. Having made a diagnosis of infantile colic by a careful history and examination, the doctor acknowledged the difficulties the mother was facing and enquired more deeply into the mother's well-being.

SYSTEM: GASTROINTESTINAL TRACT[2,18,19,21]

Recurrent Abdominal Pain

Case Study 15 : Exclude Treatable Causes by History and Examination, Do Basic Investigations Then, If Normal, Call it "Functional Abdominal Pain"[8,14,17,20,23]
Helen, a bright 10-year-old girl is brought by her parents with recurrent abdominal pain for the past 4 months. The pain often comes in the morning and the child misses many classes. The pain is not usually worse with eating, but it is worse when the girl is under stress or is anxious. There is no vomiting or constipation. There is no noticed weight loss. The social history reveals that the child has been anxious and even tense due to intense peer competition in her elite primary school.

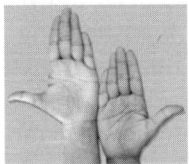

Examine the child in detail to exclude important organic causes of abdominal pain.

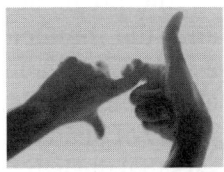

In this case, the mother's diet is a historical link.

An important examination is due next month which will then determine her continued education in that school.

All her other siblings were class toppers for that examination and the parents expect the same from her. She is described by her parents to have a tense and at certain times, obsessive personality. Her academic performance though satisfactory does not meet the expectations of her parents.

There is a family background of ill-defined headaches and peptic disorders.

Examination shows normal growth parameters. There is no fever.

Examination reveals that the abdominal pain is localized to the periumbilical area. Examination of all systems were normal. Her urine was tested to be normal.

Relevant history: 4 months of abdominal pain, no vomiting, no constipation, no weight loss, anxious, peer pressure, high parental expectations.

Relevant examination: Periumbilical pain, all other examinations are normal.

Points to note: The absence of physical symptoms in abdominal pain does not in itself exclude organic causes of abdominal pain. However, the history and physical examination taken together highlights that the patient is otherwise well, and the pain has an association with classes at school. The age of the patient, the pressure that is put on her in terms of high expectations, the description of her personality and the site of the pain suggest that one must keep the differential diagnosis of a functional abdominal pain in mind in this patient. It is the duty of any doctor to exclude organic causes of abdominal pain. Differentiate functional abdominal pain and irritable bowel syndrome from more serious underlying disorders.[18,19] Important warning signs have to be excluded in the history. Remember that a complete history and physical examination, including determination of the degree of functional interference, (like missing school) is vital. Activities of daily living such as going to school, playing games and so on must always be asked and do bear relevance to the clinical diagnosis and management. Sinister symptoms that warrant detailed investigation include history of fever, vomiting, weight loss, site of pain away from the umbilicus, bilious vomiting, blood in stool, blood in vomitus and, in the adolescent, a history suggestive of delayed or precocious puberty. Another important feature of pathological abdominal pain which is absent here is nocturnal pain.

A complete blood count, erythrocyte sedimentation rate, amylase, lipase and a urinalysis are important basic investigations that must be done before attributing symptoms to a functional cause. Abdominal ultrasonography is an investigation, without radiation hazard, that may readily be used. If all tests are normal, management could include counseling on learning to relax during times of pain and approaches for the child to stay involved in school and regular activities without undue stress or anxiety. A referral to a behavioral therapist may be useful.

SYSTEM: HEPATOBILIARY

Case Study 16: An Active Child Who is Jaundiced and Exclusively Breastfed[8,14,17,20,23]

A full-term infant, 2 weeks of age is brought by the mother with a bilirubin of 260 µmol/l. The jaundice was first noticed on day 10 of life. The baby's blood group is the same as that of the mother (O +ve) and the Glucose-6-phosphate dehydrogenase (G6PD) status is normal.

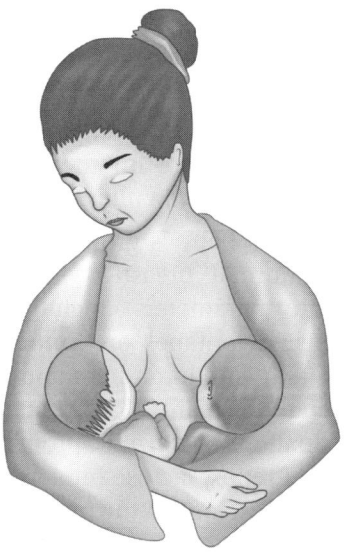

A healthy breastfeeding mother has enough breastmilk to feed her twins. Link breastmilk jaundice to a breastmilk constituent that inhibits conjugation of bilirubin.

The pregnancy and delivery had been uneventful and the mother is successfully breastfeeding her 2-week-old infant. The mother has not given anything else although adviced by the grandmother to give plenty of plain water to clear the jaundice. The mother says that the baby initially lost some weight but has now regained birth weight. She says that the child sucks well and that her breasts are often engorged.

There was jaundice which appeared on day 10 but the infant was continuously and exclusively breastfed. The stool and urine were of normal color. The mother remembers that her older child who was also exclusively breastfed was noted to be jaundiced for about a month.

Clinical examination revealed a vigorous infant with a lusty cry. Examination of all systems was entirely normal. There was noted jaundice clinically assessed to be moderate in severity.

Relevant history: Sucking well, jaundice appeared on the tenth day of life.

Relevant examination: Vigorous infant, lusty cry, jaundice.

Points to note: From history and physical examination, the infant has no evidence of any other cause of jaundice, such as hemolysis, infections, biliary atresia, or metabolic diseases. Remember that some breastfed infants develop a harmless form of jaundice (unconjugated hyperbilirubinemia) as the milk of these mothers contains 5-beta-pregnane-3-alpha, 20-beta-diol or nonesterified long chain fatty acids which competitively inhibit the conjugating enzyme, glucuronide tranferase. In some other mothers, their milk may contain a glucuronidase that contributes to the jaundice. Also remember that normal neonates lose up to 10% of their body weight in the first 10 days of life. This is then regained and from then, there is a constant rise in body weight.

Case Study 17: Breastfeeding Jaundice as Opposed to Breast Milk Jaundice[8,14,17,20,23]

A six-day-old infant who is breastfed is brought with jaundice, insufficient milk intake and poor weight gain. The child is jaundiced. The mother says that she does not feel that her breasts are engorged when she compares them to the breastfeeding experience of her older child who is now two years old. The mother also says that not much breast milk is obtained when she pumps her breasts.

She comments that she does not often change the nappies of the infant as it is usually dry. The mother and child are blood group O positive. The infant's G6PD status is normal.

The infant is alert but not very active. He is mildly dehydrated. The urine looks concentrated. There is jaundice. The anterior fontanel is not sunken. When the breastfeeding technique is observed by the doctor, he finds that the infant does not latch properly to the breast.

Relevant history: Insufficient milk, mother does not feel breast engorgement, infrequent nappy change.

Relevant examination: Mild dehydration, poor latching on breast.

Points to note: When breastfeeding is inadequate, an increase in unconjugated bilirubin secondary to an exaggerated enterohepatic circulation of bilirubin occurs. Improved milk production and intake will resolve the jaundice.

Water supplements have no effect on bilirubin and should not be given in breastfed infants. Weight loss of more than 10% from birth weight, clinical evidence of dehydration and less than five wet pampers a day are high risk factors in a neonate who is jaundiced. The doctor has to counsel on the proper technique of breastfeeding. Good attachment of baby to mother's breast is indicated by recognizable features in an infant who suckles (Refer to Chapter 6). A lactation consultant can also ideally be involved.

Case Study 18: Dehydration-Sara's Eagerness to Drink Avoided her Hospital Admission[8,14,17,20,23]

Sara, an 18-month-old girl, was brought to the emergency department of a busy district hospital by her mother, a hospital assistant. Mum says that she had 10 watery green stools and vomited five times in the previous 12 hours. She has a poor appetite but is eager to drink. She has no fever. There is no blood in the stool and the vomitus is clear yellow in color. On enquiry, her mum says that she has not passed much urine for the past 10 hours. She attends a daycare nursery where a few other children are reported to be 'unwell' with diarrhea. Sara has been previously well, with normal growth and development. Her mother had her most recent weight

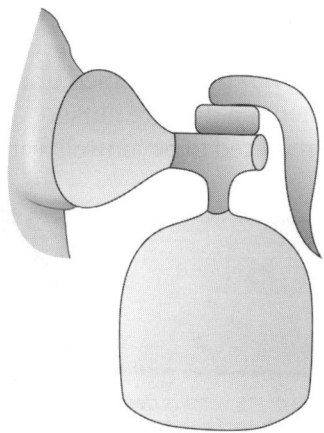

A breast pump.

records taken eight days back when she got her booster injections. Her mother did not take her for the rotavirus vaccine as it was rather expensive and not yet offered in the government vaccination schedule.

On examination, the child was thirsty and irritable. Her eyes looked sunken. The doctor in the ER records a drop in weight by 8%. The temperature was 37.5°C. The pulse rate was 160 beats/min and the pulses were weak. Her respiratory rate was 40 breaths/min. The capillary refill was less than 2 seconds. The blood pressure was normal. The skin turgor was slightly reduced as the skin pinch went back slowly. Although Sara was drinking water frequently, her mucous membranes were dry. The anterior fontanel was slightly depressed. Her abdomen was soft. Her bowel sounds were normal. As Sara was irritable but thirsty, the doctor tells the mother that she is moderately dehydrated. The doctor says that there is need to admit Sara for intravenous fluid replacement if she does not improve with oral rehydration solution. He keeps Sara in the observation room and observes her closely. The mother agrees to try oral rehydration, and the child is repeatedly offered small sips of a commercial oral rehydration solution. The child asks for her favorite glass with the little teddy bear by the side.

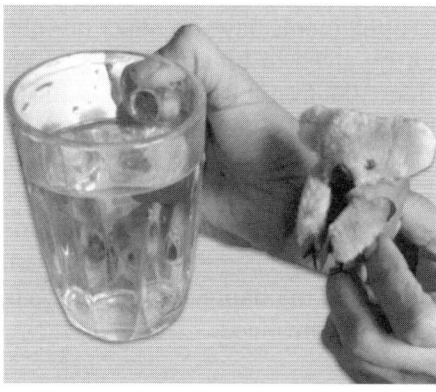

Thirst is an important compensatory mechanism in dehydration.

The mother also continues breastfeeding. During the period of observation both Sara's mum and the doctor are happy to see that Sara reaches out for the glass, cup or spoon when it is offered to her. When the cup is taken away, Sara is unhappy because she wants to drink more. They then give her as much as she can take and mum breastfeeds too.

After two hours, the vomiting settles. Sara is less irritable and happier now. Her pulse is 140 beats/min with improved volume. These positive clinical signs have negated the need for intravenous fluids. The child is discharged after 6 hours observation in hospital and the mother is advised to reintroduce Sara to her usual diet as soon as this is tolerated. The doctor thanks the mother for playing her part in avoiding another admission for the day!

He also gives the mother leaflets for the other mothers at Sara's daycare center and some advice on the rotavirus vaccination that is available at the nearest clinic. He explains to the mother that Sara is too old to be given the rotavirus vaccination which is given between 6 weeks and 8 months.

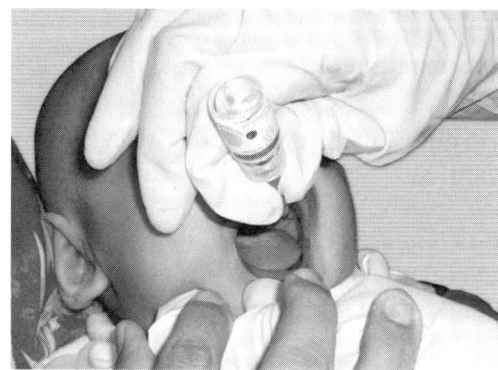

Like oral polio, rotavirus vaccination is also given by the oral route. (Photograph courtesy: Associate Professor Dr Loh Keng Yin, reprint with permission).

Relevant examination: Child thirsty and restless. The temperature was 37°C. She was irritable. The pulse rate was 160 beats/min and the pulses were weak. Her respiratory rate was 40 breaths/min. The capillary refill was less than 2 seconds. The blood pressure was normal. The skin turgor was slightly reduced. Although Sara was drinking water frequently, her mucous membranes were dry. The anterior fontanel was slightly depressed. Upon drinking in the observation room, the pulse rate decreases to 140 beats/minute and with improved volume.

Relevant history: Ten watery green stools and five vomits in the previous 12 hours. She is eating poorly but drinks eagerly, not passing much urine for the past 12 hours. She attends a daycare nursery where a few other children are reported to be 'unwell' with diarrhea.

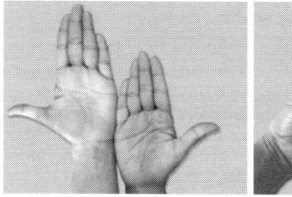 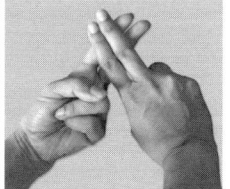

Examine the signs of the various degrees of dehydration linking closely to the history and the clinical state of the patient to arrive at the complete diagnosis.

Points to note: Sara has signs of moderate dehydration. Rotavirus is an important cause of hospitalization as a result of dehydration in children. Children with mild-to-moderate dehydration should be treated with oral rehydration solutions but to do this without resorting to intravenous therapy, you must be sure that the child is feeding well and eager to drink like Sara. In moderate dehydration, difficulty in sucking or swallowing, having to be coaxed to drink or lethargy are indications to err on the safe side and admit for intravenous therapy. Children with severe dehydration or shock need to be admitted for administration of intravenous fluids. Antimotility drugs are not indicated in children with gastroenteritis, as the possible risks outweigh the advantages. The doctor does his part in preventive health care—a duty that all doctors should not forget, regardless of how busy they are. The development of the rotavirus vaccine is of great public health benefit and should be incorporated into the government immunization schedule.

Case Study 19: An Uncooperative Child is Better Examined on the Mother's Lap[8,14,17,20,23]

A 2-month old male infant presents with an abdominal mass noted 3 days ago when the baby was given a bath. The young resident was told by the mother that the infant has been crying and is very irritable lately. The mother who is exclusively breastfeeding the infant also complains that the child feeds poorly. The mother notes that the child is warm to touch and feels that the child has become pale. The stool and urine were normal. Her prenatal ultrasound suspected oligohydramnious. The child had a spontaneous vaginal delivery at 35 weeks. The Apgar score was 8 (1 minute), 9 (5 minutes) and there were no complications except for neonatal jaundice which required phototherapy.

The review of systems was unremarkable. In particular there was no diarrhea, neither was there profuse sweating. There was no vomiting, bilious or otherwise. There was no disturbance of bowel or micturition.

On examination, the infant looked thin. He was pale. There was no jaundice. The abdominal examination was difficult as the child was irritable and refused to lie down. The doctor knelt down on her knees and examined the child who was more comfortable on the mother's lap. The mother would intermittently distract the child by familiar sounds of a rattle. Sometimes she would breastfeed the child. The doctor observed fullness in the left flank. During both superficial and deep palpation, she felt a mass in the left flank. The surface was irregular and nontender. It was ballotable. Percussion note of the mass was tympanic.

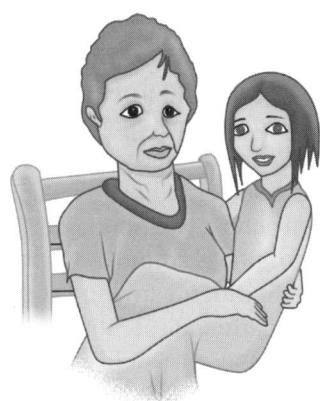

The flexibility of the pediatric physical examination—it is permitted that an uncooperative child is examined on the mother's lap or in any position the child is comfortable with.

The bowel sounds were normal. There was one small lymph node palpable in the left inguinal area. Based on the site, the ballotable feature of the mass and the cystic nature, the doctor felt that it was a mass originating from the left kidney. The history of oligohydramnios was now relevant. Reasonable differentials were considered. A plain radiograph of the abdomen and ultrasound of the abdomen were done.[21]

Relevant history: Abdominal mass. The child feeds poorly, child has become pale.

Relevant examination: A mass in the flank which was hard, irregular, nontender, tympanic, ballotable.[21]

Points to note: The patient's age, history, and physical examination are crucial in evaluating a child with an abdominal mass. The causes differ between neonates, infants and children.[18] A thorough physical examination can be difficult in the very young or uncooperative child. Various approaches to keep the child happy can be innovated in order to gain maximum information from the physical examination. For example, a parent's lap is a good substitute for the examination couch, especially with apprehensive young patients. The mother could breastfeed her child while the exposed abdomen is inspected. The infant or toddler should lie supine with the abdomen exposed for inspection of protrusion, bulging, peristaltic waves, or asymmetry. The examiner must ensure that her hands are warm so as not to discomfort the child. Cooperation of the mother by distraction can be extremely helpful for relaxing the child and abdomen. The abdominal palpation must start with light palpation of all 4 quadrants and the flank areas. On light palpation, the examination should assess for guarding or tenderness. This is followed by deep palpation. Percussion helps outline size of masses and differentiates the underlying components. Solid masses and fluid-filled cysts have a dull percussion note while air-filled structures are tympanic. This is followed by auscultation for bowel sounds.

Based on the findings, can you list the anatomical, etiological and pathological differential diagnosis. What further information would you need? You may refer to other chapters in this book including Chapter 10 to remind you of some of the typical features of renal masses to help you think of the possible differential diagnoses to consider.

SYSTEM: NERVOUS SYSTEM[24,25]

Case Study 20: A Child with Seizures without Fever[8,14,17,20,23,24]

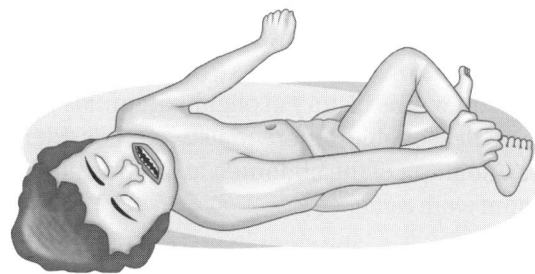

Child suffering from generalized tonic clonic seizure.

A child of nineteen months develops a generalized tonic clonic seizure not associated with fever. The mother, who observed the seizure, says that he was well for the past few days and even on the morning of the seizure. She did not notice any recent change in activity or behavior. Suddenly, as he was sitting on his chair, he experienced tonic clonic movements of his upper and lower limbs associated with uprolling of the eyeballs. There was frothing of saliva from his mouth. This lasted about 10 minutes. There was no sphincter incontinence. He was drowsy soon after the fit, in the postictal period, but after a few hours, he seemed to be his normal self. This was the first episode of such an event observed by the mother. There was no history of fever or known trauma. There is no history of drug ingestion or accidental drug overdose. The child did not have diarrhea or vomiting in the recent past. His appetite was good as usual. In the past, the child has never exhibited temper tantrums like breath holding spells.

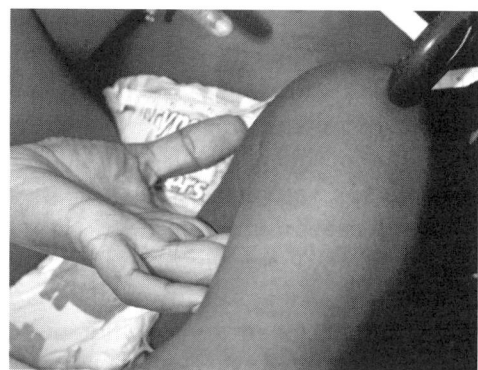

Although sometimes it is a little challenging to do in children, you must examine all reflexes in a child with seizures. The tendon reflexes in children are best elicited with a pediatric sized tendon hammer. Distract the child with a toy and talk to the child when eliciting reflexes.

In the developmental history, the mother says that this child walked and talked later than his siblings although the mother cannot remember the details of the development. The past medical history does not reveal any history of chronic or recurrent illnesses. The past surgical history is negative. There is a family history of epilepsy in the child's uncle. The uncle is on medication and is well-controlled. The parents are nonconsanguineous. There is no known family history of microcephaly or dysmorphisms, obvious abnormal skin lesions suggestive of neurocutaneous stigmata, chromosomal anomalies or known genetic problems amongst the immediate family members. There is no family history of any member requiring special schooling nor history of deafness or blindness. There is no family history of mental retardation.

The antenatal history revealed that the mother had gestational diabetes toward the later part of pregnancy and was on diet control. The birth and neonatal history revealed that the child was a product of a Cesarean section delivery and had a few documented episodes of jitteriness diagnosed to be due to hypoglycemia in the neonatal records. There was an episode of neonatal seizures. These seizures occurred only once and the child had recovered completely. The child was discharged home without medication.

On observation, the child was lying on the bed with his mother next to him. There was no specific posture to suggest hypertonia such as fisting or hypotonia such as frog leg posture. The temperature was normal. The pulse was of normal rate, rhythm and volume. The respiratory rate and blood pressure were normal. On examination, the height and weight were on the 50th centile. The COH was slightly below the 3rd percentile.

Formulation of Differential Diagnosis and Provisional Diagnosis

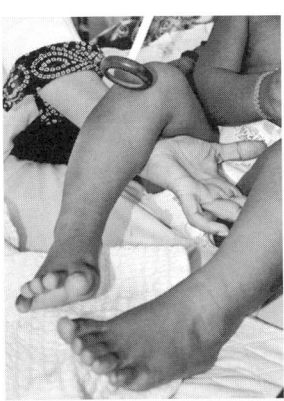

The knee jerk is elicited and compared on both limbs by observation of the contraction of the quadriceps femoris.

The anterior fontanel was closed. There was no neck stiffness. When asked for past records of growth charts including plotting of COH during vaccination visits, the mother says that the doctor never plotted the COH or growth parameters of the child during those visits, hence no previous records could be obtained. There was no noted dysmorphism such as upward slanting of the palpebral fissures or micrognathia. There were no ear or eye abnormalities noted. There were no lesions on the skin to suggest neurocutaneous stigmata. CNS examination was normal except for generalized hyper-reflexia. The plantars were downgoing. There were no cranial nerve deficits. The pupillary reflexes were normal and gross testing of vision was normal. A distraction test was normal. Examination of all other systems was unremarkable. A detailed developmental examination could not be done but a basic examination revealed a functioning level of about 12–15 months. The child was only able to stoop, stand and cruise but was unable to walk independently. He had a pincer grip, was able to put a cube in a cup but was not able to scribble or to stack up cubes (although he played with them at home). He was able to wave bye-bye, to drink from a cup but not able to imitate others or to use a spoon and a fork at 15 months. It was decided that the developmental examination had to be repeated when the child was more comfortable in the ward.

CCCC

Correlate (with other clinical signs), **C**ompare (with the reflexes in all limbs in the child), **C**apture (the abnormality), and **C**onfirm (the diagnosis).

Relevant history: Afebrile seizures, neonatal hypoglycemia, neonatal seizures, family history of epilepsy. The mother feels that this child walked and talked later than his siblings.

Relevant examination: COH below 3rd centile, no neurocutaneous lesions.

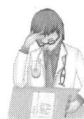

"The negatives in the history are important to narrow my differential diagnosis of afebrile seizures; I must remind myself that history-taking involves important positives and useful negatives which cannot be dismissed."

Points to note: The child had a seizure without fever. You must think of whether these seizures were caused by an intracranial event, such as infections or head injuries. Infections in this case, are unlikely, as there is no fever. Remember to exclude acute extracranial causes of seizures in the history and physical examination such as the ingestion of toxic substances, including side effects of medication, drug overdose and abnormal heart rhythms which are negative in this history and the physical examination of the pulses and pupil reactions are normal. Hypoglycemia and electrolyte imbalances are unlikely as there is no vomiting, diarrhea or anorexia and no significant past history of known illnesses such as diabetes mellitus. The absence of breath holding spells causing anoxic seizures, is a negative history obtained here. In evaluating afebrile seizures, remember to ask about the details of the seizure to someone who has observed the episode. In the developmental history, the mother uses comparison to siblings as a means of recall and feels that this child is slower in development, overall, to her other children. The developmental examination seems to indicate that there is developmental delay but this examination has to be repeated for confirmation.

How important is the neonatal history in this case? Although a definite causal relationship between neonatal seizures and an increased risk of epilepsy is not fully clear, symptomatic neonatal seizures due to hypoglycemia is a recognized factor for subsequent development of seizures. In symptomatic neonatal hypoglycemia, a higher incidence of infantile spasms and partial seizures have been reported. This emphasizes the importance of early recognition and immediate management of hypoglycemia in the neonatal period.

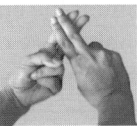

Neonatal hypoglycemia is a recognized link to microcephaly; think of other causes of microcephaly.

Microcephaly or head circumference less than 2 standard deviations from the mean for age and sex is a recognized observation in infants with neonatal hypoglycemic brain injury.[24] The importance of measuring the COH is emphasized as many of the early causes of seizures can affect brain growth. The importance of plotting growth percentiles during vaccination visits is seen here as this information is absent and comparison and study of the trends in head growth cannot be done. Any single reading of growth percentiles has limited value. The developmental examination often has to be repeated as the child is not in his familiar surroundings and is unwell. Here initial developmental testing indicates a possible developmental delay in gross motor, fine motor and social milestones. Hence the history of neonatal hypoglycemia, a COH below the 3rd percentile and developmental delay must be evaluated together in considering the possible differential diagnoses in this child.[24]

Microcephaly warrants considering a more in depth history, detailed history as well as a detailed eye and ear examination and repeating another neurodevelopmental assessment. In this case, the history of gestational diabetes and one episode of hypoglycemic fits in this child as a neonate cannot be ignored as a cause of the microcephaly and the presenting seizures.[24] A magnetic resonance imaging scan (MRI) of the brain, an electroencephalogram (EEG), baseline biochemistry, metabolic screen, TORCHES screen and where indicated, genetic testing—karyotype and molecular genetics are also done to determine the cause.[24,25]

SYSTEM: DEVELOPMENT

Case Study 21: Do You involve Anil in History-taking?[8,14,17,20,23]

Anil, the only son in a family of 4 children, an 8-year-old boy with Down syndrome is brought to the A and E with abdominal pain. He is accompanied by his mother. His mother, a chatty woman does all the talking. It seems to the doctor that she feels Anil's history will waste the doctor's time and the mother often tells Anil to be quiet when he tries to say something about how he is feeling.

His mother gives the history of how he complained of abdominal pain that morning, vomited once and had to miss school that day. She says that he has been complaining of abdominal pain the whole day, although he did not cry but was lying down most of the time that

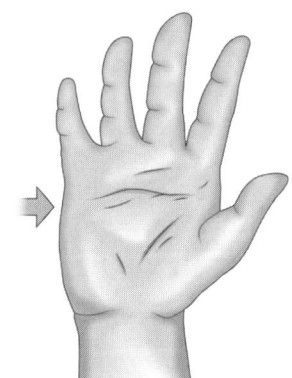

Simian crease in Down syndrome.

day. So she felt that something must be wrong, hence she brought him for an opinion.

The mother says that he talked and walked much later than all his siblings. Anil is going to a special school but the mother says that she is very disappointed with Anil's performance. The mother complains that he does not like to sit down for long enough periods for her to train him.

Past history: The mum tells the doctor that Anil has Down syndrome and she feels unlucky as she was quite young when he was conceived. The doctor never told her that Anil had Down syndrome when she had her prenatal ultrasound scans. She says that he is quite well except that whenever he gets a cough or flu he ends up with ear trouble like pain and discharge from the ears.

Developmental history: Slower in all aspects of development compared to his sisters.

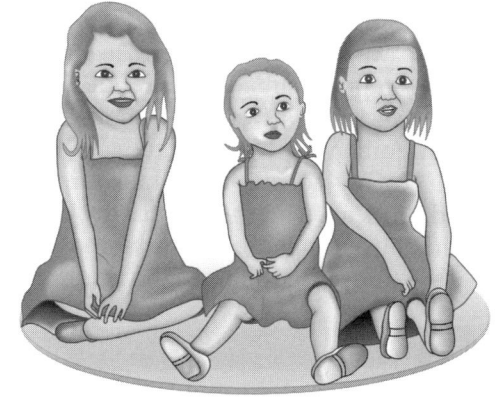

Anil's development is compared to that of his siblings.

After the mother gives her history, the doctor interjects. The doctor persists in asking Anil some questions. The nature of the pain is important to understand. The doctor also feels that for a good history, he must involve the patient in history taking. When he asks Anil a few questions, he discovers that Anil has the ability to understand him, comprehend his questions and answer rationally. The doctor gives Anil an interesting colorful ball that lights up if pressed. Anil takes it with a smile. He asks Anil direct questions. He asks Anil to show him where the abdominal pain is. Anil points to the right iliac fossa. He asks Anil where the pain was in the morning. Anil points to the umbilicus.

Be kind; be considerate. Sympathy and empathy are qualities of a good doctor

Past history: The mum tells the doctor that Anil has Down syndrome and she feels unlucky as she was quite young when he was conceived. The doctor never told her that Anil had Down syndrome when she had her prenatal ultrasound scans. She says that he is quite well except that whenever he gets a cough or a flu he ends up with ear trouble like pain and discharge from the ears.

The doctor then tells Anil that he would like to feel his tummy. Anil lies down on the examination couch. The doctor starts with inspection. He notices that there is a tendency for Anil to flex his hip and knee on lying down. All quadrants of the abdomen are moving with respiration. The doctor asks Anil to point to the area that hurts him and starts abdominal palpation furthest from the right iliac fossa. On deep palpation, the doctor notices that there is rebound tenderness at the right iliac fossa. He does not feel any masses. There is no other positive sign. After permission from Anil and with curtains drawn (as from the beginning of the examination), he inspects the genitals and the perianal region, explains to Anil that he will check that area gently with his finger, does a careful per rectal examination with a gloved finger while talking to Anil about his favorite games in school. The doctor

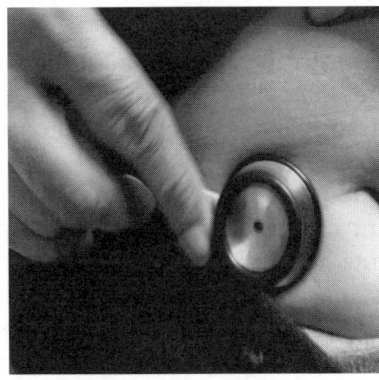

Auscultation for bowel sounds is an important part of the examination. Deduce both the differentials and a clue to apt management based on the frequency of bowel sounds that you hear.

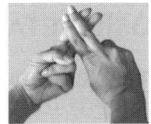

Flexion of the hip and knee when lying down is to relieve iliopsoas muscle spasm and is seen as a typical posture in an older child with acute appendicitis.

completes his examination by auscultation of the bowel sounds.

He also tells Anil that he would like to check his urine. The doctor explains in simple terms how Anil should give a midstream urine in the container he gives him. The doctor makes a clinical diagnosis of acute appendicitis. The doctor also examines all other systems before completing his physical examination.

He speaks clearly to the mother and informs her that Anil would need to be admitted. The doctor also tells the mother that Anil should not be given anything orally. The doctor calls the pediatric surgeon who will examine Anil and take the consent for surgery.

Relevant history: The presence of abdominal pain. The doctor persists in asking Anil some questions. He asks Anil direct questions. He asks Anil to show him where the abdominal pain is. Anil points to the right iliac fossa. He asks Anil where the pain was in the morning. Anil points to the umbilicus.

Relevant examination: He notices that there is a tendency for Anil to flex his hip and knee on lying down.

All quadrants of the abdomen are moving with respiration. The doctor asks Anil to point to the area that hurts him and starts of the abdominal palpation furthest from the right iliac fossa. On deep palpation, the doctor notices that there is rebound tenderness at the right iliac fossa. He does not feel any masses. There is no other positive sign.

Points to note: In pediatrics, children who are able to understand and relate their symptoms must be involved in history taking. The patient feels the pain which may not be related entirely to the parents (or in this case may not be given a chance to relate); to these children, simple open-ended questions or direct questions must be asked. Anil is a case of Down syndrome. It is not for the doctor to make any judgment on the ability of Anil to interpret or comprehend symptoms. While the incidence of mental disability is higher in children with Down syndrome, remember that their story is as important as any other in forming a diagnosis, as illustrated in this case.

SYSTEM: MUSCULOSKELETAL

Case Study 22: Correlate, Compare, Capture, and Confirm Your Findings[8,14,17,20,23]

Robin a previously well 3-year-old child has fever and pain in the left knee and hip of three days duration. The child has been limping for the past two days but now absolutely refuses to bear weight. The mother recalls that the boy did fall off his tricycle five days ago. He cried a little but after that, he walked normally soon after the fall. She applied some cream near the left upper part of the leg where she saw a small abrasion. There is no history of recent travel. There is no history of tick bite exposure, pharyngitis or enteritis. There is no history of a recent URTI or of any other illness. The child has been fully immunized. The temperature is 38.5°C. The heart rate is 145 beats/minute and the pulses are bounding. The respiratory rate is 32 breaths/minute. The blood pressure is 105/78 mm Hg.

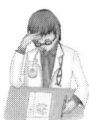

"I must obtain all the important clinical signs on observation as the child is in acute pain and may not allow me to examine him completely."

On examination: The child looks well-nourished but frightened and toxic. He sits on his mother's lap, crying in pain. There are no rashes, macules or bruises noted. He is not pale. There is no gum bleeding or palatal hemorrhages. The oral cavity is normal. There was warmth and redness of the skin overlying the left thigh. There is no sternal tenderness. The chest is clear and except for tachycardia, the CVS examination is normal. There are a few small tender lymph nodes in the inguinal area. Examination of the abdomen does not reveal hepatosplenomegaly.

The back is examined with the child sitting on mum's lap because the patient refuses to stand or bend. The spine is palpated and found to be straight with no bruises, dimples or tufts of hair seen.

Both limbs are *compared* and observed closely. There is no swelling, erythema or pain to palpation on the right ankle, knee and hip and the left ankle. The right knee and hip have full range of movement. There was no obvious muscle weakness in that leg. On the left side, distraction with a toy was required for examination. The child allows the left ankle to be examined. There was no pain, redness or swelling and had full range of movement. The left knee was examined with distraction and the mother's help. There was no pain to light palpation but the child does not allow for deeper palpation. The patient cries aloud when the left hip is touched. This finding is *correlated* to the findings on the right side. The patient is made to lie down on the mother's lap. On lying down the left leg is kept flexed and externally rotated. On lying on the mother's lap, it is found that the left hip is swollen, hot, red and very tender. Muscle power could not be tested in that leg due to the pain. Other joints are not affected. This information is necessary to *capture* accurate differential diagnosis. The gait could not be examined as the patient refuses to walk. Based on the history and physical examination, the doctor reviews his findings to *confirm* some possible differential diagnosis.

Relevant history: Age, painful limp, history of trauma.

Relevant examination: Fever, cellulitis, warmth and redness of the skin overlying the left thigh, position of left hip and finding of acute inflammation of left hip. On lying down, the left leg is kept flexed and externally rotated. While lying on the mother's lap, it is found that the left hip is swollen, hot, red and very tender.

Points to note: This is a previously well three-year-old child with history of fever and pain in one leg which resulted in limping. This progressed to total refusal to stand on the affected leg or walk. There is a history of trauma. The child was able to walk normally after the trauma; this makes a fracture unlikely. The child develops fever and severe pain of the affected limb a little later. The cellulitis of the skin could be the portal of entry of the infection. Consider septic arthritis or osteomyelitis as the most possible diagnosis. However, an incomplete or greenstick fracture will need to be excluded. Other differentials could include transient synovitis, juvenile rheumatoid arthritis or reactive arthritis. The general examination and the acuteness of the history does not suggest a lymphoproliferative disorder.

Septic arthritis is also an important differential diagnosis. This diagnosis is an emergency because if left untreated, destruction of the growth plate and avascular necrosis can result.

Investigations such as a plain radiograph of the affected joint can be helpful. Additionally, complete blood counts, a full blood picture to examine morphology of cells to exclude lymphoblasts, blood cultures, C-reactive protein, and ESR are helpful. I would emphasize that you remember to Correlate (with other clinical signs) Compare (with the other limb), Capture (the abnormality), and Confirm (the diagnosis with appropriate investigations).

REFERENCES

1. Biancaniello T. Innocent Murmurs. Clinician Update. Circulation. Available at http://circ.ahajournals.org/content/111/3/e20.full.pdf. Accessed in February 2015.
2. American Academy of Pediatrics. Committee on Nutrition. Soy protein-based formulas: recommendations for use in infant feeding. Pediatrics. 1998;1011 pt 1:149–53.
3. Brzezinski P, Sinjab AT. Pityriasis rosea in 12-month-old infant. Our Dermatol Online. 2012; 3(2): 119-122
4. Clifford TJ, Campbell MK, Speechley KN, Gorodzinsky F. Infant colic: empirical evidence of the absence of an association with source of early infant nutrition. Arch Pediatr Adolesc Med. 2002;156:1123-8.
5. Elizabeth KE. Clinical Pediatrics for Undergraduates. New Delhi: Jaypee Brothers Medical Publishers (P) Ltd; 2009.
6. Fisher RG, Boyce TG, Hugh L. Nose and Throat syndromes. Moffet's Pediatric Infectious Diseases: A Problem-oriented Approach. Lippincott William & Wilkins, 2005.
7. Garrison MM, Christakis DA. A systematic review of treatments for infant colic. Pediatrics. 2000;1061 pt 2:184–90.
8. Goel KM, Gupta DK. Hutchinson's Pediatrics, 1st edn. India: Jaypee Brothers Medical Publishers (P) Ltd; 2009
9. Harb R, Thomas DW. Conjugated Hyperbilirubinemia: Screening and Treatment in Older Infants and Children. Pediatr. Rev. 2007;28;83-91.
10. Hardjojo A, Shek LPC, Hugo PS, van Bever, Lee BW. Rhinitis in children less than 6 years of age: Current knowledge and challenges. Asia Pac Allergy. 2011;1(3):115-22.
11. Illingsworth RS. Three-months' colic. Arch Dis Child. 1954;29:165-74.
12. Kellen PE. Diaper dermatitis: Differential diagnosis and management. Can Fam Physician. 1990;36:1569-72.
13. Lucassen PL, Assendelft WJ, Gubbels JW, van Eijk JT, van Geldrop WJ, Neven AK. Effectiveness of treatments for infantile colic: systematic review. BMJ. 1998;317:171. BMJ. 1998;316:1563-9.
14. Marcdante K, Kliegman RM, Jenson HB, Behrman RE (Eds). Nelson's Essentials of Pediatrics. 6th edn. Saunders Elsevier, 2010.
15. Mason S, Swash M (Eds). Hutchinson's Clinical Methods (17th edn). A Baillere Tindall book published by Cassell Ltd; 1980.
16. Michael E, McConnell, Adkins SB III. Murmurs in Pediatric Patients: When Do You Refer? Am Fam Physician. 1999;60(2):558-64.
17. Milner AD, Hull D. Hospital Pediatrics. 3rd edn. ELBS with Churchill Livingstone. 1998.
18. Moreno MA, Furtner F, Rivara FP. Functional Abdominal Pain in Children and Adolescents. JAMA Pediatr. 2013;167(2):204.
19. Rahhal RM, Eddine AC, Bishop WP. A Child with an Abdominal Mass. Hospital Physician. 2006.pp.37-42.
20. Behrman RE (comps), Kliegman RM, Nelson WE, Vaughan VC III. (Eds). Nelson's Textbook of Pediatrics, 14th edn. Philadelphia: WB Saunders; 1992.
21. Roberts DM, Ostapchuk M, O'Brien JG. Infantile Colic. Am Fam Physician. 2004;70(4):735-40.
22. The Auscultation Assistant. University of California, Los Angeles. Available at http://www.med.ucla.edu/wilkes/ASDMain.htm. Accessed in February 2015.
23. Stephenson T, Wallace H (Eds). Clinical Paediatrics for Postgraduate Examinations. UK: Churchill Livingstone. 1991.
24. Udani V, Munot P, Ursekar M, Gupta S. Neonatal hypoglycemic brain injury—A common cause of infantile-onset remote symptomatic epilepsy. Indian Pediatr. 2009;46:127-32.
25. What are the different ways in which a genetic condition can be inherited? Available at http://ghr.nlm.nih.gov. Accessed in April 2013.

The essence of the relevant chapters in the following books have also been numbered as references in this chapter. We recommend for further reading, the rich text in these books for greater integration and deeper understanding.

1. Elizabeth KE. Clinical Pediatrics for Undergraduates. Jaypee Brothers Medical Publishers (P) Ltd, India. 2009.
2. Goel KM, Gupta DK. Hutchinson's Pediatrics, 1st edn. Jaypee Brothers Medical Publishers (P) Ltd, India. 2009.
3. Marcdante K, Kliegman RM, Jenson HB, Behrman RE (Eds). Nelson's Essentials of Pediatrics. 6th edn. Saunders Elsevier. 2010.
4. Mason S, Swash M (Eds). Hutchinson's Clinical Methods, 17th edn. A Baillere Tindall book published by Cassell Ltd. 1980.
5. Milner AD, Hull D. Hospital Pediatrics. 3rd edn. ELBS with Churchill Livingstone. 1998.
6. Behrman RE (comps), Kliegman RM, Nelson WE, Vaughan VC III. (Eds). Nelson's Textbook of Pediatrics, 14th edn. Philadelphia: WB Saunders. 1992.
7. Stephenson T, Wallace H (Eds). Clinical Pediatrics for postgraduate examinations. UK: Churchill Livingstone. 1991.

SECTION 5

'THE KNOW' FACTS

- Factual Knowledge

Chapter 14

Factual Knowledge

FACTUAL KNOWLEDGE CATEGORIZED AS 'MUST KNOW', 'GOOD TO KNOW' OR 'NICE TO KNOW'

Your factual knowledge will influence how you think. The historical and physical links will help you think through the clinical history and clinical examination. This chapter lists causes and differential diagnoses of the more common pediatric conditions.[1-29] It is hoped that further reading around the factual knowledge given in this chapter will enhance the historical and physical links you will develop, to come to a reasonable diagnosis.

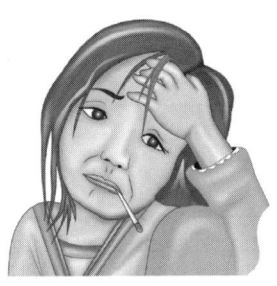

SYSTEM: FEVER IN CHILDREN

Approach to the Patient

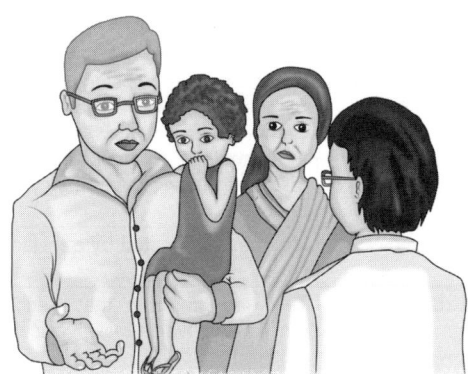

Fever is a common symptom causing parental worry.

When confronted with a child who is brought with a complaint of fever, you must:

• Ascertain that the child is febrile
• Think of the etiological causes
• Take a relevant history (following the historical links provided by the historian)
• Then, examine the child (using physical links)

"I must know".

Causes of Fever[16-27]

Fever occurring with an infection may be divided in the following causes:

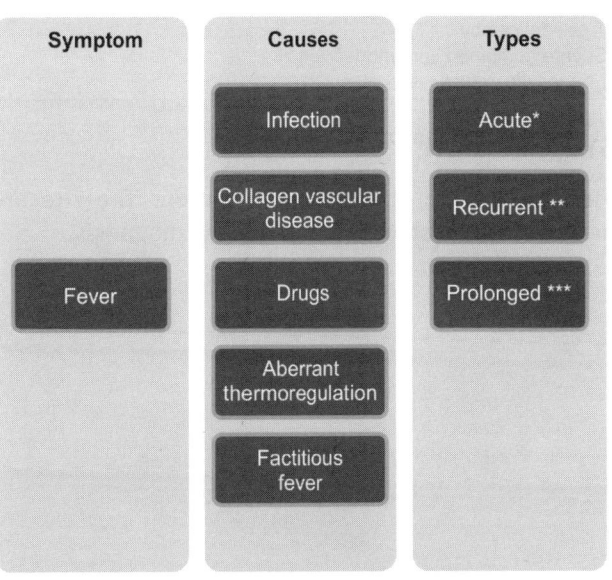

Note:
*Acute and of short duration occur very frequently in children
**Recurrent, prolonged where recurrent episodes occur with definite afebrile intervals
***Prolonged in association with a chronic disease

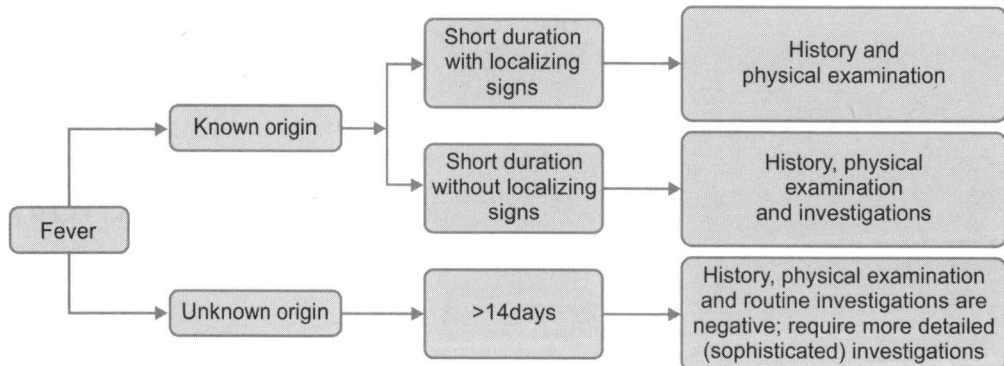

Types of Fever[8,17,18,21,25,27]

"I must know".

Differential Diagnosis to Consider in a Child with Prolonged Fever

The broad categories are the following:[21]
• Bacterial infections
• Viral infections
• Collagen vascular disease
• Parasitic infections
• Systemic fungal infections
• Malignancies
• Increased susceptibility to infection
Hypogammaglobulinemia
Selective IgA deficiency
T cell deficiency
Severe combined immunodeficiency
Phagocytic defect

SYSTEM: SKIN[8,17,18,21,25,27]

Viral rashes are common in children. The site and nature of skin rash will help make the diagnosis.

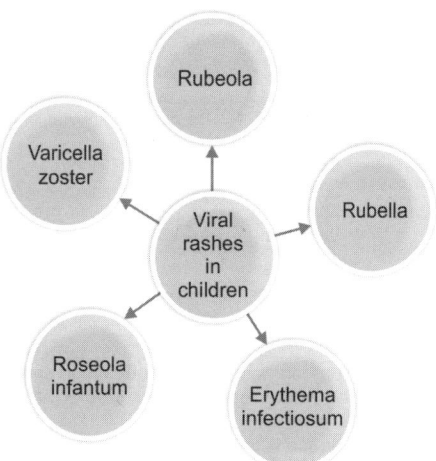

"I must know".

Viral Rashes[8,17,18,21,25,27]

Measles	Macular rash begins above hairline and spreads in cephalad to caudal manner; confluent. Rash fades from cephalad to caudal
Black measles	Rash is petechial or hemorrhagic
Modified measles	Measles is modified by the presence of antibodies
Pathognomonic sign	Koplik spots
Rubella	Discrete erythematous macular papular rash starts on face, spreads to the body, lasts for 3 days
Pathognomonic sign	Forchheimer spots, post-auricular and suboccipital lympadenopathy
Roseola infantum	A maculopapular rose colored rash, coincident with defervescence, lasts for 1–3 days
Possible complication	Hemophagocytosis syndrome. About a third of cases are associated with febrile seizures
Erythema Infectiosum	Rashes appear in 3 stages. Slapped cheek: associated with circumoral pallor. Erythematous maculopapular truncal rash, with fading gives a lacy reticulated rash
Possible complication	May be complicated by transient aplastic crises.
Varicella zoster Infection	Tiny red papules that become non-umbilicated oval tear-like vesicular lesions on a red base. Ulceration, crusting and healing of vesicles occur. New vesicles occur in crops at trunk, head and face and less frequently the arms and legs
Typical feature	A polymorphic rash, pruritis is marked when healing

Factual Knowledge

"I must know".

Where bacterial rashes are considered, you must know that the most common bacterial infection of the skin in children is **impetigo**.

It commonly affects children between two and five years of age and is very contagious. The diagnosis is usually a clinical one.

The causative organisms are the following:
- *Staphylococcus aureus*, which is the most common causative organism
- *Streptococcus pyogenes* (group A beta-hemolytic *Streptococcus*) causes fewer cases, either alone or in with *S. aureus*

The differential diagnosis will differ in the bullous and nonbullous forms as the clinical appearances are different.

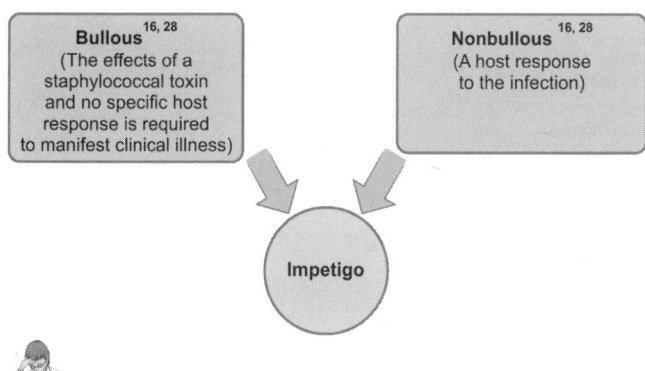

"It is good to know."

Consider these differential diagnoses in nonbullous and bullous impetigo.

Differential Diagnosis of Impetigo[4,16,21,28]

Lesions mimicking nonbullous impetigo
- Tinea
- Herpetic impetigo
- Erysipelas
- Atopic dermatitis
- Folliculitis
- Cutaneous candidiasis
- Contact dermatitis
- Insect bites
- Ecthyma
- Discoid lupus
- Scabies
- Acute febrile neutropenia
- Drug-induced eruptions

Lesions mimicking bullous impetigo
- Dermatitis herpetiformis
- Bullous pemphigoid
- Lupus erythematous
- Herpes zoster
- Hand, foot and mouth disease
- Varicella
- Pemphigus vulgaris
- Stevens-Johnson syndrome
- Bullous scabies
- Bullous erythema multiforme
- Bullous fixed drug reaction
- Toxic epidermal necrolysis
- Thermal burns and scalds

If the site of the rash involves the nappy area, you must know the *differential diagnosis of diaper dermatitis (or rash in and around the perianal area)*. Knowing this will help you ask relevant questions (develop historical links) and look for relevant signs (develop physical links).

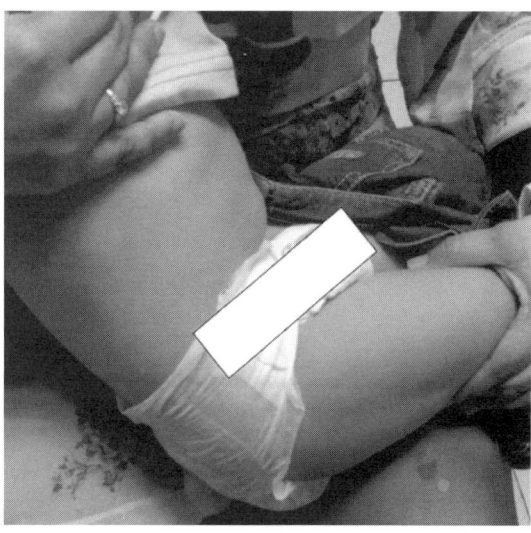

Knowledge of conditions in the diaper area must not be ignored in the pediatric patient.

Differential diagnosis of rashes in the napkin region[8,17,18,21,25,27]
• Atopic dermatitis
• Contact dermatitis
• Seborrheic eczema
• Chemical napkin dermatitis
• Candidiasis
• Impetigo
• Intertrigo
• Perianal dermatitis
• Miliaria
• Acrodermatitis enteropathica
• Kawasaki disease
• Infantile psoriasis
• Scabies
• Warts
• Tinea cruris
• Miliary tuberculosis of the skin
• Syphilis

If the rash is pruritic, knowledge of these facts is useful. Differential diagnosis of miscellaneous rashes with pruritus.[8,17,18,21,25,27]

Infective causes of pruritis
- Herpes zoster
- Varicella
- AIDS
- Infectious hepatitis
- Parasitic disease
  - Giardiasis
  - Onchocerciasis,
  - Schistosomiasis
  - Ascariasis
- Prion disease

Systemic causes of pruritis
- Conjugated hyperbilirubinemia
- Drug eruptions

Autoimmune
- Dermatitis herpetiformis (associated with celiac disease)
- Dermatomyositis

Hematologic
- Hemochromatosis
- Leukemia
- Lymphoma
- Iron deficiency anemia
- Polycythemia rubra vera
- Mastocytosis
- Plasma cell dyscrasias

Hepatobiliary
- Biliary atresia
- Choledochal cyst
- Chronic pancreatitis with obstruction of biliary tracts
- Hepatitis
- Sclerosing cholangitis
- Biliary cirrhosis
- Chronic liver disease

Malignancy
- Solid tumors with paraneoplastic syndrome

Metabolic and endocrine
- Hyper/hypothyroidism
- Hyperparathyroidism
- Diabetes mellitus
- Chronic kidney disease
- Carcinoid syndrome

Neurologic
- Cerebral abscess
- Cerebral tumor
- Multiple sclerosis
- Stroke

Drug-induced
- Drug-induced cholestasis

Dermatological causes of pruritis
- Scabies
- Urticaria
- Insect bites
- Dry skin
- Tinea
- Allergic/irritant contact dermatitis
- Atopic dermatitis
- Dermatitis herpetiformis
- Folliculitis
- Pediculosis (lice infestation)
- Sunburn
- Cutaneous T-cell lymphoma (mycosis fungoides)
- Bullous pemphigoid
- Psoriasis
- Lichen planus
- Lichen simplex chronicus
- Eczema*

"I must know."

* Eczema
- Atopic
- Contact
- Seborrheic
- Discoid
- Pompholyx

Remember that skin lesions can be a manifestation of internal diseases. For example, in a patient with bleeding in the skin, the differential diagnosis of causes of purpuric rash or bruising may be thought of as follows after a simple investigation:

Purpuric Rash: Diagnoses to Consider[8,17,18,21,25,27]

Purpuric rash with normal platelet count	Purpuric rash with low platelet count
Henoch-Schonlein purpura Glanzmann's thrombasthenia (Autosomal recessive disorder) Bernard-Soulier Syndrome (Autosomal recessive disorder) Storage pool disease Drugs • Aspirin • Furosemide • Nitrofurantoin • Heparin • Sympathetic blockers • Clofibrate • Some nonsteroidal anti-inflammatory drugs (NSAIDs) Von Willebrand disease Disseminated intravascular coagulopathy Circulating anticoagulants Liver disease Vitamin K deficiency Uremia Hereditary hemorrhagic telangiectasia Ehlers-Danlos syndrome Trauma	Idiopathic (immune) thrombocytopenic purpura Post-transfusion purpura Neonatal autoimmune thrombocytopenia Nonimmune thrombocytopenia • Hemolytic-uremic syndrome • Thrombotic thrombocytopenic purpura • Disseminated intravascular coagulopathy Thrombocytopenia–absent radii (TAR) syndrome Fanconi anemia Wiskott-Aldrich syndrome Congenital amegakaryocytic thrombocytopenia Drug reactions • Alkylating agents • Antimetabolites • Anticonvulsants • Chlorothiazide diuretics • Estrogens Autoimmune disease – SLE Infections **Viral** – Antecedent viral infection e.g. upper respiratory tract infection, dengue hemorrhagic fever, malaria, yellow fever, rickettsia infection, rubella, cytomegalovirus, herpes simplex viruses, HIV Bacterial infections - TORCH infections, meningococcal infection, leptospirosis Bone marrow infiltrations - leukemia, histiocytosis, storage diseases, neuroblastoma, myelofibrosis and granulomatosis Platelet sequestration - Kasabach-Merritt syndrome (thrombocytopenia and giant hemangioma) Acute leukemia Aplastic leukemia Metabolic diseases • Propionic acidemia • Methylmalonic acidemia

SYSTEM: ENT[8,17,18,21,25,27]

The approach to ENT problems in children must be based on knowing common problems that affect this system. Common causes are always considered first. The nature of the problem may also give you a clue to the underlying pathology. Unilateral nose bleeds may be due to nose picking whereas bilateral epistaxis is more likely to be associated with a systemic problem.

"I must know"

In the differential diagnosis of epistaxis, consider the following:[8,17,18,21,25,27]

Differential diagnosis of epistaxis[8,17,18,21,25,27]
• Trauma especially if unilateral "nose picking"
• Local and systemic infections
• Foreign bodies
• Bleeding disorders
• Neoplasms
• Idiopathic (the commonest)

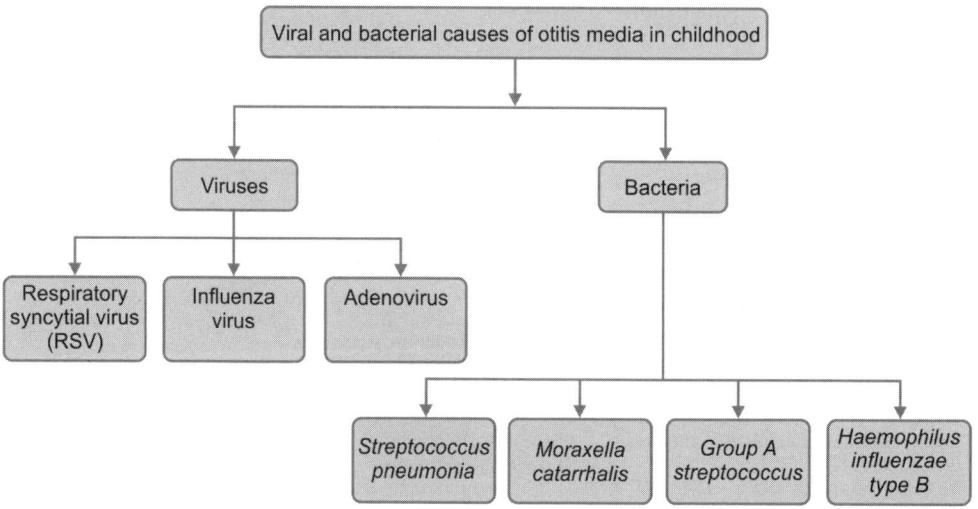

Common Etiological Causes of Otitis Media[17,21]

Otitis media is frequently seen in children.

Some problems that affect children are best thought of by the age of the patient as pediatrics covers a range of age groups and as mentioned earlier, the anatomy of the airway differs in children from adults.

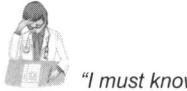
"I must know."

Differential Diagnosis, by Age of the Pediatric Patient, in Upper Airway Obstruction[8,17,18,21,25,27]

When symptoms are persistent, infections and trauma as etiological causes (which are the more common causes of diseases in children) become less likely.

In persistent symptoms, consider underlying congenital, anatomical or physiological abnormalities.

Causes of Upper Airway Obstruction[8,17,18,21,25,27]

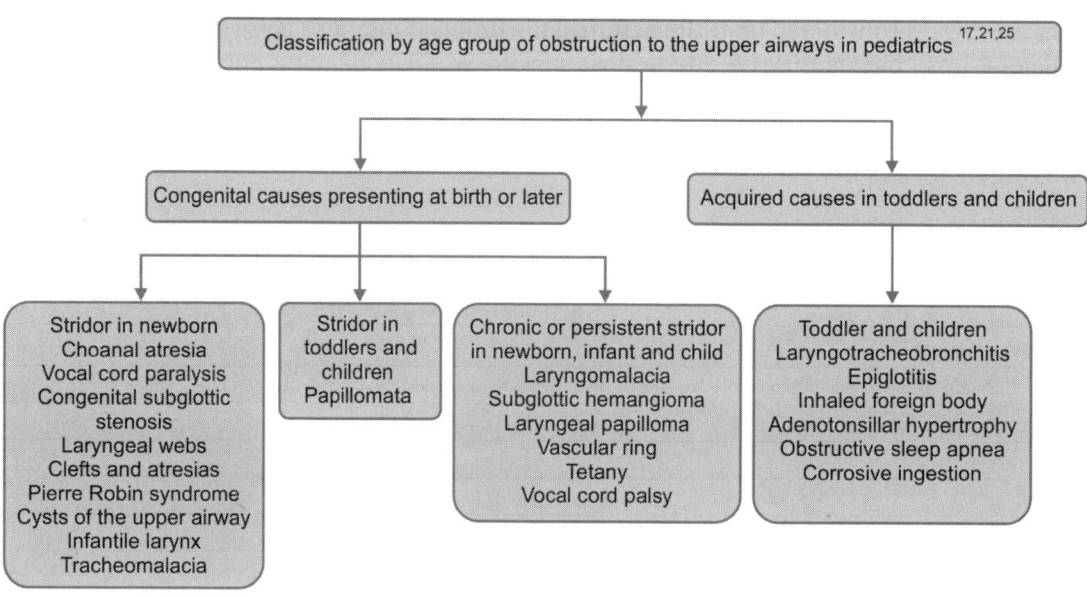

SYSTEM: RESPIRATORY[8,17,18,21,22,25,27]

Respiratory problems are common among children. Respiratory infections lead to airway obstruction and are an important cause of morbidity in children. The pediatric wards often have many respiratory cases, so you must know them well.

Obstructive Airway Disease in Children: Why Children are Anatomically and Physiologically Predisposed[8,17,18,21,22,25,27]

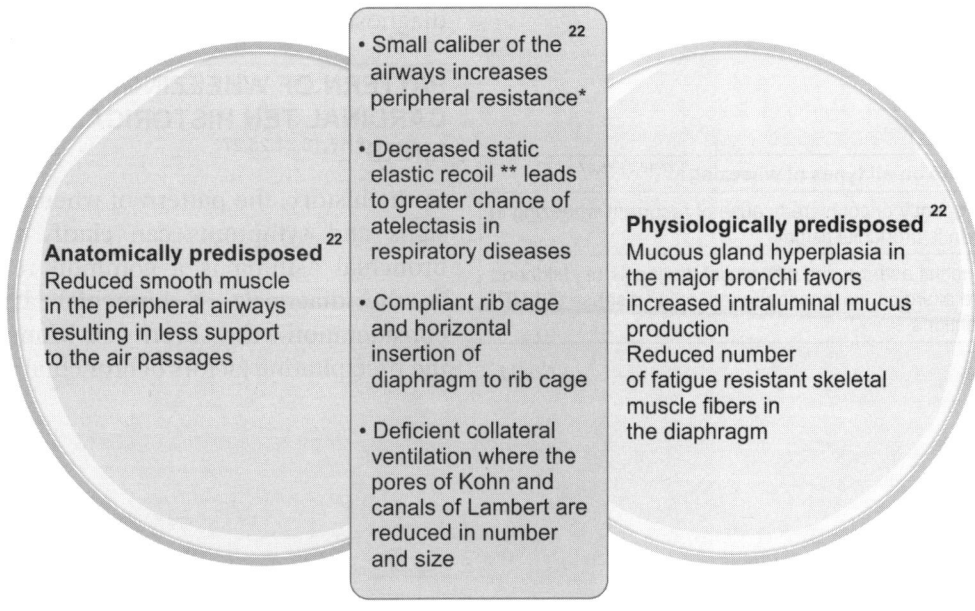

Anatomically predisposed[22]
Reduced smooth muscle in the peripheral airways resulting in less support to the air passages

- Small caliber of the airways increases peripheral resistance*[22]
- Decreased static elastic recoil ** leads to greater chance of atelectasis in respiratory diseases
- Compliant rib cage and horizontal insertion of diaphragm to rib cage
- Deficient collateral ventilation where the pores of Kohn and canals of Lambert are reduced in number and size

Physiologically predisposed[22]
Mucous gland hyperplasia in the major bronchi favors increased intraluminal mucus production
Reduced number of fatigue resistant skeletal muscle fibers in the diaphragm

* The bronchial tree is narrower up to five years of age. This results in decreased conductance rendering the infant and young child to increased incidence of small airway disease. The resistance is higher in the airways of infants compared to that of the adult; peripheral airway resistance in younger children is four times higher than adults.
** Decreased static elastic recoil causes early closure of the airways during tidal breathing with ventilation and perfusion mismatch.

Remember that when the differential diagnoses are considered, the anatomical site of the pathology must be considered. The correct terminology of the disease affecting the lower respiratory system reflects the anatomical site of the lesion and influences the etiological diagnosis.

Description and nomenclature of lower respiratory tract infection[17] (Describes bronchitis, bronchiolitis, pneumonia or a combination of any of these)
Bronchitis: is a clinical condition due to inflammation of the bronchi. The inflammation and edema narrows the airways acutely
Bronchiolitis: is a clinical condition where there is inflammation of the smaller air passages or bronchioles
Pneumonia: is a clinical condition where there is an infection of the lower respiratory tract, it affects the airways and the lung parenchyma
Pneumonitis: is a clinical condition describing inflammation of the lung with or without consolidation
Lobar pneumonia: is an infection of the lung causing pneumonia that is localized to one or more lobes
Atypical pneumonia (*Mycoplasma, Legionella* or *Chlamydia pneumonia*): is a clinical condition where the pattern of pneumonia is other than typical lobar pneumonia or bronchopneumonia
Bronchopneumonia: is a clinical condition that describes lung inflammation mainly involving the bronchioles. This is usually associated with patchy consolidation of the adjacent lobules as a result of mucopurulent exudates
Interstitial pneumonitis: is pneumonitis involving the interstitium which is composed of the alveoli and the bronchioles.

Some symptoms like wheezing as a result of lower airway obstruction are a very common manifestation of respiratory disease in children. The reasons for this have already been explained in Chapters 3 and 10. As it is a very common symptom of disease in children, analyze it with **The Cardinal Ten (Historical)**.

Wheezing: a shrill sound similar to a whistling sound due to narrowing of the lower airways.

"It is good to know."

Diagnostic points on all types of wheezing[8,17,18,21,25,27]
• The most frequently encountered cause of recurrent wheezing in young children is bronchial asthma
• Besides bronchial asthma, the differential diagnosis of childhood wheezing are allergies, gastroesophageal reflux disease (GERD) and viral infections

Contd...

Contd...

• A child's response to bronchodilators may help in distinguishing bronchial asthma from other triggers of wheezing in children
• Exclude other causes of wheezing such as congenital lesions of the lung or aspiration if it is the first time the child wheezes or if it is recurrent and unexplained. A chest X-ray is useful

Most infants and children with recurrent wheezing have or develop bronchial asthma; nevertheless, other causes should be considered in the differential diagnosis.

PATTERN OF WHEEZING: CLARIFY WITH THE CARDINAL TEN HISTORICAL AND PHYSICAL LINKS[8,17,18,21,25,27]

In the history, the pattern of wheezing and associated signs and symptoms can clarify the diagnosis. As bronchial asthma is a common respiratory disease in the diagnosis of bronchial asthma, take into consideration—the severity of bronchial asthma and the precipitating factors of bronchial asthma.

Factual Knowledge 279

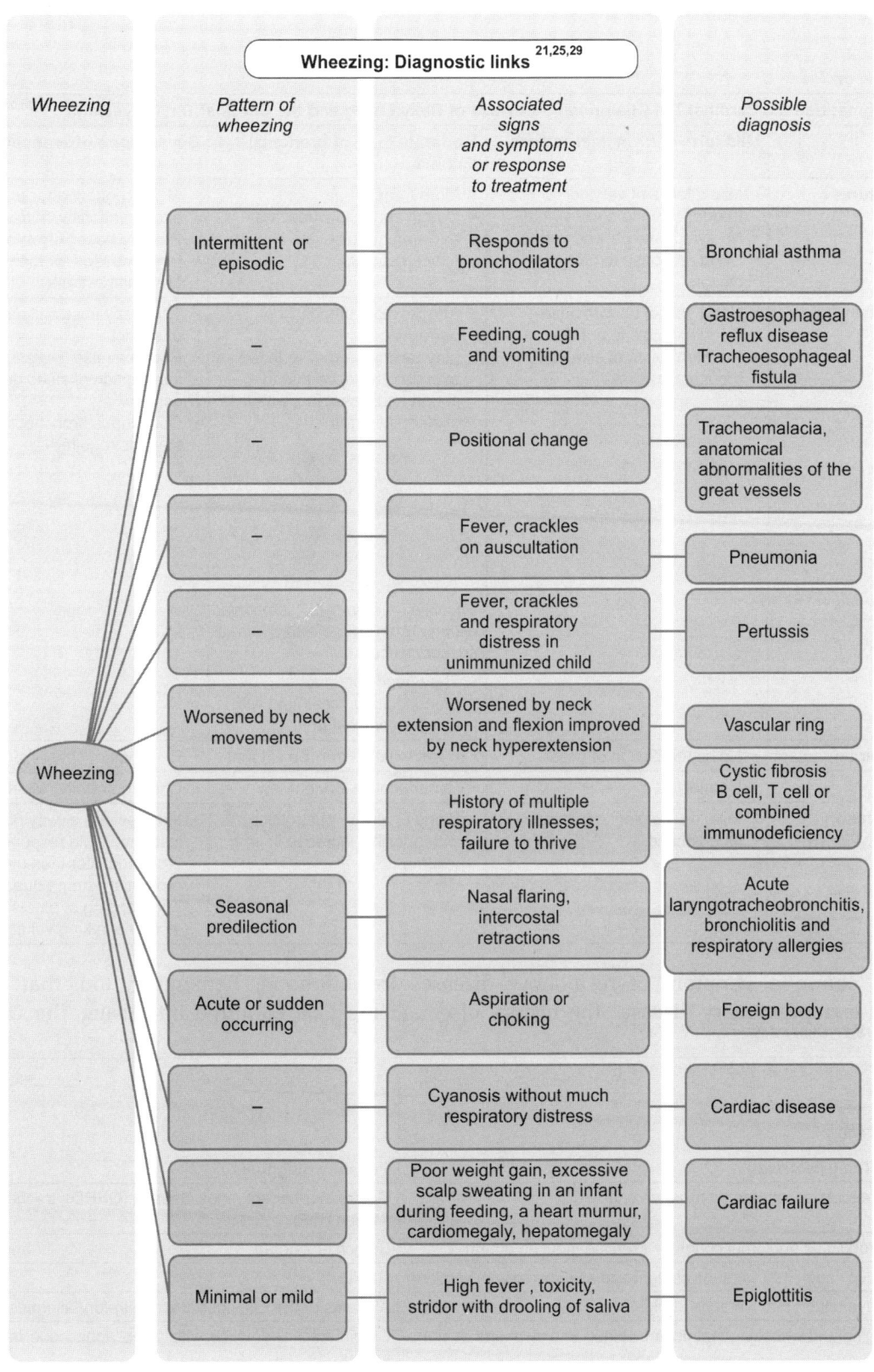

"I must know."

Bronchial asthma: Use the Cardinal Ten (Historical), Activities of Daily Living and the Cardinal Ten (Physical)[8,17,18,21,25,27]			
	Mild form of bronchial asthma	Moderate form of bronchial asthma	Severe form of bronchial asthma
Historical features	• Mild attacks of varying frequency up to once a week • No symptoms between attacks • Good response to broncho-dilators	• More frequent attacks • Cough and mild wheezing between more severe exacerbations	• More frequent attacks, more severe exacerbations with daily wheezing • Require hospitalization which is rarely needed for mild and moderate bronchial asthma
Activities of daily living	• Good school performance • Good exercise tolerance • No interruption of sleep by bronchial asthma	• Attacks may affect school performance • May be impaired or reduced exercise tolerance due to cough and wheezing, with loss of sleep at night *Effective therapy for bronchial asthma can be delivered via a spacer device.* • They need continuous bronchodilator treatment with inhaled corticosteroid	• They may miss a significant amount of school • Poor exercise tolerance and interruption of sleep due to bronchial asthma • Continuous bronchodilator and steroids required
Physical features	• No hyperinflation of chest	• Hyperinflation may be evident	• Evidence of chest deformity
Chest X-ray	• Normal	• Hyperinflation evident	• Chest deformity evident
Airway obstruction	• Mild, reversible, no increase in lung volume	• Signs of airway obstruction with possible increase in lung volume	• More severe airway obstruction, less reversible response to bronchodilator than mild or moderate bronchial asthma due to air trapping. The trapping of air also causes an increase in lung volume.

Cough is a common symptom of respiratory diseases in childhood. Remember, too, that it is also a symptom of extrapulmonary disease. The history of cough must be enquired into using **The Cardinal Ten (Historical)**.[8,17,18,21,25,27]

"I must know."

The Cardinal Ten (Historical)	Possible diagnosis
A cough after feeding accompanied by wheezing	Gastroesophageal reflux disease (GERD), tracheoesopahgeal fistula (TOF)
Chesty or unproductive nocturnal cough or exercise-induced cough	Bronchial asthma
Dry, unproductive cough that worsens at night and associated with vomiting	GERD
Dry, unproductive cough that worsens at night	Allergies of the ENT, general respiratory allergies
Snoring, coughing and wheezing that disturbs sleep and awakens at night	Craniofacial anomalies with sleep apnea due to obstruction in infants
Snoring, coughing and wheezing that disturbs sleep or awakens at night	Obstructive sleep apnea as a result of adenoids, the tonsils or both in older children

In the respiratory system also, recurrent or chronic symptoms suggest inherited diseases, congenital anomalies, or underlying susceptibility to diseases.

"I must know."

Differential diagnosis of chronic cough[8,17,18,21,25,27]
1. Recurrent aspiration secondary to tracheoesophageal fistula
2. Cystic fibrosis
3. Gastroesophageal reflux disease
4. Postnasal drip and post viral cough
5. Pertussis
6. Primary ciliary dyskinesia
7. Congenital laryngomalacia
8. Chronic sinusitis with lower respiratory tract infections
9. Foreign body
10. Bronchiectasis
11. Tuberculosis and chronic pulmonary infections
12. B cell, T cell or combined immunodeficiency
13. Cow's milk protein allergy (undiagnosed)

SYSTEM: CARDIOVASCULAR[8,17,18,21,22,25,27]

The heart sounds tell you many things about the heart. Although observation is the most important part of the physical examination, listening to the heart sounds can be informative. Auscultation of the precordium is best done when the child is calm; hence, in pediatrics, it is done soon after inspection. The first and second heart sounds can change in intensity with underlying cardiac lesions.

The 2nd Heart Sound[8,17,18,21,22,25,27]

It is important in pediatric cardiology. It is normally split and the split is greater in inspiration than in expiration due to the changes in the intrathoracic pressures.

Split 2nd Sound[8,17,18,21,22,25,27]

Why does splitting of the 2nd heart sound occur? Aortic valve closure precedes pulmonary valve closure. Other clinical findings of diagnostic importance involving the 2nd heart sound is if it is normal in intensity and has the features of normal splitting, many important conditions are excluded.

Fixed splitting means that no change of the split occurs with respiration. Reverse splitting means that the split widens on expiration.

Abnormal Heart Sounds[8,17,18,21,22,25,27]

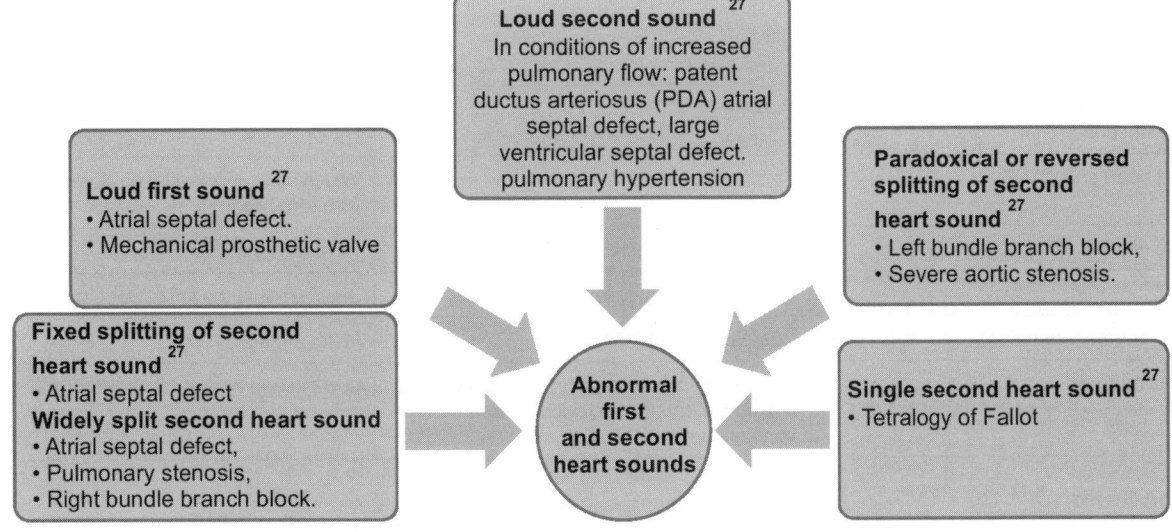

282 The Link: Pediatric History-Taking and Physical Examination

"I must know."

On auscultation of the heart, besides appreciating the first and second heart sounds, **listen for added sounds**.

A murmur is caused by turbulence of blood as blood moves through the heart during the cardiac cycle.

There are many causes of cardiac murmurs in children. Physiological or functional murmurs are murmurs that can be heard due to turbulence of blood flow without any underlying abnormality of the heart. They are common in children. Physiological murmurs are important to recognize. There are some characteristic features which have already been mentioned in Chapter 10. The 10 S features of a functional murmur can thus be determined. Some cardiac lesions like a ventricular septal defects or a patent ductus arteriosus produce murmurs that are easily distinguished from a physiological murmur. Some cardiac lesions that are more difficult to distinguish from a functional murmur include the murmur heard in an atrial septal defect (ASD). A complete history and physical examination is required.

Comparison and Differences in the Physical findings in a Functional (Innocent) Heart Murmur and an Atrial Septal Defect (ASD)[8,17,18,20,21,25,27]

These murmurs are compared because in both situations the child is clinically well.

Comparative features	Innocent murmur[8,17,18,20,21,22,25,27]	Atrial septal defect[8,17,18,20,21,22,25,27]
History	The child is asymptomatic and clinically well	Asymptomatic in childhood. If symptomatic, symptoms include: • Dyspnea, especially when exercising • Fatigue • Pedal edema in the older child • Heart palpitations or 'child's awareness of heartbeat • Frequent lung infections
Physical examination Inspection of precordium	Normal	May be normal or hyperdynamic
Auscultation First heart sound (S1)	Normal	Normal
Second heart sound (S2)	Splits and wider in inspiration than expiration	Widely split and fixed (i.e., does not change with respiration)
Systolic murmur (supine)	Increases and decreases	Increases and decreases
	Best heard at lower left sternal border	Best heard at the left upper border
Systolic murmur (standing)	Decreases in intensity	Is not affected
Diastolic murmur	If heard, the functional murmur is continuous, maximal at the supraclavicular area and is a venous hum	Low pitched across tricuspid valve area

Cardiac Failure[8,17,18,21,25,27]

Cardiac failure occurs when the myocardium is no longer able to produce the necessary cardiac output to maintain adequate tissue oxygenation. It is important to recognize. An underlying cause must be sought to complete the etiological diagnosis.

Factual Knowledge 283

The cardinal signs of heart failure
• Cardiomegaly
• Tachycardia
• Tachypnea
• Hepatomegaly
• Chest retractions especially prominent in young infants

"I must know."

Heart Failure: Signs and Symptoms[8,17,18,21,25,27]

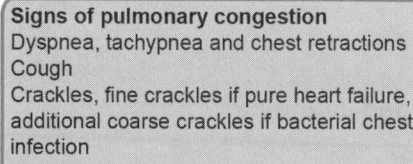

Signs of pulmonary congestion
Dyspnea, tachypnea and chest retractions
Cough
Crackles, fine crackles if pure heart failure, additional coarse crackles if bacterial chest infection
Rhonchi

Signs of systemic venous congestion
Hepatomegaly
Increased neck vein distension and pulsation—difficult to observe in infants
Peripheral edema—rare in children

Signs of impaired myocardial function
Pallor
Cardiomegaly
Tachycardia –persistent raised heart rate
    >160 beats per minute in infants
    >100 bpm in older children
Consider supraventricular tachycardia (SVT) if heart rate:
>220 beats per minute in infants
>180 beats per minute in older children
Gallop rhythm
Alteration in arterial pulse:
Weak peripheral pulses
Capillary refill > 2 seconds
Pulses paradoxus
Pulses alternans
Failure to thrive
Signs of sympathetic overdrive :
diaphoresis, peripheral vasoconstriction, irritability

SYSTEM: GASTROINTESTINAL[8,17,18,21,25,27]

Some disorders in children stem from anatomical or pathophysiological causes. Others have a psychological overlay. Constipation and soiling are examples of this etiological spectrum.

"I must know."

Differential Diagnosis of Causes of Constipation and Soiling in Children[8,10,17,18,20,21,22,25,27]
1. Behavioral
2. Nutritional
3. Anatomical
4. Neuromuscular
5. Metabolic

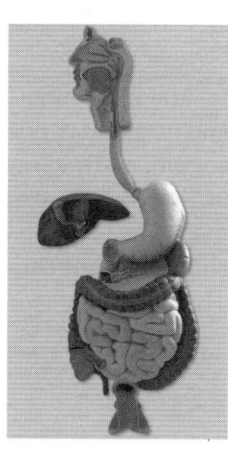

Some features in the child may suggest that a problem is more psychological than physical. Though these features are not always present or consistent, they help in guiding you to a diagnosis.

"I must know."

Constipation: Functional and organic causes[10,11,21]		
Symptoms and signs of suggestive features	Functional causes	Organic causes
Symptoms commence early, often at birth	Rare	Common
Retention posturing	Common	Rare
Passage of impacted large stool	Common	Rare
Pain or discomfort on bowel movement	Common	Common
Fecal soiling	Common	Rare

SYSTEM: HEPATOBILIARY[8,17,18,21,25,27]

Hyperbilirubinemia or elevated serum bilirubin concentrations stains the skin, sclera, mucous membranes, and body fluids yellow. This is a common symptom in pediatrics and may be a manifestation of a physiological or a pathological process.

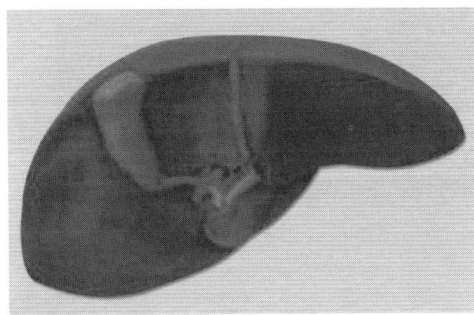

The differential diagnosis for jaundice is age specific and in children, one must be aware of the more common conditions in all age groups. It is clinically manifested in infants when the serum bilirubin concentration is more than 4–5 mg/dL (68.4–85.5 μmol/L) and in older children at concentrations more than 2–3 mg/dL (34.2–51.3 mmol/L).[9]

"I must know."

Serum Total Bilirubin is Assessed in the Laboratory as the Sum of Two Components:[9]

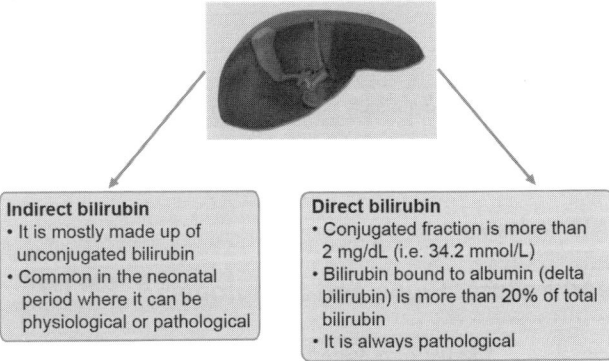

- **Indirect bilirubin**
  - It is mostly made up of unconjugated bilirubin
  - Common in the neonatal period where it can be physiological or pathological

- **Direct bilirubin**
  - Conjugated fraction is more than 2 mg/dL (i.e. 34.2 mmol/L)
  - Bilirubin bound to albumin (delta bilirubin) is more than 20% of total bilirubin
  - It is always pathological

Prolonged Jaundice[8,9,17,18,21,25,27]

Definition

When jaundice lasts for more than 2–3 weeks in the infant after birth, it is regarded as abnormal and requires additional investigation. This may be conjugated or nonconjugated.

"I must know."

Prolonged Unconjugated or Indirect Hyperbilirubinemia[8,17,18,21,25,27]

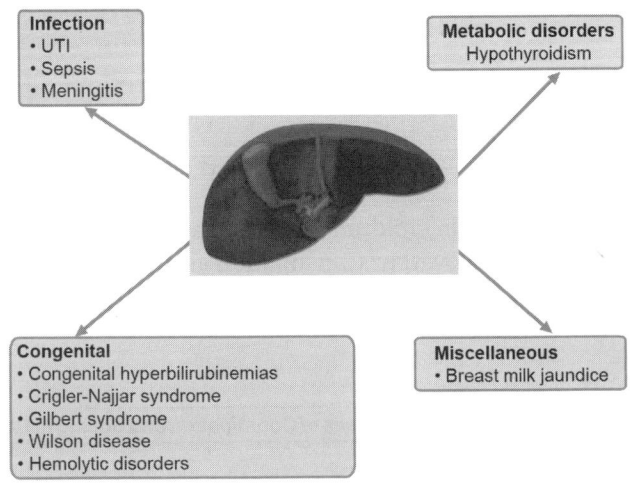

- **Infection**
  - UTI
  - Sepsis
  - Meningitis

- **Metabolic disorders**
  - Hypothyroidism

- **Congenital**
  - Congenital hyperbilirubinemias
  - Crigler-Najjar syndrome
  - Gilbert syndrome
  - Wilson disease
  - Hemolytic disorders

- **Miscellaneous**
  - Breast milk jaundice

In a jaundiced child, when the color of the stool is pale and urine dark, you must think of conjugated hyperbilirubinemia. You must know that this is always abnormal. Depending on the history and the age of the child, you will consider some differential diagnosis. Ask about all the historical links and search for the physical signs.

"I must know."

Differential Diagnosis of Conjugated or Direct Hyperbilirubinemia[8,9,17,18,21,25,27]

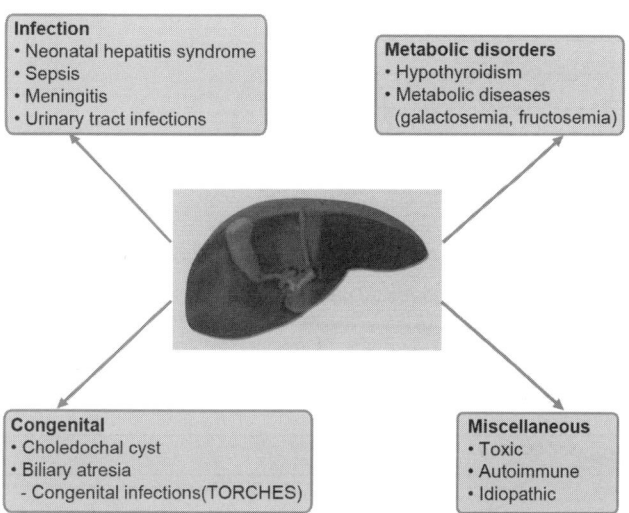

When you feel an enlarged liver, you must define its nature as well as know the causes. If you know some of the more common causes, you will be able to use appropriate physical links and look for other relevant and important signs.

"I must know."

Causes of Hepatomegaly

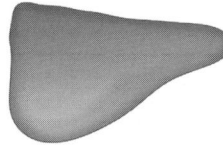

Causes of hepatomegaly with smooth hepatic enlargement[8,17,18,21,25,27]
• Infections where acute liver enlargement causes tenderness at the right hypochondrium due to acute stretching of the hepatic capsule
• Autoimmune conditions
• Chronic hemolytic anemias
• Cardiovascular causes such as constrictive pericarditis and cardiac failure
• Obstruction to biliary flow
• Metabolic or storage diseases
• Neoplastic

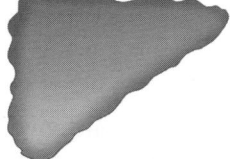

Causes of hepatosplenomegaly with irregular enlargement of the liver[8,17,18,21,25,27]
• Benign hepatic tumors
• Infections such as Echinochoccus granulosus (Hydatid disease)
• Teratoma
• Malignant hepatic tumors in infants (e.g. hepatoblastoma)
• Malignant hepatic tumors in older children (e.g. hepatocellular carcinoma)
• Prehepatic, hepatic and posthepatic causes of portal hypertension

286 The Link: Pediatric History-Taking and Physical Examination

"I must know."

Portal hypertension as a result of prehepatic causes[8,17,18,21,25,27]
Neonatal sepsis leading to umbilical vessel thrombosis
Umbilical catheter induced 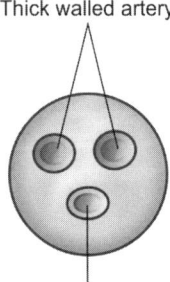 Thick walled artery Thin walled vein *Asepsis during umbilical catheterization reduces the incidence of portal vein thrombosis.*
Portal vein thrombosis
Congenital anomaly
Massive splenomegaly
Hepatic causes of portal hypertension[8,17,18,21,25,27]
Congenital hepatic fibrosis
Cirrhosis
Storage diseases like Gaucher's disease
Posthepatic causes of hypertension[8,17,18,21,25,27]
Hepatic venous blockage (Budd-Chiari syndrome)
Inferior vena cava blockage
Cardiac causes
The cardiac causes of portal hypertension are congestive cardiac failure and constrictive pericarditis. 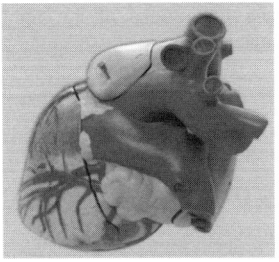

SYSTEM: RENAL[8,17,18,21,25,27]

Urinary Tract Infection in Children[3]

Urinary tract infection in the neonate is associated with symptoms and signs that are nonspecific as mentioned in Chapter 3. In this age group, it is usually part of a bacteremia due to hematogenous spread and parenteral antibiotics are needed for 10–14 days. Congenital anomalies of the renal tract whether anatomical or functional importantly contribute to the incidence of UTI in children. Vesicoureteral reflux is important to consider. In the history and physical examination, some of these factors can be elucidated.

"I must know."

Factors that predispose to UTI in children [8,17,18,21,25,27]

Age	Neonatal period
Gender	Male gender
Causes	• Obstructive lesions which may be anatomical or mechanical such as renal calculi
	• Oliguria due to prerenal, renal or postrenal causes
	• Family history of vesicoureteral reflux (VUR) or renal disease
	Congenital causes
	• Congenital or acquired anatomical anomalies, e.g. VUR
	• Functional renal abnormalities
	• Presence of foreskin in the uncircumcised male
	• Renal abnormality that is antenatally diagnosed
	Chronic diseases, e.g. hypertension, diabetes mellitus
	Spinal anomalies—congenital or acquired
	Infectious cause
	Fecal colonization
	Perineal colonization
	Instrumentation of the urinary tract
	Sexual activity in adolescence or as may sometimes occur in sexual abuse
	Suggestive or definite history of a previous UTI
	Recurrent fever of uncertain origin
	Gastrointestinal cause
	Constipation
	Abdominal mass
	Immunocompromised status
	Congenital or acquired immunocompromised states
	Functional causes
	Dysfunctional voiding

While an anatomical diagnosis will clarify that the renal system is involved and the location of the pathology within the renal tract, an etiological diagnosis is needed to commence appropriate antibiotic therapy.

"It is nice to know."

Urinary Tract Infections in Children: Etiological Agents [3,8,17,18,21,25,27]

–VE
Gram-negative rods
Escherichia coli
Proteus mirabilis
Klebsiella spp
Citrobacter spp
Enterobacter cloacae
Pseudomonas aeruginosa
Providencia stuartii
Serratia spp

Gram-negative cocci
Neisseria gonorrhoeae

+VE
Gram-positive cocci
Enterococcus spp
Streptococcus group B
Staphylococcus aureus
Staphylococcus epidermidis
Staphylococcus saprophyticus
Streptococcus group D
Streptococcus faecalis

Other pathogens
Candida spp
Chlamydia trachomatis
Adenovirus

There are some differences in the method of urine collection in children as they are dry by day at about 2 years and dry by night at about 3 years, and they obviously cannot understand instructions for the collection of urine.

Diagnostic Points [3,8,17,18,21,25,27]

Methods of urine collection

1. **Mid-stream, clean catch urine specimen**
   In this method the initial part of the stream of urine is discarded as this mainly contains periurethral bacteria
   Interpretation:
   Pure growth of a single organism $>10^5$ colonies/mL
2. **Catheterized specimen of urine**
   Interpretation:
   Pure growth of a single organism $>10^4$ colonies/mL
3. **Suprapubic aspiration of bladder for urine specimen**
   In infants, the bladder is intra-abdominal. This procedure is best done an hour after a feed
   Interpretation: Any growth is significant

Knowing risk factors in a disease is important in many ways. In the process of history taking and physical examination, specifically ask direct questions and use the relevant links. The physical examination should be complete and should focus on the risk factors for diagnosis, treatment, management including counseling and prognostication.

Nephritis in childhood is commonly caused by poststreptococcal infection. However, in the history and physical examination, do not forget to search for the other causes. Important negative history and examination contribute to the process of analytic thinking to exclude unlikely diagnosis and confirm more likely diagnosis.

"I must know."

Differential Diagnosis of Nephritis in Childhood[3,8,17,18,21,25,27]

Systemic causes	Local causes
• Infective endocarditis • Sickle cell disease • Hemolytic uremic syndrome (HUS) • "Shunt" nephritis • Goodpasture syndrome • Collagen diseases SLE, PAN, RA	• Henoch-Schönlein purpura nephritis (HSPN) • Rapidly progressive (crescentic) glomerulonephritis • Alport syndrome

Primary Nephrotic Syndrome: Possible Differentials[8,17,18,21,25,27]

• Minimal change—No changes under light microscopy but podocyte foot process fusion on electron microscopy
• Focal segmental—May develop from MCNS or as a separate entity; one-third progress to renal failure
• Membranoproliferative—Hypocomplementemia with signs of glomerular disease
• Membranous—Seen in adolescents and children with systemic infections, such as hepatitis B and C, syphilis, malaria, toxoplasmosis, leprosy, schistosomiasis, tuberculosis or lymphomas or in association with drug therapy like captopril, nonsteroidal anti-inflammatory drugs (NSAIDs), gold and penicillamine

In any disease, the typical features are the most common presentation. However, it is important to know that atypical presentations of diseases exist. When a patient presents atypically, an index of suspicion is required to make the diagnosis. Sometimes, the prognosis may not be as favorable.

Clinical Features for Non-MCNS that May Require a Renal Biopsy[8,17,18,21,25,27]

- Atypical age groups such as younger than a year and older than twelve years
- Prominent or gross hematuria
- Hypertension
- Acute renal failure
- Chronic renal disease in the family
- Evidence of systemic disease that have the potential to directly or indirectly affect the kidney
- Steroid resistance.

A disease of an organ may be primary or may be a result of other diseases or insults and may secondarily affect the organ. Hence, the knowledge of secondary causes of a disease makes it imperative that a complete physical examination be conducted in all patients. The lack of time should never be an excuse for a poor or incomplete physical examination.

Some differentials for secondary causes of nephrotic syndrome[8,17,18,21,25,27]
• Henoch-Schönlein purpura (HSP)
• Systemic lupus erythematosus (SLE)
• Quartan malaria
• Heavy metal poisoning
• Drugs—NSAIDs, gold, penicillamine, IV biphosphonates, lithium, interferon, possibly some anticancer agents

Listed differential diagnosis of other causes of hematuria[8,17,18,21,25,27]
• Congenital anomalies of the urinary tract
• Urinary calculi
• Trauma
• Renal tumors
• Thrombocytopenias, thrombasthenias or coagulopathies
• Vascular lesions of the kidney, e.g. hemangiomas, AV malformations
• Renal vein thrombosis
• Malignancies causing disseminated intravascular coagulation (DIC)

Secondary to osmotic diuresis
- Glucose —diabetes mellitus
- Urea —relieved obstructive uropathy
- Hypercatabolic states
- Chronic renal failure
- Following renal transplantation

Deficiency of ADH
- Central diabetes insipidus
- Posttraumatic
- Neoplasia
- Infections

Increased fluid intake
Behavioral or psychogenic
Primary hypothalamic causes (as occurs in the lesions in the hypothalamic thirst center)

Medications
Diuretics
Theophylline

Causes of polyuria

Nephrogenic Diabetes Insipidus
Obstructive uropathy
Inherited disorders
Sickle cell diseases
Hypercalcemia

Causes of polyuria[21]

Oliguria[8,17,18,21,25,27]

Oliguria is an important clinical sign and requires urgent management. Oliguria in children may be due to a prerenal cause like dehydration or hemorrhage or to any underlying condition that reduces renal blood flow leading to poor renal perfusion. If treated early, the kidney function is preserved. It is thus important to recognize prerenal failure. Renal causes of oliguria are due to intrinsic renal pathology or due to extrinsic renal diseases that have resulted in compromised renal function. Prerenal failure if untreated will result in renal failure. Postrenal obstructive or compressive causes must be excluded.

"I must know."

Urinalysis[21,25] Link type of renal failure to urea and electrolytes	Prerenal[21,25] • Reversible causes such as dehydration and hypovolemia due to any cause must be excluded first in prerenal causes of renal failure • Here the urine has a high osmolality and urea without much loss of sodium	Renal[21,25] Renal causes including renal parenchymal and glomerular causes lead to intrinsic renal failure
Urine osmolality	>400 mmol/kg	<350 mmol/kg
Urinary sodium	<20 mEq/L	>40 mEq/L
Renal failure index (RFI)	<1	>1
Urine/plasma osmolality	>1:2	<1:1
Urine/plasma urea ratio	>4:1	<4:1
Quantity of fractional filtered sodium excreted	<1	>1
Blood urea nitrogen: creatinine ratio	>20	<15

SYSTEM: BLOOD[8,17,18,21,25,27]

Anemia in children is an important symptom and usually reflects underlying nutritional status. Specific hematological diseases occur in children but anemia often coexists with chronic diseases which influence nutrition by impairment of appetite, absorption and utilization of nutrients. It is important to try to detect the earliest symptoms and signs of anemia. Correction of the anemia can make an important clinical difference to the growth and development of the child.

"I must know."

Main reasons for anemia in developing countries[15]
Dietary insufficiency of micronutrients
Iron
Vitamin B_{12}
Folate
Iron deficiency due to blood loss[15]
Blood loss in stool from hookworm
Blood loss in urine from schistosomiasis
Trichuris with dysentery syndrome
Hemolysis[21]
Malaria
Hemoglobinopathy
Anemia due to infection
Tuberculosis
Malaria
Hookworm

Identifying the risk factors that cause iron deficiency is important in history taking and examination. Good practice of pediatrics also entails the counseling and possible prevention of such factors in as far as possible.

"It is good to know."

Hypochromic microcytic anemia is more common in these groups:[8,17,18,21,25,27]
Malnutrition at any age
Very premature infants
Infants of diabetic mothers
Infants of anemic mothers
Exclusive breastfeeding after six months
Strict vegans
Early introduction of cow's milk (before 12 months)
Excessive cow's milk intake
No complementary feeding after 1 year
Blood loss through heavy menstruation or bloody diarrhea
Children with special healthcare needs
Parasitic infestation, e.g. *Ascaris*, *Trichuris*, hookworm[15]

"I must know."

Drugs commonly causing hemolysis in glucose-6-phosphate dehydrogenase deficiency (G6PD deficiency):[8,17,18,21,25,27]
• Aspirin (Salicylates)
• Chloroquine
• Chloramphenicol
• Cotrimoxazole
• Dapsone
• Hydrochloroquine
• Methylene blue
• Nitrofurantoin
• Nalidixic acid
• Naphthalene
• Primaquine
• Probenecid
• Sulfonamides
• Vitamin K analogues

Note: Some traditional medications, such as those taken from roots or herbs must be used with caution especially in mothers who are breastfeeding their G6PD deficient babies. These may contain oxidants that can pass through the breast milk. Application of salicylate containing medication on the skin of G6PD deficient babies must also be avoided.

The spleen enlarges in response to infections, systemic diseases, storage disorders and neoplasms. A good history and physical examination will elucidate the causes.

"I must know"

Causes of splenomegaly[21]	Reactive, compensatory, infiltrative and other causes of splenomegaly[21]
Infections	Tuberculosis Bacterial endocarditis Septicemia, brucellosis Schistosomiasis Malaria (massive splenomegaly)
Any condition that results in portal hypertension	Prehepatic, posthepatic and hepatic causes
Extramedullary hemopoiesis	Hemolytic anemias Hemoglobinopathies
Systemic diseases	Juvenile rheumatoid arthritis Systemic lupus erythematosus Malaria
Storage diseases	Mucopolysaccharidosis Niemann-Pick Langerhans cell histiocytosis
Neoplasms	Leukemias—Chronic myeloid leukemia Lymphomas
Massive splenomegaly	Tropical splenomegaly (massive splenomegaly) Chronic myeloid leukemia

SYSTEM: CHILDHOOD MALIGNANCIES[8,17,18,21,25,27]

Sometimes, childhood malignancies exist more frequently in children with inherited or genetic predispositions. Although such disorders are not common, this knowledge increases the index of suspicion for an underlying malignancy, which influences diagnosis and follow-up management.

"It is nice to know."

Childhood cancers and syndromes[7,26]	
Syndrome	Malignancy
Down syndrome or Trisomy 21	Leukemia, testicular germ cell tumors
Edward's syndrome or Trisomy 18	Wilms' tumor
Turner syndrome 45XO	Wilms' tumor, neuroblastoma, colon cancer
Klinefelter's syndrome	Germ cell tumor, lung cancer, non-Hodgkin lymphoma
Xerodema pigmentosum (autosomal recessive)	Melanoma
Syndromes associated with somatic overgrowth such as Beckwith-Wiedemann syndrome, Sotos syndrome and Simpson-Golabi-Behmel	Wilms' tumor Hepatoblastoma Neuroblasoma Pancreatoblastoma
Tuberous sclerosis (multisystem hamartomas)	Subependymal giant cell astrocytoma Small cell lung cancer Ganglioglioma Acute myelocytic leukemia

SYSTEM: ENDOCRINE[8,17,18,21,25,27]

Cretinism is a preventable cause of mental retardation. Although screening tests at birth can pick it up, you must be familiar with all its features. Detecting problems that can be corrected is an important role of a doctor, so sharpen your power of observation, a vital component of the physical examination.

"It is good to know."

Features of cretinism[21]
Coarse face
Wide fontanel
Hoarse cry
Feeding difficulties

Contd...

Contd...

Apnea
Noisy respiration
Somnolence
Mental retardation
Hypotonia
Flat nasal bridge
Macroglossia
Short broad fingers
Dry skin
Cutis marmorata
Prolonged unconjugated or indirect hyperbilirubinemia
Constipation
Distended abdomen
Cardiomegaly
Bradycardia
Cardiac murmurs

An understanding of etiology will enhance your understanding and diagnostic ability, hence the emphasis on anatomical and etiological diagnosis in history taking and physical examination.

"It is good to know."

List of differential diagnosis in the causes of congenital hypothyroidism[8,17,18,21,25,27]

Thyroid Gland

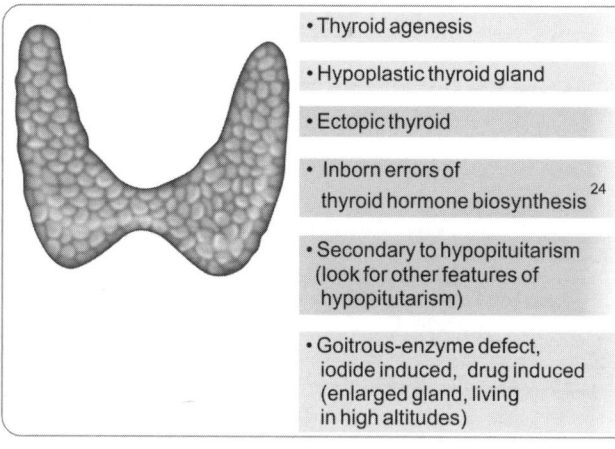

- Thyroid agenesis
- Hypoplastic thyroid gland
- Ectopic thyroid
- Inborn errors of thyroid hormone biosynthesis[24]
- Secondary to hypopituitarism (look for other features of hypopitutarism)
- Goitrous-enzyme defect, iodide induced, drug induced (enlarged gland, living in high altitudes)

Children suffer from diabetes mellitus.

"I must know."

Types of diabetes mellitus in children and adolescence[17,21]
Type 1 or insulin-dependent diabetes mellitus
Transient neonatal
Permanent neonatal
Classic type 1 of multifactorial etiology
Type 2 or noninsulin-dependent diabetes mellitus
Due to underlying diseases, e.g. cystic fibrosis, hemochromatosis
Classic adult type
Maturity onset diabetes of youth (MODY)
Mitochondrial diabetes mellitus
Drug-induced, e.g. corticosteroids
Pregnancy-induced diabetes mellitus

Neonatal hypoglycemia is important to recognize. Recognition of signs and symptoms leads to early diagnosis and treatment. This prevents childhood morbidities like mental retardation, fits and mortality; hence this knowledge is important as a tool in preventive pediatrics.

"I must know."

Diagnostic points on neonatal hypoglycemia[8,17,18,21,25,27]
The diagnosis of hypoglycemia is considered if the blood sugar level is equal to or below ≤ 2.5 mmol/L
• Symptomatic hypoglycemia is more ominous than asymptomatic hypoglycemia
• A level of <1 mmol/L is critical
Contributing etiological causes of neonatal hypoglycemia
Small for gestational age
Large for gestational age
Infant of the diabetic mother
Premature babies
Neonatal sepsis
Perinatal hypoxia due to any cause
Polycythemia due to any cause
Critically-ill babies due to any cause
Recognized syndromes associated with hypoglycemia

The growth parameters must be plotted on age and gender specific percentile charts. When short stature is encountered, a good history and thorough physical examination are vital. It is important to know the common causes.

292 *The Link*: Pediatric History-Taking and Physical Examination

"It is good to know".

Short stature other than endocrine causes[17,21]
In familial short stature
A child is short but on complete history and physical examination is found to have no underlying disease
Elicited family history of one or more relatives who are also short without underlying diseases
The bone age tallies with the chronological age
The rate of growth is normal
Constitutional delay of growth and puberty (CDGP)
This commonly occurs in boys who are otherwise healthy
An elicited history of delay in puberty and examination confirms this
An associated family history of delayed puberty
Bone age delayed and tallies with height age
The rate of growth is below the normal
Reassurance that these children will attain normal adult height and puberty without intervention

SYSTEM: CENTRAL NERVOUS SYSTEM[8,17,18,21,25,27]

The classification of epileptic seizures will help you make a differential diagnosis. It is useful to know the guidelines used in the classification. In determining seizure type, ask about the nature of the seizure, the part of the body involved and whether consciousness was lost or altered.

In the differential diagnosis of ataxia, many causes must be considered. In pediatrics, the astute mother who herself looks after the child usually gives you a reliable history, and great reliance is placed on the mother's story. However, often the mother is at work. In these cases, a knowledge of the causes of a given condition, such as ataxia, is necessary in order to ask the relevant questions. This, in turn, improves the accuracy of the diagnosis that you make and clarifies etiology.

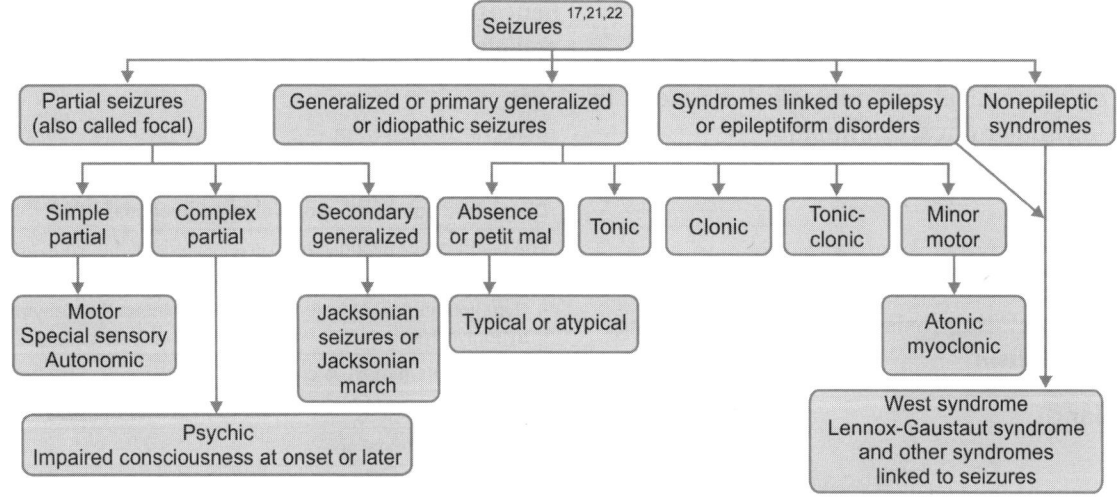

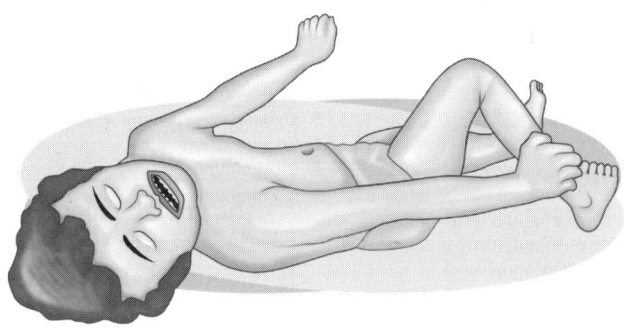

Tonic-clonic seizure

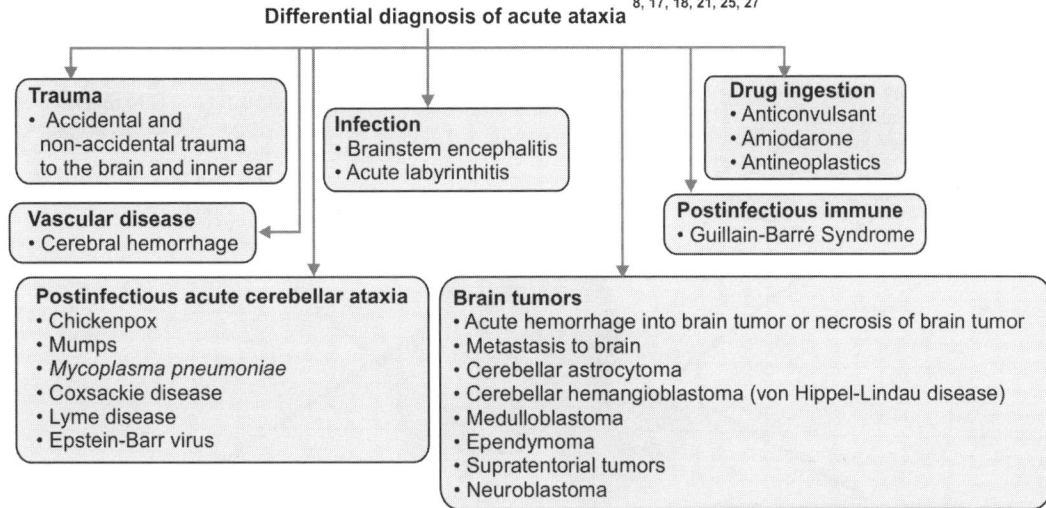

Differential diagnosis of acute ataxia [8, 17, 18, 21, 25, 27]

Trauma
- Accidental and non-accidental trauma to the brain and inner ear

Infection
- Brainstem encephalitis
- Acute labyrinthitis

Drug ingestion
- Anticonvulsant
- Amiodarone
- Antineoplastics

Vascular disease
- Cerebral hemorrhage

Postinfectious immune
- Guillain-Barré Syndrome

Postinfectious acute cerebellar ataxia
- Chickenpox
- Mumps
- *Mycoplasma pneumoniae*
- Coxsackie disease
- Lyme disease
- Epstein-Barr virus

Brain tumors
- Acute hemorrhage into brain tumor or necrosis of brain tumor
- Metastasis to brain
- Cerebellar astrocytoma
- Cerebellar hemangioblastoma (von Hippel-Lindau disease)
- Medulloblastoma
- Ependymoma
- Supratentorial tumors
- Neuroblastoma

In pediatrics, all children under 2 years of age must have their circumference of head measured and plotted on a graph appropriate for gender and age. An abnormally big head may be due to hydrocephalus. The mechanisms of hydrocephalus clarify etiology.

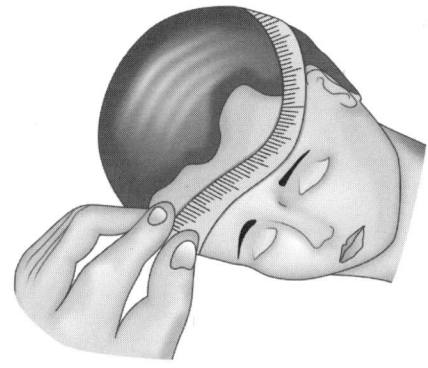

The COH or OFC is the occipitofrontal circumference

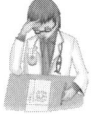

"I must know."

Causes of hydrocephalus[8,17,18,21,25,27]
• Communicating or non-communicating hydrocephalus
• Intraventricular obstruction
• Meningitis
• Congenital aqueductal stenosis
• Dandy-Walker syndrome-occlusion of exit to 4th ventricle resulting in a large 4th ventricle and cerebellar hypoplasia
• Arnold-Chiari malformation—downward displacement of cerebellar tonsils and brain stem with or without spina bifida
• Arachnoid cysts
• X-linked congenital hydrocephalus
• Neoplasm or vascular malformation
• Extraventricular obstruction
• Infection
• Post-hemorrhagic
• Leukemic infiltrates

Differential Diagnosis of Macrocephaly[8,17,18,21,25,27]

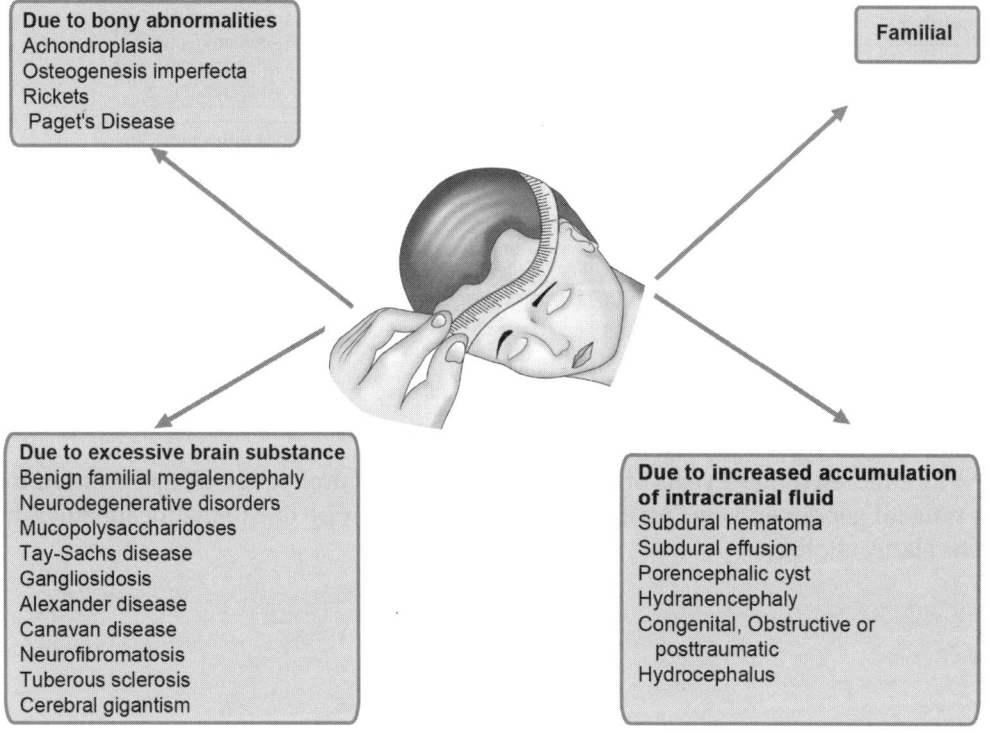

Cerebral Palsy[8,17,18,21,25,27]

As you have seen in Chapter 10, cerebral palsy has a few subtypes. The clinical manifestations are linked to the part of the brain involved in the underlying cause of the disorder.

Classification by Type of Motor Disorder[21,25,27]
• Spastic cerebral palsy (CP with hypertonic muscles associated with stiff and jerky movements)
• Dyskinetic cerebral palsy (CP with difficulty or distortion in performing voluntary movements)
• Ataxic cerebral palsy (CP associated with disorganized, clumsy or jerky movements)
• Dystonic cerebral palsy (CP with involuntary movements with prolonged muscular contraction)
• Choreoathetoid cerebral palsy (CP with involuntary purposeless or semipurposeful uncontrollable movements)
• Mixed cerebral palsy (CP with mixed features)

A history of neonatal seizures influence the child's well-being. The cause of seizures in the neonatal period must be elucidated by a detailed history.

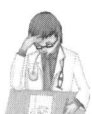
"It is nice to know."

Neonatal seizures that cause symptoms may be attributed to:[8,17,18,21,25,27]
Placental abruption (hypoxia)
Infection, such as viral encephalitis, toxoplasmosis, bacterial meningitis, rubella and syphilis
Intracranial hemorrhage (e.g. birth injury, preterm)
Congenital brain anomalies (genetic or acquired, such as tuberous sclerosis)
Acid based, blood sugar or electrolyte imbalances, including hypoglycemia, hypocalcemia or hypernatremia
Errors of metabolism, such as maple syrup urine disease, pyridoxine dependency or phenylketonuria (PKU)
Drug withdrawal, which may be seen in infants born to mothers addicted to alcohol, heroin, cocaine, methadone or barbiturates

System: Development[21,25]

Gross motor, fine motor, social development, hearing and speech are milestones that a child attains during the course of development. The etiological causes of deafness can influence other developmental milestones if the insult is early. Conductive deafness may affect speech if recurrent or uncorrected.

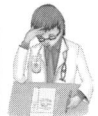

"It is good to know."

Differential diagnosis to consider in deafness (clusters)[8,17,18,21,25,27]
Syndromes and genetic causes
CHARGE syndrome
Waardenburg syndrome
Down syndrome
Treacher Collins syndrome
Intrauterine
Cytomegalovirus, syphilis congenital rubella, and toxoplasmosis
Ototoxic drugs such as aminoglycosides, loop diuretics and chemotherapeutic agents
Perinatal
Birth asphyxia
Low birth weight
Prematurity
Hyperbilirubinemia
Ototoxic drugs
Postnatal
Serous or secretory otitis media
Suppurative otitis media
Encephalitis, meningitis or meningoencephalitis
Mumps
Ototoxic drugs
Accidental or non-accidental trauma to the head or inner ear

The causes of visual impairment, if known, will require identifying other related abnormalities. Blindness can also affect fine motor development. The causes of blindness are also influenced by geographical location.

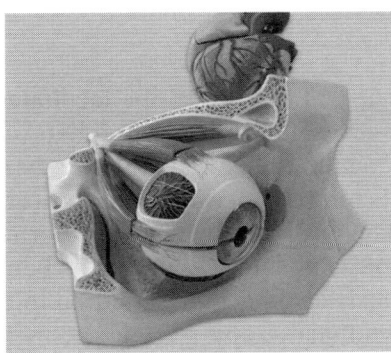

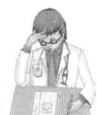

"It is good to know."

Differential diagnosis of the causes of visual impairment[8,13,17,18,21,25,27]
Severe malnutrition and vitamin A deficiency
River blindness or onchocerciasis
Glaucoma
Trachoma
Diabetes mellitus
Ocular injuries
Severe myopia
Optic atrophy
Cataracts
Optic nerve hypoplasia
Buphthalmos
Colobomata
Retinopathy of prematurity (ROP)
Chorioretinits
Leber's congenital amaurosis
Perinatal asphyxia-cortical blindness with normal pupillary light reflex

Speech delay can be due to local causes or may be part of a global developmental delay. The hearing of a child with speech delay must be checked.

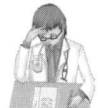

"I must know."

Differential diagnosis of causes of or resulting in speech delay[8,17,18,21,25,27]
• Hearing impairment
• Mental retardation
• Local causes such as cleft palate
• Problems with vocal cords, mouth, tongue, teeth or lungs
• Neurological dysarthrias
• Developmental language disorders
• Infantile autism
• Hyperactivity
• Psychosocial issues
• Non-accidental injury such as social and emotional deprivation

The term developmental regression has been explained in Chapter 3. It is an ominous symptom and one must discern all possible causes. A detailed history followed by a complete physical examination leads to a provisional diagnosis and often referral to a specialist is necessary.

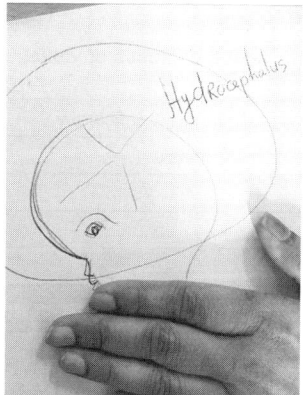

Sketch of a large head due to hydrocephalus.

Causes of developmental regression include:[8,17,18,21,25,27]
• Cerebral tumors
• Specific types of epilepsy
• Specific hematomas
• Hydrocephalus
• Metabolic and neurodegenerative disorders

Hydrocephalus: A Cause of Developmental Regression[8,17,18,21,25,27]

Inborn errors of metabolism must, sometimes, be considered in the pediatric differential diagnosis. Some diagnostic indicators and background knowledge are useful in its broad understanding and classification. Diagnostic points in inborn errors of metabolism.

Suspect inborn errors if you elicit the following in the history, physical examination and laboratory tests.
- There is a family history of other affected children, neonatal or infant deaths in siblings
- There are siblings with mental retardation or neurological disorders[26]
- Consanguinity in parents
- Neonates are unwell after a period of being seemingly healthy
- Recurrent encephalopathic episodes
- Persistent and recurrent acidosis
- Urinary ketones in an acidotic neonate
- Recurrent clinical problems despite negative routine investigation results
- The finding of unexplained thrombocytopenia or leukopenia.

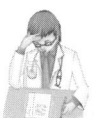

"It is good to know."

The main presentations in inborn errors of metabolism include those that present with a sudden, dramatic effect sometimes mistaken for sepsis and those that result in a more chronic presentation. A subacute presentation can also occur.

Acute and sudden presentation[12,25]
• The 'smaller' molecule group are mainly autosomal recessive. The patients who are relatively well suddenly become sick
• The toxic metabolites are primarily ammonia, amino acids, organic acids and sugars
• Disease due to small molecules often involve small organic acids, amino acids, glucose, fatty acids, nucleotides and ammonia

Chronic, more insidious presentation[12]
• The 'larger' molecule group, e.g. the storage diseases
• Their clinical features are usually multisystem, predominantly neurological, gradual in onset with chronic clinical problems
• Disease due to large molecules are usually due to aberrant synthesis or degradation of polymeric molecules, for example, glycoproteins and glycolipids

Intermediary group with subacute presentation[12]
• Intermediary metabolites can influence the activity of a biochemical pathway, due to altered transport of metabolites within the cell and or outside the cell. An example of this is primary carnitine deficiency

Autism[1,2,21]

There is an increasing awareness of this condition. Some information about this disorder is useful knowledge in general pediatrics for diagnosis, referral and counseling.

Screening[1,2,21]

Early detection of autism can be facilitated by using the trial: Checklist for Autism in Toddlers (CHAT).[1,2,21] This is a screening checklist which is based on the finding that children not exhibiting 'joint attention' or 'pretend play' at the age where they normally occur, are at risk of being later diagnosed as being autistic. Early diagnosis enables these children to be referred for interventional therapy.

Factual Knowledge

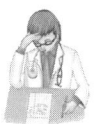

"It is good to know."

Recognized features in autism or autism spectrum disorders [1,2]

- A significant restriction in social and emotional interaction with impairment of communication

- **Features of speech**
  If speech is present, predominant features in an autistic child include:
  - Echolalia
  - Pronoun reversal
  - Nonsense rhyming

- **Features in autism**
  - Delayed speech
  - Headbanging
  - Teeth grinding
  - Rocking
  - Diminished responsiveness to pain and external stimuli
  - Self-mutilation
  - Delayed speech

- The diagnosis manifests more clearly around 3 years as 'pretend play' before this age is still within the normal development of a child and therefore cannot be discerned as abnormal

- **General behavior of the autistic child**
  - Diminished or absent eye contact
  - Mouthing objects
  - Visual scanning of hand and finger movements
  - Physically aggressive behavior, pica or putting inedible items in the mouth
  - Withdrawn and spends hours in solitary play.
  - Tantrum-like rages accompany disruptions of routine

- Reduced response to pain and a lack of startle to loud sounds

SYSTEM: MUSCULOSKELETAL [8,17,18,21,25,27]

This system is difficult to examine in an uncooperative child. Observation is very important. The observation of limb movement is often combined with elements of the neurological and developmental system in the child. Age-related angular variations of the legs must be remembered. Genu varum and genu valgum can be physiological or pathological (Refer to Chapter 10).

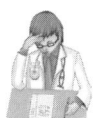

"It is good to know."

Causes of Genu Varum [6,8,17,18,21,25,27]

- Apparent genu varum
- Physiologic genu varum
- Inherited longitudinal deficiency of the tibia
- Congenital familial tibia vara or Blount's disease
- Infection
- Fracture
- Tumor
- Rickets—vitamin D deficiency or refractory (hypophosphatemia)
- Fibrocartilaginous dysplasia
- Bone dysplasia, such as achondroplasia (autosomal dominant) and metaphyseal dysplasia
- Lead or fluoride intoxication.

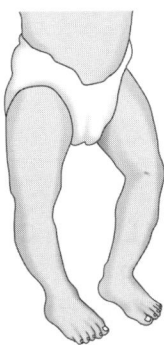

A drawing of genu varum by 10-year-old Bernard

Causes of Genu Valgum [6,8,17,18,21,25,27]

- Developmental—physiologic
- Congenital

- Iliotibial band contracture
- Fracture leading to unequal growth arrest
- Metabolic bone disease
- Trauma
- Malunion of fracture
- Infection
- Arthritis of knee due to chronic conditions such as rheumatoid arthritis, hemophilia
- Bone dysplasia—Morquio syndrome, Ollier disease (multiple enchondromatosis), multiple hereditary exostosis and multiple epiphyseal dysplasia
- Osteogenesis imperfecta.

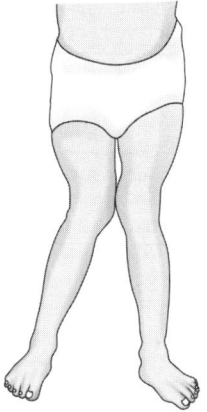

A drawing of genu valgum by 12-year-old John

The diagnosis of a child with a limp is based on the age of presentation and whether it is painful or painless. The painful limp has been discussed in Chapter 10. In a limping child, a detailed history and physical examination will indicate a probable cause; so as appropriate to the case, consider the following as differential diagnoses.

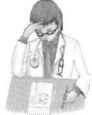

"It is good to know."

Common Causes of Limp in Children and Adolescents According to Age[8,17-19,21,25,27]

Causes that shorten the leg are more common than those that lengthen. These causes include congenital growth defects such as skeletal dysplasias and hemiatrophy, infections that involve the epiphysis (e.g. osteomyelitis), tumors, fractures that affect the growth plate or have overriding ends, Legg-Calve-Perthes disease, slipped capital femoral epiphysis (SCFE) and radiation. Lengthening of the leg can be a consequence of hemihypertrophy, in which one or more structures on one side of the body grow to be larger than the other side, vascular malformations or tumors (such as hemangioma), Wilms' renal tumor, septic arthritis, healed fractures or orthopedic surgery.

1–5 years old (Especially children who have started to walk and less than 3 years of age)[8,17-19, 21,25,27]

- Shortening of leg may be due to many factors including congenital growth deficiencies as seen in seen in hemiatrophy and skeletal dysplasias
- Trauma
- Synovitis
- Infective arthritis
- Osteomyelitis
- Developmental dysplasia of the hip
- Juvenile rheumatoid arthritis
- Spastic cerebral palsy
- Discrepancy of leg length
- Duchenne muscular dystrophy
- Diseases involving the muscles or nerves.

5–10 years old

- Trauma
- Synovitis
- Osteomyelitis
- Infective arthritis
- Developmental dysplasia of the hip
- Discrepancy of leg length
- Spastic cerebral palsy
- Duchenne muscular dystrophy
- Diseases involving the muscles or nerves
- Avascular necrosis of the proximal femoral head (Perthes disease/Legg-Calve-Perthes disease).

10–15 years old

- Trauma
- Osteomyelitis
- Infective arthritis
- Slipped upper femoral epiphysis
- Patellofemoral pain syndrome
- Discrepancy of leg length
- Diseases involving the muscles or nerves
- Developmental dysplasia of the hip
- Neoplasm, malignant or benign tumors.

Juvenile rheumatoid arthritis is also known as juvenile idiopathic arthritis. It is the commonest type of arthritis

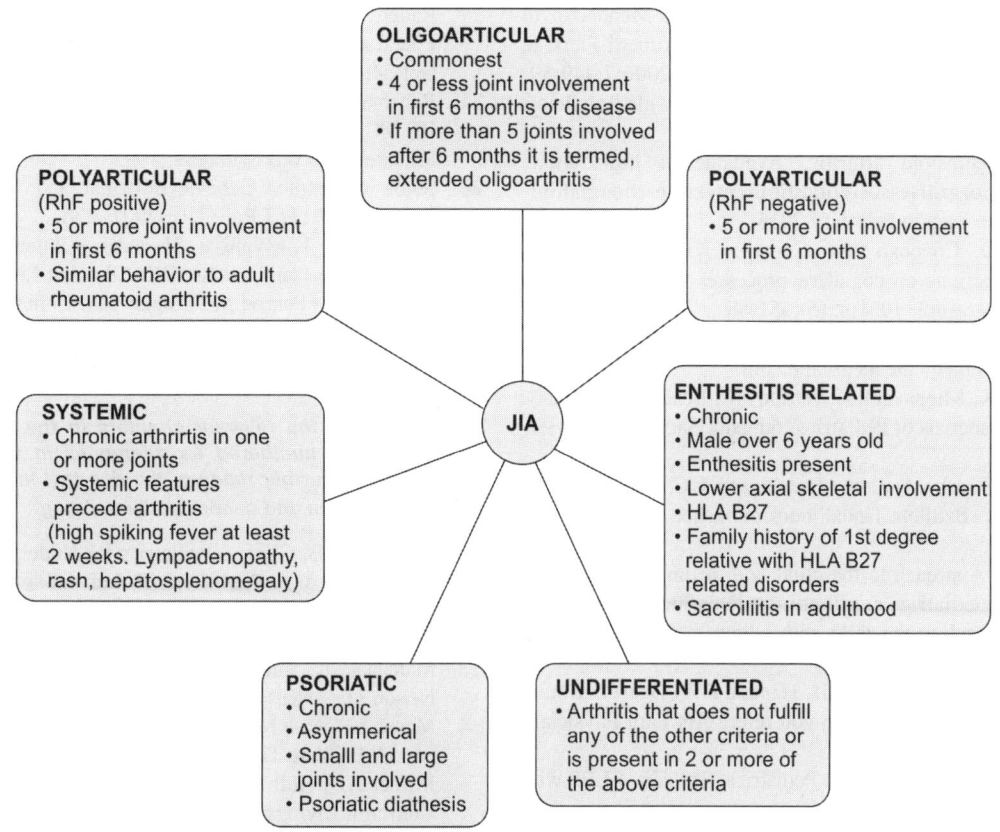

Classification of juvenile idiopathic arthritis (JIA)

in children below sixteen years of age and manifests as constant pain, swelling and stiffness.

Juvenile idiopathic arthritis or JIA is the new nomenclature used to help differentiate between the various subtypes of juvenile rheumatoid arthritis that is sometimes considered in the differential diagnosis of musculoskeletal involvement in systemic diseases.

Clinically, this disease manifests differently with predilections for gender and age group. Knowledge about this can help you to consider the various specific types of JIA in the differential diagnosis.

Diagnostic Points in Juvenile Idiopathic Arthritis[8,14,17,18,21,23,25,27]

Juvenile idiopathic arthritis (JIA) can be a cause of a limp in children which is painful in the acute stage and painless in the chronic stage.

REFERENCES

1. Autistic Spectrum Disorders. A Guide for Paediatricians in India. Available at http://autism-india.org/AFA%20Paediatrician%20booklet.pdf.
2. Baron-Cohen S, Wheelwright S, Cox A, et al. Early identification of autism by Checklist for Autism in Toddlers (CHAT). J R Soc Med. 2000;93:521-5.
3. Chon CH, Lai FC, Shortliffe LM. Pediatric urinary tract infections. Pediatr Clin N Am. 2001;48(6):1443.
4. Cole C, Gazewood J. Diagnosis and treatment of impetigo. Am Fam Physician. 2007;75(6):859-64.
5. Elizabeth KE. Clinical Pediatrics for Undergraduates. India: Jaypee Brothers Medical Publishers (P) Ltd. 2009.
6. Espandar R, Seyed Mohammad-Javad Mortazavi, Baghdadi T. Angular Deformities of the Lower Limb in Children Asian J Sports Med. 2010 Mar;1(1):46-53.
7. Ganmore I, Smooha G, Izraeli S. Constitutional aneuploidy and cancer predisposition. Available at http://www.ncbi.nlm.nih.gov/pmc/articles/PMC2657942/pdf/ddp084.pdf. Accessed in February 2015.
8. Goel KM, Gupta DK. Hutchinson's Pediatrics, 1st edn. India: Jaypee Brothers Medical Publishers (P) Ltd; 2009.
9. Harb R, Thomas DW. Conjugated hyperbilirubinemia: Screening and Treatment in Older Infants and Children. Pediatr Rev. 2007;28;83-91.
10. Hyman P. Childhood Defecation Disorders: Constipation and Soiling. Available at http://www.medschool.lsuhsc.edu.
11. Hyman P. Pediatric and Adolescent Gastrointestinal Motility and Pain Program. Available at http://www.medschool.lsuhsc.edu.

12. Inborn errors of metabolism: The flux from Mendelian to complex diseases. Brendan Lanpher, Nicola Brunetti-Pierri & Brendan Lee. Nature Reviews Genetics, June 2006;7:449-59.
13. JMJ Bull. Leading Causes of blindness. Worldwide Roodhooft Soc. Belge Ophtalmol., 2002;283:19-25.
14. Juvenile rheumatoid arthritis. Available at http://www.mayoclinic.org/diseases-conditions/juvenile-rheumatoid-arthritis. Accessed in February 2015.
15. Kvalsvig JD, Cooppan RM, Connolly KJ. The effects of parasite infections on cognitive processes in children. Ann Trop Med Parasitol. 1991;85(5):551-68.
16. Lewis LS, Steele RW. Impetigo Differential Diagnoses. Available at emedicine.medscape.com.
17. Marcdante K, Kliegman RM, Jenson HB, Behrman RE (Eds). Nelson's Essentials of Pediatrics. 6th edn. Saunders Elsevier, 2010.
18. Mason S, Swash M (Eds). Hutchinson's Clinical Methods (17th edn). A Bailllere Tindall book published by Cassell Ltd; 1980.
19. Mayson B. Approach to the child with a limp. Available at http://learnpediatrics.com/body-systems/musculoskeletal-system/approach-to-the-child-with-a-limp/. Accessed in February 2015.
20. McConnell ME, Adkins SB III, Hannon DW. Heart murmurs in pediatric patients: when do you refer? Am Fam Physician. 1999;60(2):558-65.
21. Milner AD, Hull D. Hospital Pediatrics. 3rd edn. ELBS with Churchill Livingstone. 1998.
22. Pediatric Respiratory System: Basic Anatomy & Physiology, Jihad Zahraa Pediatric Intensivist, Head of PICU, King Fahad Medical City. http://www.mecriticalcare.net/downloads/lectures/PedsBasicAnatomyPhysiology.pdf
23. RACGP JIA guidelines. August 2009.
24. Radetti G, Zavallone A, Gentili L, Beck-Peccoz P, Bona G. Foetal and neonatal thyroid disorders. Minerva Pediatr. 2002 Oct;54(5):383-400.
25. Behrman RE (comps), Kliegman RM, Nelson WE, Vaughan III VC (eds). Nelson's textbook of pediatrics (14th ed). Philadelphia: WB Saunders; 1992.
26. Sotos syndrome. Geneviève Baujat and Valérie Cormier-Daire .Orphanet J Rare Dis. 2007;2:36.
27. Stephenson T, Wallace H (eds). Clinical Pediatrics for postgraduate examinations. UK: Churchill Livingstone; 1991.
28. Stulberg DL, Penrod MA, Blatny RA. Common Bacterial Skin Infections. Am Fam Physician. 2002;66(1):119-25.
29. Weiss LN. The Diagnosis of Wheezing in Children. Am Fam Physician. 2008;15;77(8):1109-14.

The essence of the relevant chapters in the following books have also been numbered as references in this chapter. We recommend for further reading, the rich text in these books for greater integration and deeper understanding.

1. Elizabeth KE. Clinical Pediatrics for Undergraduates. Jaypee Brothers Medical Publishers (P) Ltd, India. 2009.
2. Goel KM, Gupta DK. Hutchinson's Pediatrics, 1st edn. Jaypee Brothers Medical Publishers (P) Ltd, India. 2009.
3. Marcdante K, Kliegman RM, Jenson HB, Behrman RE (Eds). Nelson's Essentials of Pediatrics, 6th edn. Saunders Elsevier. 2010.
4. Mason S, Swash M (Eds). Hutchinson's Clinical Methods, 17th edn. A Bailllere Tindall book published by Cassell Ltd. 1980.
5. Milner AD, Hull D. Hospital Pediatrics, 3rd edn. ELBS with Churchill Livingstone. 1998.
6. Behrman (comps) RE, Kliegman RM, Nelson WE, Vaughan VC III (Eds). Nelson's Textbook of Pediatrics, 14th ed. Philadelphia: WB Saunders. 1992.
7. Stephenson T, Wallace H (Eds). Clinical Pediatrics for postgraduate examinations. UK: Churchill Livingstone. 1991.

Index

A

Abdomen 172
    auscultation of 176
    distended 291
    palpation of 173
    percussion of 175
Abdominal distension 38
Abdominal mass 174
Abdominal pain 21, 30, 40, 257
    causes of 257
    functional 32, 257
    surgical causes of 31
Abdominal wall, anterior 172
Acholic stools 35
Acne neonatorum 228
Addison's disease 162
Adenoids 99
Adenoma sebaceum 198
Adenovirus 287
Adolescents 131
Afebrile seizures 263
Air pollution, chronic 26
Airway
    disease in children 277
    problems 63
Alagille's syndrome 35
Alcohol 61, 92
Allergic history 93, 122
Allergic rhinitis 29
Allergy
    reduce 98
    to cow's milk protein 53
Alopecia 81, 157
Alpha-fetoprotein 62
Alport's syndrome 84
Alström syndorme 197
Amino acid disorders 18
Aminopterin 61, 92
Amiodarone 103
Anal orifice 167, 216
Anaphylactic reaction 118
Androgen secreting tumors 52
Anemia
    regardless of cause, symptoms of severe 54
    to infection 289
Anencephaly 59
Ankle
    jerk 186
    swelling of 37
Anoxic seizures 42
Anticonvulsants 103

Antimalarials 104
Antitrypsin deficiency 85
Anxiety 50
Apgar score 62
Aphthous ulcers 160
Apnea 291
Appetite 34, 35, 56
Ariboflavinosis 81
Arm 215
    span 144
Arterial venous 160
Arthralgias 22
Ascaris 289
Ascorbic acid 81
Aspirin 103, 290
Asplenia 116
Asthma 253
    history of 252
Ataxia 50, 187
Atenolol 104
Athetosis 184
Atrial septal defect 36, 255, 282
Autism 79, 296
Autosomal recessive disorders 84, 86
Avirulent vaccine 112
Awaiting splenectomy 116

B

Bacille calmette-güerin 109
    vaccine 102
Back, examination of 166
Bacteria 112, 113
Baldness, posterior 157
Bardet-Biedl syndrome 197
Beckwith-Wiedemann syndrome 59
Behavioral disorders 90
Behavioral problems 88
Beriberi 81
Biceps jerk 186
Bifid 147
Bifidus factor 98
Bigeminal pulse 147
Biliary
    atresia 165
    cirrhosis 165
Bilious vomiting 21
Bilirubin encephalopathy 66
Bioterrorism agents 94
Biotin 81
Biotinidase deficiency 18
Birth asphyxia, causes of 62, 63
Birth history, history of 121
Bitot's spots 155

Bladder 175
Bleeding disorder 54, 86, 115
Blindness 72
Blood 289
    disease 55
    group 58
    pressure 145, 146, 153
        measuring 145
Bloody vomitus 21
Bone
    conduction 194
    dysplasia 298
Bottle feeding 173
Bowel habits 33, 40
    abnormal 89
Bradycardia 147
Brain
    development 90
Breast 233
    abnormalities of 233
    development 217
    engorgement 233
    milk 96-99, 100, 112
        cells 99
        cellular defenses in 98
        components in 98
        function in 98
        jaundice 259
        leukocytes 98
        lymphocytes 99
        protect allergy 98
        protect atopy 98
        protect diseases 96
        protection 97, 100
        regulate lymphocytes 98
        viruses in 103
    pump 259
        to breast milk 102
    types of 233
Breastfeeding 96, 118, 173
    benefits to
        baby 97
        mother 97
    history 80, 102
    jaundice 259
    long-term benefits of 102
    protection against diseases 102
Breath
    holding 42
    spells 42, 90
    shortness of 21
    sounds 169
        abnormal 170
        abnormalities in 170

Breathlessness 21
Bronchial asthma 253, 278
Bronchial breath sounds 170
Bronchiectasis 165
Bronchopneumonia 277
Bronchopulmonary dysplasia 80
Bruising 23
B-tetanus toxoid 102
Buccal mucosa 215
Budd-Chiari syndrome 286
Bull's neck 164
Buphthalmos 295

C

Café au lait spots 198, 229
Canadian-born 4
Candida ablicans 161, 167
Cannabis 104
Capillary nevi 229
Cardiac
    abnormality 227
    apex 171
    causes 286
    failure 37, 282
    murmurs 291
        causes of 282
Cardinal signs 283
Cardiovascular system 21, 35, 178, 179, 218
Carpenter syndrome 197
Cartilage 224
Cataract 159, 295
Celiac disease 165
Central nervous system 41, 63, 87, 218, 227, 292
Central precocious puberty 52
Cephalopelvic disproportion 62
Cerebellar signs 187, 219
Cerebral palsy 141, 294
Cerebral tumors 79, 296
Cerebrospinal fluid 183
Ceroid lipofuscinosis 79
Chest
    circumference 145
    infections 21, 23
    pain 21, 37
        uneasiness in 26
Chewing, abnormalities 234
Child protection 6
Child with ambiguous genitalia 51
Child with
    fever, history of 14
    limp 48
    skin lesions 246
Child's heart 137
Child's lungs 168
Childhood
    behavioral disorders 90

cancers 290
    malignancies 290
Chlamydia trachomatis 61, 287
Chloramphenicol 103, 290
Chloroquine 290
Cholera 94, 116
Chorioretinits 295
Chronic diseases 9, 17, 86, 287
Ciliary dyskinesia 281
Cirrhosis 165
Citrobacter spp 287
Clonus 186
Clostridium perfringens 113
Clostridium tetani 113
Cobalamin binding protein 98
Codominance 85
Cohen syndrome 197
Cold
    chain 109
    intolerance 22
Collapsing pulses 147
Coloboma 231
Colostral immunoglobulin A 98
Colostrum 97
Coma 50
Common respiratory symptoms 24
Complement cascade 98
Complete pediatric history 120
Congenital
    adrenal hyperplasia 18, 51, 52, 85
    cardiac
        defects 63
        diseases 160
        lesions 36, 37
    cataracts 231
    causes 287
    dislocation of hip 234
    glaucoma 231
    heart disease 18, 165
    hydrocele 167
    hypothyroidism 18
        causes of 291
    laryngomalacia 281
    myopathies 65
    neuromuscular disease 63
    syphilis 167
Consciousness, loss of 23
Constipation 21, 22, 23, 34, 291
    causes of 283
Contagious diseases 17
Corrigan pulse 147
Corynebacterium diphtheriae 113
Cotrimoxazole 290
Cough 21, 23, 24, 29, 37
    diagnosis of chronic 281
    types of 21, 168
Coumarin 61, 92
Cow's milk 79, 93

allergies 79
    in infancy 98
    diet 80
    protein
        allergies 33, 34, 257
        intolerance 257
Coxsackievirus B 61
Cranial meningocele 166
Cranial nerve 182, 189, 219
    anatomy 192
    III 190
    IV 190
    testing 192
    VI 190
Craniotabes 157
Craving, abnormal 89
Crigler-Najjar syndrome 65
Crohn's disease 162
Crouzon syndrome 158
Crying 88
    during feeding 22
    type of 88
Cutaneous perfusion 153
Cutis marmorata 228, 291
Cyanosis, severe chronic 165
Cyclophosphamide 61
Cystic fibrosis 18, 35, 165, 252, 281
Cystic hygromas 163, 164
Cysts 164
    types of 161
Cytokines
    actions of 101
    benefits of 101
Cytomegalovirus 61, 103

D

Dacrocystoceles 231
Dacryostenosis 231
Daily living
    activities of 9, 24
    in children, activities of 9
Dapsone 103, 290
Deafness 44, 72
Deficit hyperactivity disorder 90
Dehydration
    degree of 153
    Sara's eagerness 259
    severe 158
    signs of 153
Delivery, history of 58, 59, 121
Dengue 94
Dental caries 20
Dermatitis 81
Diabetes mellitus 226, 291, 295
    drug history in 50
    food history in 50
    types of 291

Diarrhea 21, 23, 33, 260
    incidence of 97
Diastolic murmur 282
Dicrotic pulse 147
Dietary 79, 121
Diethylstilbestrol 61, 93
Diphtheria 109
Diplopia 50
Disease
    complications of 132
    severity of 10
Dizziness 21
Dorsalis pedis 146
Down syndrome 62, 150, 151, 158, 264, 265, 290
    facies 214
Drug
    allergy 91
    history 91, 122
    in newborn 92
    in young child 92
    interactions 92
    social 104
    therapy of lactating mother 104
    usage 104
Dry skin 291
Dubin-Johnson syndrome 66
Dysdiadochokinesia 188
Dyskinesias 184
Dysmorphic child 90
Dysphagia 23, 34
Dysplasia of hip 185
Dyspnea 37, 41
Dystonia 184
Dysuria 22, 40

E

Ear 20, 28, 159, 199, 218, 219
    discharge 21, 28
    in febrile child 249
    normal 232
    pain 21, 28
    pits 232
    ringing sensation in 20
    tags 232
Eczema 198, 253, 274
    atopic 93, 167
Edema 40
Edward's syndrome 290
Eggs 93
Ehlers-Danlos syndrome 158, 164
Elucidates disease, etiology of 19
Empyema 165
Encephalocele 166
Endocrine
    causes 292
    system 22, 48, 151
ENT symptoms 29

Enterobacter cloacae 287
Enterococcus spp 287
Enteroviruses 61
Environmental history 26
Epilepsy, types of 79, 296
Epiphora 230
Epithelial pearl 230
Epstein-Barr virus 103
Erythema infectiosum 272
Erythema toxicum 228
Escherichia coli 61, 287
Estriol 62
Ethanol 104
Exacerbating factors 23
Eye 199, 218, 219, 230
    contact 23
    itching of 29
    lazy 23
    movements, abnormal 23
    observation of 158
    of newborn
        abnormalities of 230
        types of 230
    redness of 29
    tearing of 29
Eyelid edema 230

F

Face 198
Facial appearance 157, 214
Facial nerve 193
Facies, abnormal 158
Fainting 21
Fat-soluble vitamin deficiencies 81
Fatty acid oxidation disorder 18
Fauces 215
Febrile child 161
    with rash 244
Feeding
    color changes with 21
    difficulties 22
    history 26, 36, 79, 121
    poor 21
    positions 97
    problem 79
Feet 215, 234
Fetal hypoxia, causes of 60
Fever 20, 22, 23, 40, 43, 148, 244, 252
    causes of 271
    in children 271
    types of 272
Finger 166
    short broad 291
    tips 166
Fistulae 164
Fits 42
Flat nasal bridge 291
Flatulence 33

Fluconazole 104
Fluoroquinolones 103
Folate 81
Folic acid binding protein 98
Fontanel 153
    posterior 183
Food 49
    allergies 79
    poisoning 94
Food-borne 94
Foremilk 97
Free fatty acids 98
Fungal 61

G

Gait 218
    abnormalities 48
Galactosemia 18
Gastroesophageal reflux disease 22, 281
Gastrointestinal
    cause 287
    diseases of 96
    symptoms, causes of 20
    system 21
    tract 19, 30, 98, 257
Gastroschisis 59
Gene 83
Genetic syndromes 49
Genital mycoplasma 61
Genital region 177, 217
Genitalia 199, 216, 225, 233
    abnormalities of 233
    development of external 217
    types of 233
Genitourinary system 22, 38
Genitourinary tract, infections of 60
Genu valgum 47
    causes of 297
    physiological 47
Genu varum 47, 297
    causes of 297
    physiological 47
German measles 58
Gestational age 62, 69, 71, 223, 225
    large for 226
Giddiness 44
Gilbert's syndrome 66
Glaucoma 295
Global Immunization Programs 116
Glossopharyngeal nerve 194
Glucose-6-phosphate dehydrogenase 258
Goiter 51
Gonococcal conjunctivitis 231
Gram-negative cocci 287
Gram-positive cocci 287
Gray baby syndrome 65
Great arteries, transposition of 36
Green nasal discharge 21

Group B streptococci 61
Growth charts 141
Growth pattern 22
Growth rates 141
Grunting cry 149
Gums 215
    bleeding 20
    examination of 162
    swollen 20, 162
Gut-associated lymphoid tissue 99

H

Haemophilus influenzae 102, 183
Hair 198, 214, 225
    abnormalities of 157
    examination of 157
    line, low 157
    problems 23
    texture 157
Hands 215, 234
Harlequin color change 229
Harrison's groove 156
Harrison's sulcus 169
Head 20, 156, 198, 218, 219
    banging 89
    circumference 140
    trauma 22
Headache 50
Hearing 28
    decreased 20
    test for 196
Heart 178, 199, 224
    disease 252
    failure 283
        signs of 283
        symptoms of 283
    murmur 254
    rate 63
    sound
        abnormal 281
        first 282
        second 282
Heartburn 22, 34
Heat intolerance 22
HEEEADSSS technique 131
Hemangioma 164, 198
Hematemesis 21
Hematochezia 22
Hematological abnormality 54
Hematological system 54, 56
Hematomas 296
Hematuria 22
    causes of 288
Hemoglobinopathies 18
Hemolysis 289
Hemolytic anemia 65
    chronic 158

Hemolytic jaundice 134
Hemophilia 115
Hepatic causes of portal hypertension 286
Hepatic venous blockage 286
Hepatitis
    A 116
    B 58, 61, 103
        vaccination 113
    C 61, 103
Hepatobiliary 284
Hepatoblastoma 285
Hepatocellular carcinoma 285
Hepatocellular jaundice 134
Hepatomegaly with smooth hepatic enlargement, causes of 285
Hepatomegaly, causes of 285
Herpes simplex 61, 103
Hind milk 97
Hips 234
Homocystinuria 18
Hookworm 289
Human chorionic gonadotropin 62
Human herpes virus 6 103, 245
Human immunodeficiency virus 61, 68, 103, 112
    infection 115
Human papilloma virus 117
Hurler syndrome 158
Hyaline membrane disease 64
Hydatid disease 285
Hydration 214
Hydrocephalus 79, 296
    causes of 293
Hydrochloroquine 290
Hyperacusis 81
Hyperbilirubinemia 284, 285
Hypertension
    causes of 286
    chronic 225
Hypocalcemia 226
Hypochromic microcytic anemia 289
Hypochromotrichia 155
Hypoglossal nerve 195
Hypoglycemia
    signs of 50
    symptoms of 50
Hypomagnesemia 226
Hypopigmented macules 198
Hypothermia 224
Hypothesis
    formulation of 16
    of clubbing 165
Hypotonia 81, 291
Hypoxia 62

I

Illness, chronic 71, 72

Immune cells 98
Immune system 98
Immunity, adaptive 107
Immunization 1, 106
    active 107
    before 109
    history 26, 121
    in preterm infants 115
    passive 107
    reactions to 113
Immunoglobulin 107
    G 98
Infant
    cry 149
    full-term 224
    post-term 225
    preterm 224
Infantile
    colic 257
    psoriasis 273
    reflexes 235
    seborrheic dermatitis 246
Infections 17
Infectious cause 287
Infectious diseases 23
Inflammatory bowel disease 165
Influenza 111
    for nasal influenza vaccine 112
    vaccine 117
    virus 100
Innate immunity 107
Insulin dependent diabetes mellitus 102
Intellectual disabilities 90
Intensity of pain 32
Intermittent fever 148
Interstitial pneumonitis 277
    severe 165
Intramuscular route of vaccination 114
Intrapartum causes 62
Intrauterine growth restriction 61, 68, 71
Intrauterine infections 68
Intraventricular hemorrhage 80
Iodine, radioactive 61, 92
Iron 289
    deficiency 80
Isotretinoin 61, 92

J

Japanese encephalitis vaccine 117
Jaundice 35, 176, 259
    child 175
    history of 35
    in breastfed babies 66
    obstructive 134
    physiological 66
    prolonged 284
Jaw 218
Juvenile idiopathic arthritis 299

K

Kawasaki disease 273
Kayser-Fleischer rings 159
Kernig's sign 183
Kidney
    disease 225
    examination of 174
Killed vaccines 109
Klebsiella spp 287
Klinefelter's syndrome 212, 290
Klippel-Feil syndrome 164
Knee jerk 186
Knock knees 156
Kwashiorkor 155

L

Labor and delivery, related to 62
Lactoferrin 98
Lactoperoxidase 98
Lamotrigine 103
Laron's syndrome 158
Laron-type dwarfism 158
Leber's congenital amaurosis 295
Leg 215
    swollen 135
Limb 218, 225
    abnormalities 47
    deformities 47
    pain 47
    paresis 44
    posture 219
    weakness 47
Linea nigra 229
Lips 159, 215
Lithium 61, 92
Live attenuated vaccine 112
Live vaccines 109, 111
Liver 175, 199
    disease, chronic 173
    palpation of 173
Lobar pneumonia 277
Loud sounds 22
Low grade fever 248
Lower limb 188
    muscle 185
Lucy-Driscoll syndrome 65
Lung disease 165
    chronic 252
Lymphangioma 164
Lymphocytes 98, 99
Lymphoid system 99
Lymphoid tissue 100
Lysozymes 98

M

Macroglossia 291
Macrophages 98, 99
Malaria 61, 94, 289
Male child inspection 177
Male infant 251
Male inspection 217
Malnutrition 72
Mammary tumor virus 103
Maple syrup urine disease 18
Marasmus 154, 155
Marfan's syndrome 144, 158, 212
Massive splenomegaly 290
Maternal diabetes mellitus 59
Maternal drug information 103
Maternal immunization status 61
Maternal infections 226
    affecting fetus 61
    consequences of 62
Maternal medical complications 61
Maternal medications 61, 226
Maternal surgery 61
Mature milk 97
Measles 109, 112, 272
Meconium aspiration syndrome 62
Meconium, components of 62
Megaloblastic anemia 81
Melena 22
Meningomyelocele 59
Menstrual period, last 223
Mental confusion 50
Mental retardation 158, 291
Metabolic derangement 226
Metabolic disorders 296
Metabolic neurodegenerative disorders 79
Metabolism, inborn errors of 296
Methemoglobinemia 161
Methylene blue 290
Metronidazole, high-dose 103
Microcytic anemia 81
Micropenis 167
Microtia 232
Micturition habits, abnormal 89
Mid-arm circumference 144
Middle ear infection 250
    symptoms of 250
Migraine 43
Miliaria 273
    neonatorum 228
Milk feeds, dilution of 34
Minocycline 103
Misoprostol 61, 92
Mitochondrial diseases 79
Mitochondrial inheritance 85
Molecular weight, low 87
Moloney murine leukemia virus 103
Morquio syndrome 298
Mother's description 23
Mouth 20, 219, 230
    breathing 20
Mucins 98
Mucopolysaccharidosis 79
Mucosal immunity 112
Mucosal-associated lymphoid tissue 99, 100
Mucous membrane 153, 162, 213
Multiple congenital anomalies 59
Multiple enchondromatosis 298
Multiple epiphyseal dysplasia 298
Multiple hereditary exostosis 298
Mumps 109, 112
Munchausen's syndrome 90
Murmur detected, history of 21
Murmur, pathologic 181
Muscle
    power 186
    tone 63, 185, 218
    weakness 22
Musculoskeletal pain 45
Musculoskeletal system 22, 45, 219
Myalgias 22
Myasthenia gravis 65
Mycobacterium 61
Mycoplasma infections 56
Myelomeningocele 166
Myoclonus 184
Myopia, severe 295

N

Nail 166, 225
    changes 166
    problems 23
Nalidixic acid 290
Naphthalene 290
Nasal
    beans 249
    discharge 29
    influenza 109
    obstruction 29
Nasogastric tube 176
Nasolabial seborrhea 81
Nasopharyngeal-associated lymphoid tissue 100
Nausea 21, 33, 43, 50
Neck 215
    examination of 162
    pain 21
    stiffness 183
Necrotizing enterocolitis 80
Neisseria gonorrhoea 61, 287
Neonatal complications of IDM 226
Neonatal hypoglycemia 263, 291
    causes of 291
Neonatal infections 97
Neonatal jaundice 65
    history of 65
Neonatal period 121
    history of 58
Neonatal seizures 263
Neonatal sepsis 67, 68

Neonate, normal full-term 224
Neoplasms 290
Nephritis in childhood 288
Nephrotic syndrome 159, 288
  causes of 288
Nerve
  abducent 190
  accessory 195
  acoustic 194
  auditory 194
Nervous system 181, 262
Neural tube defects 59, 81
Neurocutaneous stigmata 85, 141
Neurodegenerative disorders 296
Neurodevelopmental system 181
Neurological event 41
Neurological system 22
Neuropathy 81
Neutrophils 98, 99
Nevus flammeus 229
Newborn 223-225
  normal 227
  period 18
  reflexes 235
Niacin 81
  deficiency 155
Nicotine 61, 104
Night blindness 155
Nikolsky's sign 206
Nitrofurantoin 104, 290
Nocturnal enuresis
  primary 89
  secondary 89
Nocturnal pain 258
Noisy breathing 21, 29
Noisy respiration 291
Non-accidental injuries 46
Nonproductive cough 252
Nonsteroidal anti-inflammatory drugs 103, 288
Noonan syndrome 151
Nose 20, 28, 29, 159, 218, 220
  bleeds 29
Nutrition 59, 214
Nutritional status in child 154

O

Occipitofrontal circumference 140
Ocular injuries 295
Olfactory nerve 189, 192
Oligohydramnios 59
  causes of 60
Oligosaccharides 98
Oliguria 176, 289
Ollier disease 298
Omphalocele 59
Onchocerciasis 295
Ondigestive tract 20

Optic atrophy 295
Optic nerve 189, 192
  hypoplasia 295
Oral cavity 159, 215
Oral polio 109
  vaccine 112
Oral vaccines 112
Organic acid disorders 18
Orthopnea 37
Otitis media
  acute 248
  causes of 276
  symptoms of 28

P

Pain
  aggravation of 32
  during urination 40
  relief of 32
Pale stools 35
Palmar grasp 235
Palms 166
Palpable pulses 153
Parasitic infestations 155
Paresthesia 50
Paroxysmal nocturnal dyspnea 21
Parvovirus 61
  infections 56
Patent ductus arteriosus 36, 161
Peanuts 93
Pediatric diabetes mellitus 49
Pediatric enquiry 8
Pediatric heart 181
Pediatric history 3, 4, 13, 124
  components of 69
Pediatric physical examination 129, 137, 211
Pediculosis capitis 163
Pellagra 81
Penicillamine 61, 92
Penis 217
Perianal dermatitis 273
Periorbital edema 176
Periorbital swelling 40
Peripheral blood 160
Peripheral cyanosis 160
Peripheral hypotonia 185
Peripheral neuropathy 81
Permanent congenital hypothyroidism 50
Perspiration 50
Petechiae 23
Peutz-Jeghers syndrome 162
Peyer's patches 99
Pharynx 215
Phenobarbitone 103
Phenylketonuria 18
Phenytoin 61, 92
Photophobia 23

Placental anomalies 60
Plantar reflex 187
Platelet-derived growth factor 165
Pleiotropy 83
Pneumonia, atypical 277
Polio 112
Poliomyelitis 61
Polychlorinated biphenyls 87
Polycythemia 227
Polydactyly 234
Polydipsia 22
Polygenic inheritance 84
Polyhydramnios 59
  causes of 59
  history of 24
Polysaccharide vaccine 117
Polyuria 22
  causes of 288
Poor weight gain 22
Port wine stains 229
Portal hypertension, causes of 285
Postpartum causes 63
Potter syndrome 60
Prader-Willi syndrome 197
Precocious puberty 22, 51
Pregnancy 59
  age 59
  history of 58, 59
  with plasma protein 62
Premature birth 80
Premature neonate 224
Prepregnancy history 58
Pressure ulcers 23
Primaquine 61, 103, 104, 290
Primitive reflexes 235
Probenecid 290
Progesterone 61
Proteus mirabilis 287
Providencia stuartii 287
Proxy 90
Pruritis 23
Pseudomonas aeruginosa 287
Pubertal assessment 178
Puberty, delayed 22
Pubic hair 178, 217
Pulmonary blood flow
  decrease in 37
  increase in 36
Pulmonary disease, Chronic 26
Pulmonary disorder 63
Pulmonary infections, chronic 281
Pulse rate 146, 147, 153
Pulses paradoxus 147
Pulses parvus et tardus 147
Pulsus alternans 147
Pupillary light reflex 192
Pyridoxine 81
  deficiency 155

Q

Quinine 61, 103, 104

R

Rabies 109
Rectal examination 176
Reflexes, abnormal 187
Regurgitation, complications of severe 33
Relapsing fever 148
Relieve breathlessness 21
Remittent fever 148
Renal
　biopsy 288
　diseases 41, 47
　disorders 63
Respirations 63, 153
Respiratory
　diseases of 96
　distress 227
　infections, protection from 100
　rate 147, 168, 224, 249
　system 21, 24, 277
Retinal hemorrhages 230
Retinoic acid 93
Retinopathy of prematurity 295
Retractile testes 167
Rhesus isoimmunization 59
Rhinorrhea 29, 248
Rhonchi 170
Riboflavin 81
　deficiency 155
Rinne's test 194
River blindness 295
Romberg's test 188
Roseola infantum 272
Rotavirus 109, 117
　diarrheas 100
Rubella 58, 61, 103, 109, 112, 272
Rubinstein-Taybi syndrome 197
Runny nose 20

S

Sacral edema 166
Saddle back fever 148
Salicylates 290
Salmonellosis 94
Sara's daycare center 260
Sarcoma virus 103
Scabies 273
School going age 52
Screaming episodes 22
Scurvy 81
Sebacious gland hyperplasia 228
Seborrheic dermatitis 229
Seizure 42, 44, 81
　activity 23
　type 44
Sense of position 188

Serum total bilirubin 284
Sexual activity, history of 22
Shell fish 93
Shigellosis 94
Sickle cell anemia 18
Simian crease 234
Sinus 29, 164
　in children 29
　pneumatization of 29
Skin 23, 52, 159, 198, 213, 219, 224, 225
　lesions 85
　　diagnosis of 53
　rashes 66
　　types of 228
　system 272
　turgor 153
Sleep disturbances 88
Sleep pattern 90
Smallpox 94
Sneezing 29, 248
Snoring 20
Social habits 59
Sodium valproate 61
Soiling in children 283
Solo syndrome 151
Somnolence 50, 291
Sotos syndrome 197
Soybean 93
Speech 78
　disturbance 44
Spina bifida 59
　occult 166
Spinal anomalies 287
Spinal column disease
　lateral 81
　posterior 81
Spinal cord transaction 62
Spinal meningocele 166
Spine
　and back 215
　examination of 166
Spleen 175
　palpation of 174
Splenic dysfunction 116
Splenomegaly, causes of 290
Spontaneous vaginal delivery 255
Squints 230
Staggering 44
Staphylococcal infections 167
Staphylococcus 94
　aureus 287
　epidermidis 287
　saprophyticus 287
Stevens Johnson syndrome 206
Still's murmur 181
Stooling habits 21
Storage diseases 290
Strawberry nevus 229

Streptococcus faecalis 287
Streptococcus group B 287
Streptococcus group D 287
Streptococcus pneumoniae 183
Streptococcus pyogenes 273
Streptomycin 61
Stroke 50
Subconjunctival hemorrhage 230
Subcutaneous injections 114
Subdural hematomas 79
Sucking well 259
Suckling blister 228
Sulfamethoxazole 103
Sulfasalazine 104
Sulfisoxazole 103
Sulfonamides 290
Supinator jerk 186
Supine 282
Suture closure, abnormalities in 157
Swallowing, abnormalities 23
Swallowing, difficulty in 34
Sweating 21
Sweet smell 5
Syncope 38, 41
Syphilis 58
Systemic diseases 290
Systemic symptoms 252
Systolic murmur 282

T

Talipes equinovalgus 234
Taphylococcus aureus 273
Tears 153
Teenage or adolescent patient 130
Teeth 215
Telangiectasia 198
Temper tantrums 88, 89
Temperament 90
Teratogenic drugs 92
Testes 217
　undescended 167
Testosterone-like drugs 61, 93
Tetanus 109
Tetracycline 61, 93, 103
Tetralogy of Fallot 36
Thalidomide 61, 93
Thiamine 81
　deficiency 155
Thorax 168, 169, 216
　palpation of 171
　percussion of 171
Throat 20, 28, 29
　sore 21
Thrombocytopenia 115
Thumb sucking 89
Thyroglossal cysts 164
Thyroid
　disease 51

disorders 50
gland 291
masses 164
Thyrotrophin receptor stimulating antibodies 51
Tinnitus 29, 44
Todd's paralysis 245
Toddlers 130
Tongue 160, 215, 218
    for state of hydration 161
    soreness of 20
Tonic-clonic seizure 292
Tonsils 99, 215
Torso ratios 144
Torticollis 164
Toxic goiter 163
Toxic shock syndrome 205
Toxoid 107, 112, 113
Toxoplasmosis 61
Tracheoesophageal fistula 59
Trachoma 295
Transient congenital hypothyroidism 51
Transitional milk 97
Transmitted sounds 169
Transplacental protection 100
Trauma 22, 46, 61
    history of recent 32
Trembling 50
Triceps jerk 186
Trichuris 289
Tricuspid atresia 36
Trigeminal nerve 193
Trimethoprim 103
Trunk 219
Trypanosomiasis 61
Tuberculosis 112, 281, 289
Turner's syndrome 164, 290
Twin pregnancies 59
Typhoid 109
    vaccine 117
Typical respiratory symptoms 24

U

Ulcers 20

Umbilical cord 232
Upper airway obstruction, causes of 276
Upper limbs incoordination 188
Upper respiratory
    diseases 5
    illness 252
Ureaplasma 61
Urinary tract infection in children 286, 287
Urine 35
    color of 39
    frequency 39
    in maple syrup disease 5

V

Vaccinating children 115, 116
Vaccination techniques 109
Vaccination, anatomical sites of 114
Vaccine 107
    types of 112
Vaginal bleeding 61
Vagus 194
Valproate 93
Varicella vaccine 116
Varicella zoster 61, 112
    infection 272
Vascular malformations 164
Vasovagal syncope 41
Vector-borne diseases 94
Ventrogluteal injection 115
Vernix caseosa 229
Vertigo, benign positional 42
Vestibulocochlear nerve 194
Vibrio cholerae 113
Viral 61
    infections 253
    rashes 272
Virus 112, 113
Vision, change in 20
Visual
    acuity 189, 192
    disturbance 44
    field 189
    impairment, causes of 295

Vitamin
    A 81
        deficiency 80, 155, 295
    B deficiency 155
    B1 81
    B12 81, 98, 289
    B2 81
    B3 81
    B6 81
    C deficiency 156
    D 61, 81, 93
        deficiency 80, 156
        resistant rickets 84
    deficiencies 81
    E 81
        deficiency 80, 156
    K 81
        analogues 290
        deficiency 80, 156
Vitiligo 81
Vomiting 22, 29, 33, 50
    without blood 21

W

Water intake 49
Water-Hammer pulses 147
Weakness 50
Weber's test 194
Wheeze 21, 38
Wheezing
    history of 26, 27
    types of 278
White nasal discharge 21
Williams syndrome 179
Wilson's disease 158
Wizened facies 158
World Allergy Organization 91

X

Xerodema pigmentosum 290
Xerosis conjunctivae 155
Xerosis cornea 155

Y

Yellow fever 94, 111, 112